AF597866

Sexually Transmitted Diseases and Adverse Outcomes of Pregnancy

WITHDRAWN

Sexually Transmitted Diseases and Adverse Outcomes of Pregnancy

EDITORS

Penelope J. Hitchcock, D.V.M., M.S.
Sexually Transmitted Diseases Branch
Division of Microbiology and Infectious Diseases
National Institute of Allergy and Infectious Diseases
National Institutes of Health, Bethesda, Maryland 20892

H. Trent MacKay, M.D., M.P.H.
Contraception and Reproductive Health Branch
Center for Population Research
National Institute of Child Health and Human Development
National Institutes of Health, Bethesda, Maryland 20892

Judith N. Wasserheit, M.D., M.P.H.
Division of STD Prevention
National Center for HIV, STD, and TB Prevention
Centers for Disease Control and Prevention, Atlanta, Georgia 30333

ASSOCIATE EDITOR

Roberta Binder, Ph.D.
Sexually Transmitted Diseases Branch
National Institute of Allergy and Infectious Diseases
National Institutes of Health, Bethesda, Maryland 20892

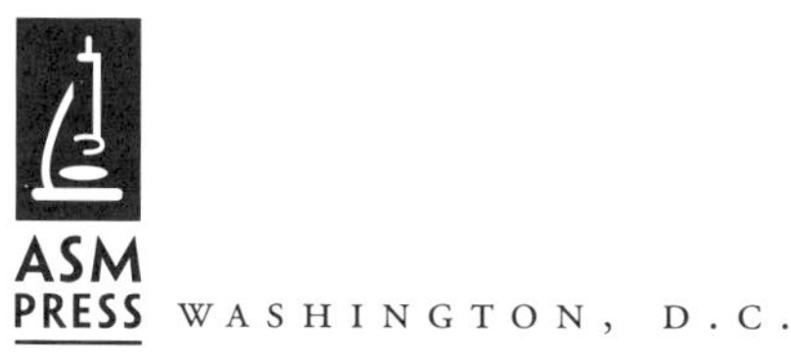

ASM PRESS WASHINGTON, D.C.

Copyright © 1999 American Society for Microbiology
1325 Massachusetts Ave., NW
Washington, DC 20005-4171

Library of Congress Cataloging-in-Publication Data

Sexually transmitted diseases and adverse outcomes of pregnancy / editors, Penelope J. Hitchcock, H. Trent MacKay, Judith N. Wasserheit ; associate editor, Roberta Binder.
p. cm.
Includes bibliographical references and index.
ISBN 1-55581-132-9
1. Pregnant women—Diseases. 2. Sexually transmitted diseases. 3. Generative organs, Female—Infections. 4. Communicable diseases in pregnancy. 5. Pregnant women—Health and hygiene. I. Hitchcock, Penelope J. II. MacKay, H. Trent. III. Wasserheit, Judith N.
[DNLM: 1. Pregnancy Complications, Infectious—etiology. 2. Sexually Transmitted Diseases—complications. 3. Pregnancy Outcome. WQ 256 S518 1999]
RG572.S49 1999
618.3—dc21
DNLM/DLC
for Library of Congress 99-11079
CIP

UNIVERSITY
COLLEGE LONDON
LIBRARY

All Rights Reserved
Printed in the United States of America

System no: 218062

CONTENTS

CONTRIBUTORS

William W. Andrews, Center for Obstetric Research, Department of Obstetrics and Gynecology, Division of Maternal-Fetal Medicine, University of Alabama at Birmingham, Birmingham, AL 35233

Ann M. Arvin, Department of Pediatrics, G-312, Stanford University School of Medicine, 300 Pasteur Drive, Stanford, CA 94305

Thomas M. Becker, Department of Public Health and Preventive Medicine, Oregon Health Sciences Center, 3181 S.W. Sam Jackson Park Road, CB-669, Portland, OR 97201-3098

Consuelo M. Beck-Sagué, Division of AIDS, STD and TB Laboratory Research and Office of Minority Health, National Center for Infectious Diseases, Centers for Disease Control and Prevention, Mailstop G-39, B-1, Room 6421, 1600 Clifton Road, N.E., Atlanta, GA 30333

Robert H. BonDurant, Department of Population Health and Reproduction, University of California, Davis, Davis, CA 95616

William J. Britt, Department of Pediatrics and Department of Microbiology, University of Alabama at Birmingham, 1600 7th Avenue South, Suite 752, Birmingham, AL 35233

Zane A. Brown, Department of Obstetrics and Gynecology, RH-20, University of Washington, 1959 Pacific Avenue, Seattle, WA 98195

Gail H. Cassell, Drug Discovery Research and Clinical Investigation, Lilly Research Laboratories, Eli Lilly and Company, Indianapolis, IN 46285

Lynette B. Corbeil, Department of Pathology, University of California, San Diego, 200 W. Arbor Drive, San Diego, CA 92103-8416

David A. Eschenbach, Department of Obstetrics and Gynecology, University of Washington, Box 356460, Seattle, WA 98195

Ronald S. Gibbs, Department of Obstetrics and Gynecology, University of Colorado Health Sciences Center, 4200 E. 9th Avenue, Box 198, Denver, CO 80262

Robert L. Goldenberg, Center for Obstetric Research, Department of Obstetrics and Gynecology, University of Alabama at Birmingham, 560 Old Hillman Building, 618 South 20th Street, Birmingham, AL 35233-7333

Michael G. Gravett, Division of Reproductive Sciences, Oregon Regional Primate Research Center; Department of Obstetrics and Department of

Gynecology, Legacy Emanuel Hospital and Health Center; and Oregon Health Sciences University, Beaverton and Portland, Oregon

Joseph A. Hill, Department of Obstetrics, Gynecology and Reproductive Biology, Division of Reproductive Medicine, Harvard Medical School, Brigham and Women's Hospital, 75 Francis Street, Boston, MA 02115

Sharon L. Hillier, Department of Obstetrics, Gynecology and Reproductive Sciences, Magee-Women's Hospital, University of Pittsburgh, 300 Halket Street, Pittsburgh, PA 15213

Robert B. Jones, Department of Medicine, Indiana University School of Medicine, Emerson Hall 435, 545 Barnhill Drive, Indianapolis, IN 46202-5124

Gareth E. Jones, Moredun Research Institute; present address, YAbA Ltd., Pentlands Science Park, Bush Loan, Penicuik EH26 0PZ, United Kingdom

Michael S. Kramer, Department of Pediatrics and Department of Epidemiology and Biostatistics, McGill University Faculty of Medicine, Montreal, Quebec, Canada

H. Trent MacKay, National Institute of Child Health and Human Development, National Institutes of Health, Bethesda, MD 20892

Howard Minkoff, Department of Obstetrics and Gynecology, State University of New York-Brooklyn, 450 Clarkson Avenue, Box 24, Brooklyn, NY 11203-2098

Stephen A. Morse, Division of AIDS, STD and TB Laboratory Research and Office of Minority Health, National Center for Infectious Diseases, Centers for Disease Control and Prevention, Mailstop G-39, B-1, Room 6421, 1600 Clifton Road, N.E., Atlanta, GA 30333

Miles J. Novy, Division of Reproductive Sciences, Oregon Regional Primate Research Center, and Department of Obstetrics and Department of Gynecology, Oregon Health Sciences University, Beaverton and Portland, Oregon

Pablo J. Sánchez, Division of Neonatal-Perinatal Medicine and Division of Pediatric Infectious Diseases, University of Texas Southwestern Medical Center at Dallas, 5323 Harry Hines Boulevard, Dallas, TX 75235-9063

Michael St. Louis, Centers for Disease Control and Prevention, Atlanta, GA 30333

Richard L. Sweet, Department of Obstetrics, Gynecology and Reproductive Sciences, University of Pittsburgh School of Medicine, Magee-Women's Hospital, 300 Halket Street, Pittsburgh, PA 15213-3180

Pål Wolner-Hanssen, Department of Obstetrics and Gynecology, University Hospital of Lund, S-225-85 Lund, Sweden

Amy Yuan, Center for Obstetric Research, Department of Obstetrics and Gynecology, Division of Maternal-Fetal Medicine, University of Alabama at Birmingham, Birmingham, AL 35233

PREFACE

The United States has the highest rates of sexually transmitted diseases (STDs) in the developed world. The majority of these infections are silent or cause symptoms so indolent that the victim does not seek health care. Despite the absence of overt symptoms, however, disease progression occurs. Chronic sequelae of STDs are associated with significant morbidity, mortality, and health care costs.

For the most part, the impact of these infections on reproductive health and quality of life is under-appreciated. In some cases, the link between STDs and chronic disease is not understood (e.g., only recently has human papillomavirus infection been recognized as the cause of cervical cancer). Ironically, sometimes the link is known but, for cultural or social reasons, it may not be acknowledged (for example, a woman with pelvic inflammatory disease [PID] may not be told that sexually transmitted gonorrhea and chlamydial infection are the most common causes of primary PID). Women and their infants bear the burden of STDs disproportionately. In part this reflects biological, gender-based differences, such as the anatomic vulnerability of the female genital tract. This burden also reflects social and cultural differences, such as a lower economic status of women. However, as parents, men and women both are particularly vulnerable in one aspect of reproductive health: the ability to conceive and bear healthy children. Adverse outcomes of pregnancy are costly; the emotional and financial burden can be enormous for the family and for the health care system.

Some STDs are familiar causes of adverse pregnancy outcomes as reflected by neonatal health: congenital syphilis, neonatal herpes, recurrent laryngeal papillomatosis, ophthalmia neonatorum, and congenital HIV infection are examples. However, one of the most neglected research areas is the role of STDs in first- and second-trimester miscarriage, stillbirth, low birth weight, premature rupture of membranes, and premature birth. Primarily because we have not conducted extensive research in this area, we don't know what we don't know. In other words, we haven't found what we haven't sought. For example, *Chlamydia trachomatis* was first isolated from the genital tract of humans in 1964, yet the role of chlamydial infection in ectopic pregnancy has only emerged in the present decade. There are many unanswered questions about chlamydial infection and pregnancy—for instance, how might undiagnosed, untreated chlamydial endometritis affect conception? The emerging link between STDs and adverse pregnancy outcomes offers exciting possibilities for prevention of these sequelae through primary and secondary prevention of STDs both before and during pregnancy.

The STD Program Staff of the National Institute of Allergy and Infectious Disease (NIAID) and the Centers for Disease Control and Prevention (CDC) National Center for HIV, STD and TB Prevention have worked together on an initiative for STDs and adverse pregnancy outcomes. The ongoing collaboration began in 1994 with a workshop that brought together a group of experts to review the existing knowledge on STDs and pregnancy and to provide insight about a research agenda. The collaboration has also produced this monograph, the purpose of which is to focus attention on this problem and to encourage scientists with diverse backgrounds to work together on multidisciplinary research on STDs and adverse outcomes of pregnancy.

The chapters of this book summarize the existing knowledge about STDs and adverse outcomes of pregnancy, identify gaps in knowledge, and highlight potential areas of new research. Experts have written chapters on disease etiology, including epidemiology, microbiology, and clinical aspects; veterinary diseases and laboratory animal models for research; the biology of host susceptibility to infection; and methodology for perinatal research.

We owe thanks to many people who have helped with this effort. We wish to thank the investigators/authors; they are pioneers in this field and deeply committed to this problem. Special thanks go to the STD Program Staff at the CDC for help in organizing the workshop, and to the STD Program Staff at the NIAID for compiling this volume. The staff at ASM Press have been extraordinarily helpful and patient, and their efforts are truly appreciated.

Finally, to those who care enough to read this volume, we thank you in advance for your interest, support, and work. We recognize that your efforts to fund and carry out the research, to write the papers, to change policy, and to legislate change will move us closer to our collective goal: having and raising healthy children. It is the most important thing that we do.

The Editors

1
Pregnancy Outcomes Related to Sexually Transmitted Diseases

Robert L. Goldenberg, William W. Andrews, Amy Yuan, H. Trent MacKay, and Michael St. Louis

The relationship between pregnancy outcome and maternal colonization with sexually transmitted bacterial and viral organisms has been studied for many years (Alexander, 1984; Wendel and Wendel, 1993). The more classic sexually transmitted diseases, syphilis, gonorrhea, herpes, trichomonas, and *Chlamydia* infection, are almost always transmitted between adults by sexual contact. The majority of human immunodeficiency virus (HIV) infections in reproductive-age women are transmitted sexually. However, there are other maternal infections that are not easily classifiable. Group B *Streptococcus*, hepatitis B virus, cytomegalovirus, and the organisms associated with bacterial vaginosis, such as the mycoplasmas, *Gardnerella vaginalis*, *Bacteroides*, and *Mobiluncus* species, are all found more commonly in sexually active women than in non-sexually active women, but their mode of transmission is often not apparent.

MEASUREMENT OF PREGNANCY OUTCOME

There are many different types of adverse outcomes of pregnancy which have been attributed to maternal infection. First, it should be noted that several sexually transmitted diseases, such as gonorrhea and chlamydia, have been associated with a failure to achieve pregnancy, predominantly through fallopian tube damage. Additionally, fallopian tube damage secondary to chlamydia and gonorrhea is the leading cause of ectopic preg-

---

Robert L. Goldenberg, William W. Andrews, and Amy Yuan, Center for Obstetric Research, Department of Obstetrics and Gynecology, Division of Maternal-Fetal Medicine, University of Alabama at Birmingham, Birmingham, AL 35233. **H. Trent MacKay,** National Institute of Child Health and Human Development, Bethesda, MD 20892. **Michael St. Louis,** Centers for Disease Control and Prevention, Atlanta, GA 30333.

Sexually Transmitted Diseases and Adverse Outcomes of Pregnancy
Edited by P. J. Hitchcock, H. T. MacKay, J. N. Wasserheit, and R. Binder
©1999 American Society for Microbiology, Washington, D.C.

nancy, which complicates close to 100,000 pregnancies in the United States each year (Lawson et al., 1988).

The specific definitions of the most important adverse pregnancy outcomes are as follows: abortion is defined in most states as a pregnancy that terminates or is terminated before 20 weeks gestational age, while a stillbirth is usually defined as a fetus born at 20 weeks gestational age or more with no heartbeat or respiratory effort. A liveborn infant is generally defined as an infant born at any gestational age with a heartbeat or respiratory effort. Death of a liveborn infant can occur in the neonatal period (in the first 28 days of life) or in the postneonatal period (between 28 days and 1 year of age). An infant death is defined as the death of a liveborn baby which occurs before 1 year of age, i.e., the sum of neonatal and postneonatal deaths. Perinatal mortality is frequently defined as the sum of fetal and neonatal deaths, although other definitions are used. There are many definitions of morbidity, but handicap frequently includes children with blindness, deafness, cerebral palsy, or mental retardation (usually defined by an IQ cutoff less than 70 or 75 [Allen, 1984]).

EARLY PREGNANCY LOSS

The incidence of first-trimester spontaneous abortion is highly dependent upon how one defines pregnancy. By the standard obstetric definition, which would include a missed period and a positive urinary pregnancy test between 4 and 6 weeks after the last period, approximately 15 to 20% of all pregnancies end in spontaneous miscarriage. The etiology of these miscarriages is generally secondary to maldevelopment of the ovum and associated chromosomal abnormalities. It is very rare to spontaneously abort a normally developing fetus during the first trimester. In fact, most of the pathologic material from spontaneous abortions fails to demonstrate any fetal tissue whatsoever. In some reports, maternal infections such as syphilis, rubella, or HIV infection have been associated with early spontaneous abortion. However, there is little evidence that these diseases play an important role in first-trimester abortion (Speroff et al., 1994).

Second-trimester abortions, i.e., those which occur between weeks 12 and 20 of pregnancy, differ substantially from first-trimester abortions in that a fetus is nearly always present. Spontaneous second-trimester abortions occur in approximately 1 to 2% of all pregnancies, and they have a tendency to repeat in subsequent pregnancies. Although the etiology of these losses is often less clear than for those which occur at other times, second-trimester losses certainly include those due to anomalous fetuses, some with chromosomal abnormalities, and those which occur secondary to uterine malformations, incompetent cervix, and leiomyomata. However, most of the spontaneous second-trimester losses occur in the face of a normal uterus and a normally developed fetus. In those cases, there is either "spontaneous" labor or rupture of membranes, leading to delivery, or fetal death, which ultimately leads to delivery. Obstetric complications such as twin pregnancy, placental abruption, the presence of maternal anti-cardiolipin antibodies or the lupus anticoagulant, and fetal growth retardation are also associated with spontaneous pregnancy losses between 12 and 20 weeks gestation. However, the relative importance of these etiologies is not well quantified (Speroff et al., 1994).

Since the etiology of so many of the second-trimester losses is not clear, and since a majority of them are associated with spontaneous labor and ruptured membranes, there is ample room to hypothesize that intrauterine infection, which has been implicated in both of these complications of pregnancy, may also be an important etiologic component of spontaneous second-trimester losses. Indeed, chorioamnionitis has frequently been described, and there are numerous case reports of amniotic fluid infection during this gestational age period. Additionally, isolation of microorganisms from pregnancy products has been reported to be more common in women with spontaneous mid-trimester pregnancy loss than in women with induced abortions (Andrews et al., 1995; Gibbs et al., 1992).

STILLBIRTH

Fetal deaths which occur after 20 weeks gestation complicate approximately 1% of all births in the United States. The fetal death rates are approximately twice as high for African American women as for Caucasian women. For women of all ethnic groups, the stillbirth rates have been decreasing slowly over the last three decades. There is reasonably good evidence that the various types of fetal monitoring programs, including fetal heart monitoring, biophysical profile, and fetal kick counts, and improved medical care, such as that which is now given to women with hypertension and diabetes, have been responsible for a significant reduction in term fetal deaths in the last two decades. Because of the reduction in term stillbirths over the last several decades, most stillbirths now occur in the preterm gestational ages. In a recent multicenter study, approximately half of the stillbirths occurred prior to 28 weeks gestational age and another one-third occurred between 28 and 37 weeks (Copper et al., 1994). In that study and in a number of others, the etiology of many of the stillbirths was not clear. However, many of the early-gestational-age fetuses died in conjunction with spontaneous preterm labor or rupture of the membranes. Placental histologic changes consistent with chorioamnionitis are found frequently in association with these early stillbirths, and these mothers are also more likely to develop postpartum endometritis. Therefore, there is substantial reason to believe that intrauterine infection may contribute to the etiology of many stillbirths as an initiator of preterm labor, as an initiator of ruptured membranes, or as an initiator of fetal death which ultimately results in the birth of a stillborn infant. Certainly syphilis, parvovirus, rubella, toxoplasmosis, and group B *Streptococcus* are proven causes of stillbirth (Donders et al., 1993; Fletcher and Gordon, 1990; Ingall et al., 1995; Minkoff et al., 1984).

NEONATAL DEATH

Neonatal deaths are defined as those which occur within the first 28 days of life. In most Western countries, these deaths occur in 4 to 8 neonates per 1,000 live births. In general, about 70% of these deaths are associated with a preterm birth and 25% are associated with a major congenital anomaly; the remainder are due to asphyxia, sepsis, meconium aspiration, birth trauma, and rarer conditions such as immune or nonimmune hydrops. Infection as a specific cause of neonatal death occurs predominantly in preterm infants and is often part of the picture which includes respiratory distress syndrome, intraventricular hemorrhage, and necrotizing enterocolitis. Group B *Streptococcus* is one of the most common organisms implicated in systemic neonatal infection, but many other organisms, including those which normally colonize the vagina and those which are acquired in the nursery, have also been implicated in sepsis-related neonatal deaths (Schuchat et al., 1990; Rouse et al., 1994).

POSTNEONATAL DEATHS

Postneonatal deaths occur in approximately 3 to 4 infants per 1,000 live births. Sudden infant death syndrome is the most common etiology, while congenital anomalies, accidents, and infection account for most of the other deaths. Infection-related causes of postneonatal mortality include meningitis, pneumonia, and diarrhea. Although deaths from these causes are rare for infants born to middle-income women in Western countries, they are more frequently seen in rural areas and among the poor. In underdeveloped countries, infection may cause up to several hundred deaths per 1,000 live births.

GROWTH RETARDATION

Fetal growth retardation is generally defined as a birth weight less than the 10th percentile birth weight for gestational age. However, the standards used to define the 10th percentile birth weight for gestational age are highly variable and often do not apply to the population being evaluated (Goldenberg et al., 1989). Also, because the measures of gestational age used for defining the standard are so variable, it is difficult to compare rates of growth retardation from one time interval to another or from one study to another. Growth retardation has many etiologies, including low maternal height, low maternal weight, smoking, preeclampsia, congenital anomalies, and intrauterine infection. With changes in obstetric recommendations about maternal weight gain over the last several decades, it appears that the rate of growth retardation is decreasing.

Nearly all infections of the mother and fetus have been associated with growth retardation, but it is unknown whether maternally transmitted infections other than those which infect the fetus early and directly, such as rubella, toxoplasmosis, cytomegalovirus, and syphilis, actually cause growth retardation. However, because most growth retardation in developed countries appears to be associated with below-average maternal size, poor nutritional status, various adverse health behaviors, and hypertension, it is unclear what portion of the growth retardation in developed countries will be explained by an infectious etiology. Growth retardation has been associated in many (but not all) studies with an increased risk of neonatal death and neurological disability (Chard et al., 1993).

LONG-TERM DISABILITY

In addition to mortality, a wide range of permanent structural and neurological morbidity has been associated with maternally transmitted infectious diseases. These include structural congenital anomalies with a defect in one or more organs; structural or functional damage to the brain, resulting in decreased cognitive ability, mental retardation, or both; and a motor disorder such as a diminution of fine or gross motor skills or an increase in spasticity or athetosis such as that associated with cerebral palsy. These morbidities, in addition to blindness, deafness, and hydrocephalus, have all been associated with infectious diseases (Alberman and Stanley, 1984).

Mental retardation is another outcome measure of great importance but one whose prevalence in the population is difficult to determine with certainty. Prevalence is undoubtedly influenced by definition, timing of testing, and many other factors. Babies born prematurely, babies with low birth weight, and babies born following intrauterine growth retardation are all at greater risk for the development of mental retardation regardless of the definition. However, most babies with these diagnoses will eventually have IQs within the normal range. However, it is clear that the socioeconomic status and educational background of the parents greatly influence the ultimate rate of mental retardation in the population (Goldenberg et al., 1996a). While perinatal infections such as group B *Streptococcus*, herpes simplex virus, and cytomegalovirus infections, syphilis, and toxoplasmosis all are demonstrated causes of mental retardation, infection-initiated preterm birth, which will be described in detail, appears to be a more important cause of mental retardation from the overall public health perspective (Alexander and Harrison, 1983; Henderson and Weiner, 1995; Goldenberg et al., 1997).

We emphasize that because many of these outcomes occur only rarely and first become apparent later in life, perinatal researchers often use surrogate measures of adverse outcome, such as preterm birth, growth retardation, and low birth weight, or the continuous measures of mean birth weight and mean gestational age to define adverse pregnancy outcome. However, if an infant is born early or small but lives and suffers no long-term neurological handicap, no adverse outcome has occurred. Against this background, the goals of most pregnant women and their medical providers include the birth of a normal-sized living infant at or near term who is healthy and free of medical or neurological impairments, and with all this accomplished at a reasonable economic cost.

ECONOMIC COST

As mentioned above, the final outcome to be considered is economic cost; it is apparent that the costs associated with many of the adverse outcomes of pregnancy mentioned can be very high. For example, a 24-week newborn, if it survives, can easily spend 4 months in the newborn intensive care unit at costs ranging between $1,000 and $2,000 per day, for a total hospital cost of over $200,000. It is estimated that the total annual cost of prematurity in the United States today is between two and four billion dollars. Many of the cost estimates are based on infants who survive, and they do not include the considerable economic costs generated to care for preterm infants that ultimately die before discharge. The cost of caring for a severely handicapped child might be as much as $40,000 per year, with a lifetime economic burden in the millions of dollars for a single individual. Virtually any program that achieves a significant decrease in the preterm birth rate or the rate of major neurological handicap, therefore, will be cost-effective.

Timing of Transmission and Sequelae

There are many definitions of "prenatal," "perinatal," and "intrapartum" in use today. In this discussion, "prenatal" refers to the period between conception and the events leading to delivery, "perinatal" refers to the time between the onset of labor or rupture of membranes and approximately 1 month after delivery, and "intrapartum" refers to the period between the onset of labor and delivery. The numerical values used for infection and transmission rates and the percentage of infected infants with various sequelae used in the tables are based on a wide variety of sources with widely discrepant estimates (Goldenberg et al., 1997). These differences may reflect differences in study design, laboratory methods, population (race and socioeconomic status or size of study population), or case definition.

Table 1 describes the timing of the fetal or neonatal acquisition of the various infectious organisms. *Treponema pallidum*, the agent of syphilis, is

Table 1 Adverse outcomes associated with direct fetal or neonatal infections

Infection	Usual timing of transmission[a]		Usual adverse outcome[a]				
	Prenatal	Intrapartum	Systemic infection without sequelae	Eye disease or blindness	Perinatal death	Neurological sequelae	New-onset postneonatal illness and death
Bacterial vaginosis	−	−	−	−	−	−	−
Chlamydia	−	+	+	+	−	−	+
Cytomegalovirus infection	+	+	+	+	+	+	+
Gonorrhea	−	+	−	+	−	−	−
Hepatitis B	−	+	−	−	−	−	+
Herpes	±	+	+	+	+	+	−
HIV infection	+	+	−	−	−	±	+
Syphilis	+	±	+	−	+	+	+
Trichomoniasis	−	−	−	−	−	−	−

[a] +, common; ±, occurs but is not common; −, occurs rarely if at all.

usually acquired after the first trimester but can be acquired at any time during the pregnancy or at delivery. *Neisseria gonorrhoeae*, *Chlamydia trachomatis*, and hepatitis B virus rarely infect the fetus in the prenatal period and are almost never found in the uterus before rupture of the membranes (Alexander and Harrison, 1983; Alger et al., 1988; Elliott et al., 1990; McDonald et al., 1991, 1992). Instead, the fetus generally acquires these organisms as it passes through the birth canal. Fetal infections with herpes simplex virus rarely occur before the rupture of the membranes (Whitley and Hutto, 1985; Whitley et al., 1991). Instead, the vast majority of transmissions occur after the rupture of the membranes or in the intrapartum period. Transmission rates to the fetus vary depending on whether the infection is primary or recurrent. Neonatal HIV infection may be acquired prenatally, but studies of second-trimester abortuses suggest that early in utero infection is rare. Rouzioux et al. (1995), using a mathematical model, estimated that one-third of the transmissions occur in the last 2 weeks of pregnancy and two-thirds occur in the intrapartum period. Women with HIV infection whose membranes rupture more than 4 h before delivery or who undergo vaginal delivery were, in some studies, more likely to transmit this infection to their neonates (Minkoff et al., 1995; Mandelbrot et al., 1996; Mayaux et al., 1995; Newell et al., 1994).

Timing of the Onset of Disease

Many of the infants infected with a specific organism during fetal life or during delivery and who manifest disease will do so in the neonatal period. These include most of the infants infected with herpes simplex virus, *T. pallidum*, or *N. gonorrhoeae*. However, for many others, the disease will not become apparent for months or years. For example, while the ophthalmologic damage caused by *N. gonorrhoeae* and *C. trachomatis* becomes apparent within several days or weeks after birth, the pneumonia associated with chlamydial infection generally occurs months after delivery (Cohen et al., 1990; Schachter et al., 1986). The deafness associated with neonatal cytomegalovirus is often not apparent until later in childhood, and the neurological sequelae of fetal or neonatal infections with *Toxoplasma*, cytomegalovirus, rubella virus, herpes simplex virus, group B *Streptococcus*, and *T. pallidum* are often not apparent until later as well (Fowler et al., 1992; Hardy et al., 1984). The most important outcome in HIV-infected neonates, childhood AIDS, does not appear until after the perinatal period. The chronic hepatitis resulting from perinatal infection with hepatitis B virus is usually not symptomatic in the neonatal period, and the late sequelae of perinatal hepatitis B infection, including cirrhosis and hepatocellular carcinoma, generally occur decades later (Sweet, 1990; Snydman, 1985).

Transmission of Organisms to the Fetus and Newborn

Since the influences of maternally transmitted organisms on adverse outcomes of pregnancy are generally presented individually, it may be instructive to compare their effects. For each organism, Table 2 indicates the approximate maternal prevalence in the U.S. population and the approximate number of mothers and their infants infected in the four million births per year in the United States. Also displayed in this table is the approximate number of U.S. infants each year who have specific types of sequelae associated with fetal or infant infection. The potential excess in preterm births attributable to various infections and the sequelae associated with those preterm births are discussed below.

The prevalence of maternal disease is estimated for some infections. Syphilis and HIV infections are currently found in approximately 0.15 to 0.2% of pregnant women in the United States (Gwinn et al., 1991; Davis et al., 1995). *N. gonorrhoeae*, hepatitis B virus, and *Trichomonas* infections are found in 1 to 2% of all pregnant women, and *Chlamydia* is found in about 5% (Mason and Brown, 1980; McGregor and French, 1991; Whitley et al., 1991; Stagno et al., 1986; Stagno, 1995; Judson, 1985). Maternal infection with herpes simplex virus or bacterial vaginosis is found in approximately 20% of pregnant women. Cytomegalovirus infection is estimated to occur in about one-third of all pregnant women. When translated into the total U.S. population, this means that there are approximately 6,000 to 8,000 pregnant women per year with syphilis or HIV infection, about 40,000 pregnant women per year with gonorrhea or hepatitis B virus infection, about 80,000 pregnant women with *Trichomonas* infection, perhaps 200,000 pregnant women with chlamydia, and approximately 800,000 pregnant women per year with herpes simplex virus infection or bacterial vaginosis. It is estimated that approximately 1.3 million pregnant women are infected with cytomegalovirus. Again, these numbers are our best estimates for infection for the entire population of pregnant women who give birth in the United States each year. Subpopulations of women who have markedly higher and lower prevalences have been described. For both herpes simplex virus and cytomegalovirus, it is assumed that previous infection, as defined serologically, is associated with persistent infection, and for that reason the number of pregnant women infected increases over time.

Some or most of the exposed infants of infected mothers, depending upon the disease, become infected (Table 2). These rates of infection range from 0.2% for herpes simplex virus to 3% for cytomegalovirus, and 25 to 40% for *T. pallidum*, hepatitis B virus, and HIV. If routine ophthalmic prophylaxis is not used, approximately 50% of the infants of infected mothers will acquire gonorrhea or chlamydia ophthalmic infections. However, with prophylaxis as practiced in most developed countries, gonococcal ophthalmia is rare and chlamydial conjunctivitis is much reduced. Translating these

Table 2 Estimated effect of direct fetal and neonatal infection with various STDs on adverse outcomes of pregnancy each year in the United States[a]

Maternal infection	Approximate maternal prevalence (%)	No. of mothers infected	No. of infants infected (%)[b]	No. of adverse outcomes of fetal or neonatal infection			
				Neonatal disease without sequelae	Perinatal death	Neurological sequelae	New-onset postneonatal illness and death
Bacterial vaginosis	20.0	800,000	0 (0)	0	0	0	0
Chlamydia	5.0	200,000	100,000 (50.0)	±[c]	0	0	20,000
Cytomegalovirus infection	33.0	1,300,000	40,000 (3.0)	500	300	2,000	5,000
Gonorrhea	1.0	40,000	20,000 (50.0)	±	±	±	0
Hepatitis B	1.0	40,000	12,000[d] (30.0)	0	0	0	4,000
Herpes	20.0	800,000	1,200 (0.15)	400	400	400	0
HIV infection	0.2	8,000	2,000[e] (25.0)	0	0	0	2,000
Syphilis	0.2	8,000	3,200 (40.0)	1,200	1,000	1,000	0
Trichomoniasis	2.0	80,000	0 (0)	0	0	0	0

[a] Assuming 4,000,000 births per year.
[b] Percentage with respect to the number of mothers infected.
[c] ± Occurs but rarely.
[d] Without neonatal hepatitis B immunoglobulin.
[e] Without maternal zidovudine.

numbers into the U.S. birth population, it can be seen that approximately 1,500 to 3,000 infants each year will be infected with herpes simplex virus, *T. pallidum*, or HIV, about 12,000 will be infected with hepatitis B virus, about 40,000 will be infected with cytomegalovirus, and 120,000 will be infected with *Chlamydia*. Infants are virtually never infected with *Trichomonas.* Manifestation of bacterial vaginosis in the infant is unknown. However, neonatal infections with *Ureaplasma urealyticum*, *Mycoplasma hominis*, various *Bacteroides* spp., *Gardnerella*, or other bacterial vaginosis-related organisms have been reported (Harrison et al., 1983).

Adverse Outcomes Associated with Maternal-Fetal-Neonatal Transmission

The next several columns in Table 2 show potential outcomes associated with fetal and perinatal infection with each of the organisms. These are estimates of outcomes achieved with current medical practices. From the existing literature, it is estimated that of the 3,200 infants infected with syphilis at the time of birth, approximately 1,000 will be stillborn or will die as neonates and about 1,000 will have long-term neurological or other sequelae. Approximately 1,200 of these 3,200 infants will live and will not have apparent long-term sequelae. With gonorrhea, assuming no ophthalmologic disease because of prophylaxis, there will be few major sequelae in infants as a result of neonatal infection. For the 100,000 infants infected with *Chlamydia* at birth, again assuming no long-term ophthalmologic sequelae because of prophylaxis, it is estimated that there will be approximately 20,000 cases of chlamydial pneumonia, nearly all of which will regress spontaneously or respond to antibiotics; however, a small portion of the affected infants will develop chronic respiratory disease (Schachter et al., 1986). Without immunoprophylaxis, approximately 4,000 of the 12,000 infants infected with hepatitis B virus at birth will ultimately develop cirrhosis or hepatocellular carcinoma (Sweet, 1990; Zeldis and Crumpacker, 1995). These numbers should be substantially reduced with routine neonatal hepatitis B immunoglobulin prophylaxis and vaccination. Of the 1,200 infants infected at birth with herpes simplex virus, an estimated 400 will die during the perinatal period, approximately 400 will have neurological sequelae, and 400 will have neonatal disease but no long-term sequelae (Whitley et al., 1991). Of the 40,000 infants infected with cytomegalovirus, approximately 7% will have signs of disease in the neonatal period. Of these 2,800 infants, 300 will die and 2,000 will have major neurological sequelae. Later in life, an additional 5,000 infants will suffer significant hearing loss associated with the cytomegalovirus infection (Stagno, 1995). It is estimated that without maternal and infant prophylaxis, 2,000 infants per year in the United States will be infected with HIV. It is assumed that each of these 2,000 infants will ultimately manifest AIDS and die. With zidovudine prophylaxis, approximately 70% of these infections and deaths could be prevented (Connor et al., 1994).

LOW BIRTH WEIGHT AND PRETERM BIRTH

Low birth weight, defined as a weight of less than 2,500 g, includes preterm infants as well as infants who are growth retarded. Low birth weight occurs in approximately 6% of all Caucasian babies and in approximately 12 to 13% of all African American babies in the United States. This is an easier pregnancy outcome measure to obtain than is preterm birth, because the date of conception is often difficult to determine. This is because the date of the last menses either is not known or is an unreliable predictor of gestational age. Nevertheless, preterm birth, defined by the World Health Organization as a birth occurring at less than 37 weeks gestation, complicates approximately 11% of all births in the United States. African American mothers have about twice the rate of preterm birth as Caucasian mothers. Overall, there has been no change or even a small increase in the rate of preterm birth in recent decades (Creasy, 1993).

The research focus is on preterm births that occur between viability (at about 23 weeks gestation) and 30 or 32 weeks gestation (Allen et al., 1993). More than 60% of the neonatal deaths and much of the short-term morbidity as well as long-term neurological disability occur in the babies born in this gestational age range. In most studies, approximately 40 or 50% of all preterm births follow spontaneous onset of labor with intact membranes (Tucker et al., 1991). The rate of spontaneous labor resulting in preterm delivery has remained basically unchanged, despite public health and medical interventions introduced over the last several decades. Approximately 20 to 25% of preterm births are associated with the physician's decision to intervene in the pregnancy, usually because of a maternal or fetal medical emergency. Maternal conditions that indicate preterm delivery include preeclampsia, other severe medical diseases, growth retardation, or evidence of fetal hypoxia. Here, the goal of early delivery is to avoid significant maternal morbidity and mortality or to prevent a fetal death. Somewhere between 25 and 40% of all preterm births follow spontaneous rupture of the fetal membranes. In those cases, labor generally ensues within 24 to 48 h. At the earliest gestational ages, a latent period of 1 or 2 weeks or more commonly occurs between rupture of membranes and delivery.

One of the major findings associated with spontaneous preterm rupture of the membranes is infection of the fetal membranes, called chorioamnionitis. Bacterial infection of the membranes and placenta prior to membrane rupture has been implicated as an etiology of premature rupture of the membranes (Gibbs et al., 1992). For years, there has been substantial histological evidence that the birth of babies weighing less than 1,000 g is associated with chorioamnionitis (Guzik and Winn, 1985; Mueller-Heubach et al., 1990). In recent years, evidence obtained by Hillier et al. (1991), Watts et al. (1992), Cassell et al. (1993b), and others suggested that specific organisms, such as *Ureaplasma*, *Mycoplasma*, *Gardnerella*, *Bacteroides*, and *Mobiluncus* species, can be found associated with this histologic chorioamnionitis. Although these organisms can be found in the normal vagina, they dominate the vaginal flora in women with bacterial vaginosis.

Survival of preterm babies is highly dependent on gestational age. Survival is now about 30% at week 23 of gestation, 50% at week 25, and 90% at week 28 (Copper et al., 1993). Recent decreases in infant mortality reflect improved survival of very preterm babies. In fact, it is rare for the older preterm babies, i.e., those born at or beyond 32 weeks, to die. The improvement in survival, especially at the more advanced preterm gestational ages, has been so great in recent years that nearly 60% of all neonatal deaths now occur in infants born weighing less than 1,000 g. These infants are also at substantial risk for long-term handicap, with about 25% having either cerebral palsy or other major impairment (McCormick, 1985; Hack and Fanaroff, 1993).

Probably more important than the specific deaths associated with neonatal sepsis is the likely association of spontaneous preterm delivery with intrauterine infection. There is a rapidly accumulating body of evidence that spontaneous preterm labor, especially when it occurs very early in gestation (i.e., earlier than 28 weeks), occurs in association with bacterial infection of the upper genital tract (Andrews et al., 1995; Gibbs et al., 1992). Infections of the decidua, fetal membranes, and amniotic fluid have been associated with preterm delivery. Support for this infectious etiology is partially derived from data linking the presence of pathogens in both the amniotic fluid and chorioamnion with spontaneous labor in women with intact membranes who are otherwise free of clinical signs or symptoms of infection (Krohn et al., 1991). The majority of these reports include cultures of amniotic fluid obtained by amniocentesis. However, recent studies have also implicated microbial infection of the chorioamnion as an important potential etiology of spontaneous preterm labor. In fact, women in spontaneous labor are twice as likely to have microbial infection of the chorioamnion as of the amniotic fluid (Cassell et al., 1993a). Importantly, there is an inverse relationship between a positive chorioamnion or amniotic fluid culture and the gestational age at delivery for women with spontaneous labor (Watts et al., 1992). That is, the earlier the gestational age, the higher the likelihood that there will be associated microbial infection of the upper genital tract (Cassell et al., 1993b). Indeed, studies now implicate chorioamnion infection as a potential cause of up to 80% of the very early spontaneous preterm births.

One of the difficult questions related to genital tract infections is whether they are causally associated with preterm birth. With virtually each of these organisms, a range of associations has been reported, varying from none to strong. In total, however, it appears that spontaneous preterm birth (defined as a birth following labor or rupture of the membranes) occurs more frequently in women with than without infection. However, even though gonorrhea, chlamydial infection, and other sexually transmitted diseases are usually found more frequently in women who have a spontaneous preterm birth, these women have other risk factors as well. Furthermore, most studies claiming an association between various infections and preterm birth have not considered many of these confounding variables. As an example, gonorrhea has been associated with spontaneous preterm birth in a number of studies (Elliott et al., 1990). Almost none of these adjusted for most risk factors, especially for the presence of bacterial vaginosis (Donders et al., 1993). Therefore, while it is likely that maternal gonorrhea infection is associated with an independent two- or threefold risk for spontaneous preterm birth, this conclusion is not certain. As distinguished from the organisms associated with bacterial vaginosis, the gonococcus is rarely found in the amniotic fluid or the fetal membranes in women who give birth prematurely. Syphilis is widely reported to be associated with a twofold increase in the risk of preterm birth, and this relationship is relatively consistent in most studies (Ingall et al., 1995).

Chlamydial infection has been associated with prematurity in some studies but not in others, with the majority of the studies showing no increased risk (Martin et al., 1982; Martius et al., 1988). Sweet et al. (1987), however, reported that women who had *C. trachomatis* infection and immunoglobulin M (IgM) antibodies were more likely to experience a spontaneous preterm birth than were women who had *C. trachomatis* infection and IgG, but not IgM, antibodies. In the Preterm Prediction Study, women tested for *C. trachomatis* at 24 weeks gestation had about twice as many preterm births associated with the presence of this organism as uninfected women did (Andrews et al., 1997). However, after adjusting for other risk factors, this association was no longer significant, contributing to the continuing uncertainty about whether chlamydial infection plays a causative role in preterm birth. Several antibiotic treatment studies report a reduction in the number of preterm births of the infants of women who had chlamydial infection. However, these studies were generally not randomized, and most were performed without knowledge of whether bacterial vaginosis or other sexually transmitted diseases were present. Many women who have chlamydial infection also have bacterial vaginosis, and in studies in which treatment of chlamydial infection appeared to reduce the rate of preterm birth, the effects of treatment on bacterial vaginosis may have played a role in the observed rate of reduction (Lamont et al., 1986; Gravett et al., 1986).

Vaginal infection with *Trichomonas vaginalis* has been associated with preterm birth in some but not all studies. The largest and most recently published study confirmed that women infected with *T. vaginalis* have a 30% increased risk of preterm birth (Cotch et al., 1997). Many of the other sexually transmitted diseases, such as HIV, hepatitis B, and genital herpes simplex virus infections, have been associated with an increased risk for spontaneous preterm birth in some but not most studies. In general, the evidence for a causative link between maternal infection with these organisms and spontaneous preterm birth is poor (Goldenberg et al., 1997).

Bacterial Vaginosis and Preterm Birth

Bacterial vaginosis is extremely common, being found in approximately 25 to 40% or more of African American women and in approximately 10 to 15% of Caucasian women (Eschenbach, 1993; Goldenberg et al., 1996b; Meis et al., 1995). More than 15 studies show an association between bacterial vaginosis and spontaneous preterm birth. Bacterial vaginosis seems to be more associated with early preterm birth (<32 weeks) rather than late preterm birth (33 to 36 weeks). Furthermore, two randomized and blinded antibiotic treatment trials demonstrate a reduction in the incidence of spontaneous preterm births of infants born to women at high risk for premature delivery (Hauth et al., 1995; Morales et al., 1994). Because of its frequency in populations at risk for preterm birth and the 1.5- to 3-fold-increased risk for spontaneous preterm birth, as many as 40% of early spontaneous preterm births, especially to African American women, may be attributable to bacterial vaginosis (Goldenberg et al., 1998; Fiscella, 1995, 1996). It should also be pointed out, however, that bacterial vaginosis could be a marker for another unrecognized condition which may be the etiology of the poor pregnancy outcome (Romero et al., 1989). For example, some investigators believe that bacterial vaginosis is an imperfect marker for an upper genital tract infection or endometritis caused by various bacterial vaginosis-related organisms (Hameed et al., 1984; Gray et al., 1992). Therefore, the prematurity attributed to bacterial vaginosis or reduced by its treatment may instead be related to an associated upper genital tract infection (Krohn et al., 1995; Korn et al., 1995; Hillier et al., 1988). Culturing for a vaginal colonization of individual bacterial vaginosis-associated organisms including *U. urealyticum* has not proven useful in predicting which women will have a preterm birth (Carey et al., 1991).

As discussed above, it is not absolutely clear whether maternal infections such as gonorrhea, syphilis, chlamydial infection, group B streptococcal infection, or trichomoniasis result in preterm birth. The data supporting the notion that bacterial vaginosis is associated with spontaneous preterm birth are more solid, especially with two trials of bacterial vaginosis treatment showing substantial reductions in the preterm birth rates (Hauth et al., 1995; Morales et al., 1994). Although the relationships are uncertain, based on our assessment of the literature, we assumed that gonorrhea is associated with a threefold increase in the preterm birth rate and that syphilis, chlamydial infection, and bacterial vaginosis infections are each associated with a twofold increase in preterm birth. The twofold-increased risk of preterm birth associated with bacterial vaginosis is more certain. From these numbers and the rates of maternal infection, assuming a 10% rate of prematurity in the general population, the excess number of preterm births per year in the United States associated with maternal infection with each organism can be calculated (Table 3). As an example, if 40,000 pregnant women in the United States are infected per year with gonorrhea, and if these women have a 30% instead of a 10% rate of spontaneous preterm birth, maternal gonorrhea infection may be associated with an estimated 8,000 excess preterm births. For the 3,200 women with syphilis, assuming a twofold increase in preterm births, approximately 320 excess preterm births owing to syphilis may occur in the United States each year. Assuming a twofold increase in preterm births, as many as 20,000 excess preterm births may be expected for the 200,000 mothers with chlamydial infection each year. Applying the same logic to maternal bacterial vaginosis infections and assuming a twofold increase in preterm births associated with bacterial vaginosis, an excess of 80,000 preterm births can be expected for the 800,000 women with bacterial vaginosis.

The last two columns in Table 3 show the estimated number of perinatal deaths and infants with major neurological handicaps associated with maternal infections and preterm births if one makes the assumption that 5% of the preterm infants die and 5% are neurologically handicapped with such conditions as blindness, hydrocephalus, mental retardation, or cerebral palsy. If these assumptions are correct, prematurity secondary to maternal gonococcal infections may be responsible for approximately 400 perinatal deaths and 400 episodes of long-term neurological sequelae. Through its influence on preterm birth, syphilis would be responsible for an additional 16 perinatal deaths and for 16 episodes of long-term neurological sequelae. Chlamydial infection might account for as many as 1,000 excess perinatal deaths and 1,000 episodes of long-term disability. Maternal bacterial vaginosis, because of its prevalence in the population and an associated twofold increase in preterm birth, may be responsible for approximately 80,000 excess preterm births, 4,000 perinatal deaths, and 4,000 episodes of long-term neurological sequelae. We emphasize that most of these adverse outcomes associated with preterm birth occur without fetal or neonatal infection.

SUMMARY

Fetal or neonatal infections with the agents of sexually transmitted diseases—*T. pallidum*, herpes simplex virus, and HIV—may have devastating

Table 3 Estimated effect of various sexually transmitted diseases on adverse outcomes of pregnancy through their effect on preterm birth[a]

Maternal infection	Approximate maternal prevalence (%)	No. of mothers infected	Estimated increase in preterm birth (fold)[b]	Estimated no. of excess preterm births	Adverse outcomes linked to preterm birth[c]	
					No. of perinatal deaths	No. of neurological sequelae
Bacterial vaginosis	20.0	800,000	2	80,000	4,000	4,000
Chlamydia	5.0	200,000	2	20,000	1,000	1,000
Cytomegalovirus infection	33.0	1,300,000	—[d]	—	—	—
Gonorrhea	1.0	40,000	3	8,000	400	400
Hepatitis B	1.0	40,000	—	—	—	—
Herpes	20.0	800,000	—	—	—	—
HIV infection	0.2	8,000	—	—	—	—
Syphilis	0.2	8,000	2	400	20	20
Trichomoniasis	2.0	80,000	1.3	—	—	—

[a] Assuming 4,000,000 U.S. births per year.
[b] Based on best available data in untreated women.
[c] Assuming 5% deaths and 5% neurological sequelae.
[d] —, insufficient evidence for a causative relationship.

effects, including death and long-term (neurological) disability. In the United States, between 1,000 and 2,500 infants per year die or are severely damaged as a result of each of these infections. In contrast to these relatively rare outcomes, approximately 400,000 infants are born prematurely each year; more than 20,000 of these die in the fetal or the neonatal period, and another 20,000 have neurological sequelae. If the projected effect on preterm birth by bacterial vaginosis and the other organisms proposed here is correct, as many as 100,000 preterm births and 5,000 or more of the deaths, as well as a similar number of the major disabilities, may be associated with maternal infections. Since bacterial vaginosis can be treated and since there are already two treatment trials showing a reduction in the incidence of spontaneous preterm births to women with bacterial vaginosis, it would seem that the greatest potential for reducing adverse outcomes of pregnancy associated with maternal infection lies in preventing or treating bacterial vaginosis. However, it is important to point out that the two published bacterial vaginosis treatment trials that have demonstrated a significant reduction in the incidence of spontaneous preterm birth were conducted with women who were at high risk for preterm birth, because of a history of preterm birth (Hauth et al., 1995; Morales et al., 1994). Therefore, the potential for preventing prematurity by screening and treatment for bacterial vaginosis should be demonstrated in the general population (including low-risk women) before a universal screening and treatment program is instituted for all pregnant women. A multicenter trial sponsored by the National Institute of Child Health and Human Development and the National Institute of Allergy and Infectious Diseases to evaluate this situation is under way.

The prevalence of maternal infections varies in different populations, as does the percentage of infants infected; only a small proportion of infected infants have measurable morbidity or mortality. Nevertheless, it is reasonable to estimate the relative effect of various maternally transmitted diseases on adverse pregnancy outcome. By comparing the effect of direct transmission of specific organisms on adverse outcomes with the effect on overall outcome through an increase in the rate of preterm births, it should be possible to establish some basis for allocation of resources to future research as well as intervention programs aimed at reducing adverse outcomes of pregnancy. Finally, an appreciation of the effect of bacterial vaginosis on outcomes of pregnancy associated with preterm birth gives bacterial vaginosis a greater public health importance than has been attributed to it in the past.

REFERENCES

Alberman, E., and F. Stanley. 1984. Guidelines to the epidemiological approach, p. 27–31. *In* F. Stanley and E. Alberman (ed.), *Clinics in Developmental Medicine* no.

87. *The Epidemiology of the Cerebral Palsies.* Spastics International Medical Publications, Lavenham, Suffolk, United Kingdom.

Alexander, E. R. 1984. Maternal and infant sexually transmitted diseases. *Urol. Clin. North Am.* **11:**131–139.

Alexander, E. R., and H. R. Harrison. 1983. Role of *Chlamydia trachomatis* in perinatal infection. *Rev. Infect. Dis.* **5:**713–719.

Alger, L. S., J. C. Lovchik, J. R. Hebel, L. R. Blackmon, and M. C. Crenshaw. 1988. The association of *Chlamydia trachomatis, Neisseria gonorrhoeae,* and group B streptococci with preterm rupture of the membranes and pregnancy outcome. *Am. J. Obstet. Gynecol.* **159:**397–404.

Allen, M. 1984. Developmental outcome and followup of the small for gestational age infant. *Semin. Perinatol.* **8:**123–156.

Allen, M. C., P. K. Donohue, and A. E. Dusman. 1993. The limit of viability—neonatal outcome of infants born at 22 to 25 weeks' gestation. *N. Engl. J. Med.* **329:**1597–1601.

Andrews, W. W., and the MFMU Network. 1997. The preterm prediction study: association of mid-trimester genital chlamydia infection and subsequent spontaneous preterm birth. *Am. J. Obstet. Gynecol.* **176:**151. (Abstract.)

Andrews, W. W., R. L. Goldenberg, and J. C. Hauth. 1995. Preterm labor: emerging role of genital tract infections. *Infect. Agents Dis.* **4:**196–211.

Carey, J. C., W. C. Blackwelder, R. P. Nugent, M. A. Matteson, A. V. Rao, D. A. Eschenbach, M. L. F. Lee, P. J. Rettig, J. A. Regan, K. L. Geromanos, D. H. Martin, J. G. Pastorek, R. S. Gibbs, K. A. Lipscomb, and the Vaginal Infections and Prematurity Study Group. 1991. Antepartum cultures for *Ureaplasma urealyticum* are not useful in predicting pregnancy outcome. *Am. J. Obstet. Gynecol.* **164:**728–733.

Cassell, G., W. W. Andrews, J. C. Hauth, G. Cutter, W. Hamrick, K. Baldus, and K. Walters. 1993a. Isolation of microorganisms from the chorioamnion is twice that from amniotic fluid at cesarean delivery in women with intact membranes. *Am. J. Obstet. Gynecol.* **168:**462. (Abstract.)

Cassell, G. H., J. C. Hauth, W. W. Andrews, G. Cutter, and R. L. Goldenberg. 1993b. Chorioamnion colonization: correlation with gestational age in women delivered following spontaneous labor versus indicated delivery. *Am. J. Obstet. Gynecol.* **168:**464. (Abstract.)

Chard, T., A. Yoong, and M. Macintosh. 1993. The myth of fetal growth retardation at term. *Br. J. Obstet. Gynaecol.* **100:**1076–1081.

Cohen, I., J. C. Veille, and B. M. Calkins. 1990. Improved pregnancy outcome following successful treatment of chlamydial infection. *JAMA* **263:**3160–3163.

Connor, E. M., R. S. Sperling, R. Gelber, P. Kiselev, G. Scott, M. D. O'Sullivan, R. VanDyke, M. Bey, W. Shearer, R. L. Jacobson, E. Jimenez, E. O'Neill, B. Bazin, J. F. Delfraissy, M. Culnane, R. Coombs, M. Elkins, J. Moye, P. Stratton, and J. Balsley, for the Pediatric AIDS Clinical Trials Group Protocol 076 Study Group. 1994. Reduction of maternal-infant transmission of human immunodeficiency virus type 1 with zidovudine treatment. *N. Engl. J. Med.* **331:**1173–1180.

Copper, R. L., R. L. Goldenberg, R. K. Creasy, M. B. DuBard, R. O. Davis, S. S. Entman, J. D. Iams, and S. P. Cliver. 1993. A multicenter study of preterm birth weight and gestational age specific neonatal mortality. *Am. J. Obstet. Gynecol.* **168:** 78–84.

Copper, R. L., R. L. Goldenberg, M. B. DuBard, R. O. Davis, and the Collaborative Group on Preterm Birth Prevention. 1994. Risk factors for fetal death in Caucasian, African American and Hispanic women. *Obstet. Gynecol.* **84:**490–495.

Cotch, M. F., J. G. Pastorek, R. P. Nugent, S. L. Hillier, R. S. Gibbs, D. H. Martin, D. A. Eschenbach, R. Edelman, J. C. Carey, J. A. Regan, M. A. Krohn, M. A. Klebanoff, A. V. Rao, and G. G. Rhoads. 1997. *Trichomonas vaginalis* associated with low birth weight and preterm delivery. The Vaginal Infections and Prematurity Study Group. *Sex. Transm. Dis.* **24:**361–362.

Creasy, R. K. 1993. Preterm birth prevention: where are we? *Am. J. Obstet. Gynecol.* **168:**1223–1230.

Davis, S. F., R. H. Byers, L. M. Lindegren, M. B. Caldwell, H. M. Karon, and M. Gwinn. 1995. Prevalence and incidence of vertically acquired HIV infection in the United States. *JAMA* **274:**952–955.

Donders, G. G., J. Desmyter, D. H. De Wet, and F. A. Van Assche. 1993. The association of gonorrhea and syphilis with premature birth and low birthweight. *Genitourin. Med.* **69:**98–101.

Elliott, B., R. C. Brunham, M. Laga, P. Piot, J. O. Ndinya-Achola, M. Maitha, M. Cheang, and F. A. Plummer. 1990. Maternal gonococcal infection as a preventable factor for low birth weight. *J. Infect. Dis.* **161:**531–536.

Eschenbach, D. A. 1993. History and review of bacterial vaginosis. *Am. J. Obstet. Gynecol.* **169:**441–445.

Fiscella, K. 1995. Race, perinatal outcome, and amniotic infection. *Obstet. Gynecol. Surv.* **51:**60–66.

Fiscella, K. 1996. Racial disparities in preterm births: the role of urogenital infections. *Public Health Rep.* **111:**104–113.

Fletcher, J. L., and R. C. Gordon. 1990. Perinatal transmission of bacterial sexually transmitted diseases. I. Syphilis and gonorrhea. *J. Fam. Pract.* **30:**448–456.

Fowler, K. B., S. Stagno, R. F. Pass, W. J. Britt, T. J. Boll, and C. A. Alford. 1992. The outcome of congenital cytomegalovirus infection in relation to maternal antibody status. *N. Engl. J. Med.* **326:**663–667.

Gibbs, R. S., M. D. Romero, S. L. Hillier, D. A. Eschenbach, and R. L. Sweet. 1992. A review of premature birth and subclinical infection. *Am. J. Obstet. Gynecol.* **166:** 1515–1528.

Goldenberg, R. L., G. R. Cutter, H. Hoffman, J. M. Foster, K. G. Nelson, and J. C. Hauth. 1989. Intrauterine growth retardation: standards for diagnosis. *Am. J. Obstet. Gynecol.* **161:**271–277.

Goldenberg, R. L., M. B. DuBard, S. P. Cliver, K. G. Nelson, K. Blankson, S. L. Ramey, C. T. Ramey, H. J. Hoffman, and A. Herman. 1996a. Pregnancy outcome and intelligence at age five years. *Am. J. Obstet. Gynecol.* **175:**1511–1515.

Goldenberg, R. L., M. A. Klebanoff, R. Nugent, M. A. Krohn, S. Hillier, and W. W. Andrews. 1996b. Bacterial colonization of the vagina during pregnancy. *Am. J. Obstet. Gynecol.* **174:**1618–1621.

Goldenberg, R. L., W. W. Andrews, A. C. Yuan, H. T. MacKay, and M. E. St. Louis. 1997. Sexually transmitted diseases and adverse outcomes of pregnancy. *Clin. Perinatol.* **24:**23–41.

Goldenberg, R. L., J. D. Iams, B. M. Mercer, P. J. Meis, A. H. Moawad, R. L. Copper, A. Das, E. Thom, F. Johnson, D. McNellis, J. Roberts, M. Miodovnik, J. P. Van Dorsten, S. N. Caritis, G. R. Thurnau, and S. F. Bottoms. 1998. The Preterm Prediction Study. The value of new vs. standard risk factors in predicting early and all spontaneous preterm birth. *Am. J. Public Health* **88:**233–238.

Gravett, M. G., H. P. Nelson, T. DeRouen, C. Critchlow, D. A. Eschenbach, and K. K. Holmes. 1986. Independent associations of bacterial vaginosis and Chlamydia trachomatis infection with adverse pregnancy outcome. *JAMA* **256:**1899–1903.

Gray, D. J., H. B. Robinson, J. Malone, and R. B. Thomson, Jr. 1992. Adverse outcome in pregnancy following amniotic fluid isolation of Ureaplasma urealyticum. *Prenatal. Diagn.* **12:**111–117.

Guzik, D. S., and K. Winn. 1985. The association of chorioamnionitis with preterm delivery. *Obstet. Gynecol.* **65:**11–15.

Gwinn, M., M. Pappaioanou, J. R. George, W. H. Hannon, S. C. Wasser, M. A. Redus, R. Hoff, G. F. Grady, A. Willoughby, A. C. Novello, L. R. Petersen, T. J. Dondero, and J. W. Curran. 1991. Prevalence of HIV infection in childbearing women in the United States. *JAMA* **265:**1704–1708.

Hack, M., and A. A. Fanaroff. 1993. Outcomes of extremely immature infants—a perinatal dilemma. *N. Engl. J. Med.* **329:**1649–1650.

Hameed, C., N. Tejani, U. L. Verma, and F. Archbald. 1984. Silent chorioamnionitis as a cause of preterm labor refractory to tocolytic therapy. *Am. J. Obstet. Gynecol.* **149:**726–730.

Hardy, P. H., J. B. Hardy, E. E. Nell, D. A. Graham, M. R. Spence, and R. C. Rosenbaum. 1984. Prevalence of six sexually transmitted disease agents among pregnant inner-city adolescents and pregnancy outcome. *Lancet* **ii:**333–337.

Harrison, H. R., E. R. Alexander, L. Weinstein, M. Lewis, M. Nash, and D. A. Sim. 1983. Cervical *Chlamydia trachomatis* and mycoplasmal infections in pregnancy: epidemiology and outcomes. *JAMA* **250:**1721–1727.

Hauth, J. C., R. L. Goldenberg, W. W. Andrews, M. B. DuBard, and R. L. Copper. 1995. Reduced incidence of preterm delivery with metronidazole and erythromycin in women with bacterial vaginosis. *N. Engl. J. Med.* **333:**1732–1736.

Henderson, J. L., and C. P. Weiner. 1995. Congenital infection. *Curr. Opin. Obstet. Gynecol.* **7:**130–134.

Hillier, S. L., J. Martius, M. Krohn, N. Kiviat, K. K. Holmes, and D. A. Eschenbach. 1988. A case-control study of chorioamnionic infection and histologic chorioamnionitis in prematurity. *N. Engl. J. Med.* **319:**972–978.

Hillier, S. L., M. A. Krohn, N. B. Kiviat, D. H. Watts, and D. A. Eschenbach. 1991. Microbiologic causes and neonatal outcomes associated with chorioamnion infection. *Am. J. Obstet. Gynecol.* **165:**955–961.

Ingall, D., P. J. Sanchez, and D. M. Musher. 1995. Syphilis, p. 529–564. *In* J. S. Remington and J. O. Klein (ed.), *Infectious Diseases of the Fetus and Newborn Infant*, 4th ed. The W. B. Saunders Co., Philadelphia, Pa.

Judson, F. N. 1985. Assessing the number of genital chlamydial infections in the United States. *J. Reprod. Med.* **30:**269–272.

Korn, A. P., G. Bolan, N. Padian, M. Ohm-Smith, J. Schachter, and D. V. Landers. 1995. Plasma cell endometritis in women with symptomatic bacterial vaginosis. *Obstet. Gynecol.* **85:**387–390.

Krohn, M. A., S. L. Hillier, M. L. Lee, L. K. Rabe, and D. A. Eschenbach. 1991. Vaginal bacteroides species are associated with an increased rate of preterm delivery among women in preterm labor. *J. Infect. Dis.* **164:**88–93.

Krohn, M. A., S. L. Hillier, R. P. Nugent, M. F. Cotch, J. C. Carey, R. S. Gibbs, and D. A. Eschenbach, for the Vaginal Infection and Prematurity Study Group. 1995. The genital flora of women with intraamniotic infection. *J. Infect. Dis.* **171:**1475–1480.

Lamont, R. F., D. Taylor-Robinson, M. Newman, J. Wigglesworth, and M. G. Elder. 1986. Spontaneous early preterm labour associated with abnormal genital bacterial colonization. *Br. J. Obstet. Gynaecol.* **93:**804–810.

Lawson, H. W., H. K. Atrash, A. F. Saftlas, A. L. Franks, E. L. Finch, and J. M. Hughes. 1988. Ectopic pregnancy surveillance, United States, 1970–1978. *Morbid. Mortal. Weekly Rep.* **39**(SS-4):9–17.

Mandelbrot, L., M.-J. A. Mayaux, A. Bongain, A. Berrebi, Y. Moudoub-Jeanpetit, J.-L. Benifla, N. Ciraru-Vigneron, J. Le Chenadec, S. Blanche, and J. F. Delfraissy. 1996. Obstetric factors and mother-to-child transmission of human immunodeficiency virus type 1: the French perinatal cohorts. *Am. J. Obstet. Gynecol.* **175:**661–667.

Martin, D. H., L. Koutsky, D. A. Eschenbach, J. R. Daling, E. R. Alexander, J. K. Benedetti, and K. K. Holmes. 1982. Prematurity and perinatal mortality in pregnancies complicated by maternal Chlamydia trachomatis infections. *JAMA* **247:**1585–1588.

Martius, J., M. A. Krohn, S. L. Hillier, W. E. Stamm, K. K. Holmes, and D. A. Eschenbach. 1988. Relationships of vaginal lactobacillus species, cervical *Chlamydia trachomatis*, and bacterial vaginosis to preterm birth. *Obstet. Gynecol.* **71:**89–95.

Mason, P. R., and I. M. Brown. 1980. *Trichomonas* in pregnancy. *Lancet* **ii:**1025–1026.

Mayaux, M. J., S. Blanche, and C. Rouzioux, J. Le Chenadec, V. Chambrin, G. Firtion, M. D. Allemon, E. Vilmer, N. C. Vigneron, J. Tricoire, F. Guillot, C. Courpotin, and the French Pediatric HIV Infection Study Group. 1995. Maternal factors associated with perinatal HIV-1 transmission: the French cohort study—7 years of follow-up observation. *J. Acquired Immune Defic. Syndr. Hum. Retrovirol.* **8:**188–194.

McCormick, M. C. 1985. The contribution of low birth weight to infant mortality and childhood morbidity. *N. Engl. J. Med.* **312:**82–90.

McDonald, H. M., J. A. O'Loughlin, P. Jolly, R. Vigneswaran, and P. J. McDonald. 1991. Vaginal infection and preterm labour. *Br. J. Obstet. Gynecol.* **98:**427–435.

McDonald, H. M., J. A. O'Loughlin, P. Jolly, R. Vigneswaran, and P. J. McDonald. 1992. Prenatal microbiological risk factors associated with preterm birth. *Br. J. Obstet. Gynecol.* **99:**190–196.

McGregor, J. A., and J. I. French. 1991. *Chlamydia trachomatis* infection during pregnancy. *Am. J. Obstet. Gynecol.* **164:**1782–1788.

Meis, P. J., R. L. Goldenberg, J. D. Iams, B. Mercer, A. Moawad, D. McNellis, J. Roberts, A. Das, R. Copper, E. Thom, F. Johnson, W. Andrews, and the NICHD MFMU Network. 1995. Vaginal infections and spontaneous preterm birth. *Am. J. Obstet. Gynecol.* **172:**548.

Minkoff, H., A. N. Grunebaum, R. H. Schwarz, J. Feldman, M. Cummings, W. Crombleholme, L. Clark, G. Pringle, and W. M. McCormack. 1984. Risk factors for prematurity and premature rupture of membranes: a prospective study of the vaginal flora in pregnancy. *Am. J. Obstet. Gynecol.* **150:**965–972.

Minkoff, H., D. N. Burns, S. Landesman, J. Youchah, J. J. Goedert, R. P. Nugent, L. R. Muenz, and A. D. Willoughby. 1995. The relationship of the duration of ruptured membranes to vertical transmission of human immunodeficiency virus. *Am. J. Obstet. Gynecol.* **173:**585–589.

Morales, W. J., S. Schorr, and J. Albritton. 1994. Effect of metronidazole in patients with preterm birth in preceding pregnancy and bacterial vaginosis: a placebo-controlled, double-blind study. *Am. J. Obstet. Gynecol.* **171:**345–349.

Mueller-Heubach, E., D. N. Rubinstein, and S. S. Schwarz. 1990. Histologic chorioamnionitis and preterm delivery in different patient populations. *Obstet. Gynecol.* **75:**622–626.

Newell, M.-L., and the European Collaborative Study. 1994. Perinatal findings in children born to HIV-infected mothers. *Br. J. Obstet. Gynaecol.* **101:**136–141.

Romero, R., M. Sirtori, E. Oyarzun, C. Avila, M. Mazor, R. Callahan, V. Sabo, A. P. Athanassiadis, and J. C. Hobbins. 1989. Infection and labor. V. Prevalence, microbiology, and clinical significance of intra-amniotic infection in women with preterm labor and intact membranes. *Am. J. Obstet. Gynecol.* **161:**817–824.

Rouse, D. J., R. L. Goldenberg, S. P. Cliver, G. R. Cutter, S. T. Mennemeyer, and C. A. Fargason, Jr. 1994. Strategies for the prevention of early-onset neonatal group B streptococcal sepsis: a decision analysis. *Obstet. Gynecol.* **83:**483–494.

Rouzioux, C., D. Costagliola, M. Burgard, S. Blanche, M. J. Mayaux, C. Griscelli, and A. J. Valleron. 1995. Estimated timing of mother-to-child human immunodeficiency virus type I transmission by use of a Markov model. *Am. J. Epidemiol.* **142:**1330–1337.

Schachter, J., M. Grossman, R. L. Sweet, J. Holt, C. Jordan, and E. Bishop. 1986. Prospective study of perinatal transmission of Chlamydia trachomatis. *JAMA* **255:**3374–3377.

Schuchat, A., M. Oxtoby, S. Cochi, R. K. Sikes, A. Hightower, B. Plikaytis, and C. V. Broome. 1990. Population-based risk factors for neonatal group B streptococcal disease: results of a cohort study in metropolitan Atlanta. *J. Infect. Dis.* **162:**672–677.

Snydman, D. R. 1985. Hepatitis in pregnancy. *N. Engl. J. Med.* **313:**1398–1401.

Speroff, L., R. H. Glass, and N. G. Kase. 1994. *Clinical Gynecologic Endocrinology and Infertility*, 5th ed., p. 841–851. The Williams & Wilkins Co., Baltimore, Md.

Stagno, S. 1995. Cytomegalovirus, p. 312–353. *In* J. S. Remington and J. O. Klein (ed.), *Infectious Diseases of the Fetus and Newborn Infant*, 4th ed. The W. B. Saunders Co., Philadelphia, Pa.

Stagno, S., R. F. Pass, G. Cloud, W. J. Britt, R. E. Henderson, P. D. Walton, D. A. Veren, F. Page, and C. A. Alford. 1986. Primary cytomegalovirus infection in pregnancy: incidence, transmission to fetus, and clinical outcome. *JAMA* **256:**1904–1908.

Sweet, R. L. 1990. Hepatitis B infection in pregnancy. *Obstet. Gynecol. Rep.* **2:**128–139.

Sweet, R. L., D. V. Landers, C. Walker, and J. Schachter. 1987. Chlamydia trachomatis infection and pregnancy outcome. *Am. J. Obstet. Gynecol.* **156:**824–833.

Torfs, C. P., B. van den Berg, F. W. Oechsli, and S. Cummins. 1990. Prenatal and perinatal factors in the etiology of cerebral palsy. *J. Pediatr.* **116:**615–619.

Tucker, J. M., R. L. Goldenberg, R. O. Davis, R. C. Baker, C. L. Hauth, and J. Owen. 1991. Etiologies of preterm birth in an indigent population: Is prevention a logical expectation? *Obstet. Gynecol.* **77:**343–347.

Watts, D. H., M. A. Krohn, S. L. Hillier, and D. A. Eschenbach. 1992. The association of occult amniotic fluid infection with gestational age and neonatal outcome among women in preterm labor. *Obstet. Gynecol.* **79:**351–357.

Wendel, P. J., and G. D. Wendel, Jr. 1993. Sexually transmitted diseases in pregnancy. *Semin. Perinatol.* **17:**443–451.

Whitley, R. J., and C. Hutto. 1985. Neonatal herpes simplex virus infections. *Pediatr. Rev.* **7:**119.

Whitley, R., A. Arvin, C. Prober, L. Corey, S. Burchett, S. Plotkin, S. Starr, R. Jacobs, D. Powell, A. Nahmias, C. Sumaya, K. Edwards, C. Alford, G. Caddell, S. J. Soong, and the National Institute of Allergy and Infectious Diseases Collaborative Antiviral Study Group. 1991. Predictors of morbidity and mortality in neonates with herpes simplex virus infections. *N. Engl. J. Med.* **324:**450–454.

Zeldis, J. B., and C. S. Crumpacker. 1995. Hepatitis, p. 805–834. *In* J. S. Remington and J. O. Klein (ed.), *Infectious Diseases of the Fetus and Newborn Infant*, 4th ed. The W. B. Saunders Co., Philadelphia, Pa.

HOST FACTORS

2
Vaginal Ecology in Pregnancy

Sharon L. Hillier

The vaginal ecology of pregnant women does not differ substantially from that of women who are not pregnant. However, studies conducted over the last decade have established that most of the organisms that infect amniotic fluid or cause chorioamnionitis are derived from the lower genital tract. In addition, recent studies have established that some organisms that are considered part of the normal vaginal microflora are associated with an increased risk of preterm or low-birth-weight delivery or both when they are present at high density in the vagina. Both group B *Streptococcus* and *Escherichia coli* have been linked with preterm or low-birth-weight delivery and are known to invade the chorioamnion directly and cause chorioamnionitis. Other vaginal microorganisms that are part of the normal flora, including those associated with bacterial vaginosis, have been linked to an increased risk of preterm birth, amniotic fluid infection, and chorioamnionitis. In contrast, high-density vaginal colonization by *Lactobacillus* species has been linked to a decreased risk of most adverse outcomes of pregnancy. Similarly, women with *Lactobacillus*-predominant flora have also been demonstrated to experience infections with *Neisseria gonorrhoeae*, *Chlamydia trachomatis*, and *Trichomonas vaginalis* less frequently. Thus, the constituents of the normal vaginal ecosystem influence the risk of preterm or low-birth-weight delivery, amnionitis, chorioamnionitis, or postpartum infections or all of these.

NORMAL VAGINAL ECOLOGY OF PREGNANCY

The vaginal microbial flora of pregnant women, like that of nonpregnant women, is diverse. In two recent studies, the vaginal microflora was

---

Sharon L. Hillier, Department of Obstetrics, Gynecology and Reproductive Sciences, Magee-Womens Hospital, University of Pittsburgh, Pittsburgh, PA 15213.

Sexually Transmitted Diseases and Adverse Outcomes of Pregnancy
Edited by P. J. Hitchcock, H. T. MacKay, J. N. Wasserheit, and R. Binder
©1999 American Society for Microbiology, Washington, D.C.

assessed in cross-sectional groups of 85 (Hillier et al., 1993) and 126 (Puapermpoonsiri et al., 1996) normal pregnant women. Vaginal fluid specimens were obtained on swabs. As shown in Table 1, lactobacilli were recovered from nearly all of the women, usually at concentrations in excess of 10 million CFU/g of vaginal fluid. H_2O_2-producing lactobacilli were recovered from 61% of the women who had *Lactobacillus*-predominant microflora. Obligately anaerobic gram-negative rods and cocci were recovered from nearly all of the women as well but at 1,000-fold lower concentrations. The most common isolate of anaerobic gram-negative rods recovered from the vagina was *Prevotella bivia*, which was recovered from 61% of the women. *Candida albicans* was recovered from 31% of the women, while group B *Streptococcus* and *E. coli* were recovered from 15 to 17%. *Ureaplasma urealyticum* was a frequent vaginal isolate, recovered from 78% of the pop-

Table 1 Vaginal microflora of 85 pregnant women having *Lactobacillus*-predominant flora who gave birth at term[a]

Organism	Frequency (% of women)	Concn (CFU/ml)
Facultative bacteria		
Lactobacillus species	96	$10^{7.0}$
Gardnerella vaginalis	61	$10^{7.2}$
Coagulase-negative staphylococci	89	$10^{4.0}$
Viridans streptococci	55	$10^{4.7}$
Enterococcus species	39	$10^{5.1}$
Group B *Streptococcus*	15	$10^{4.2}$
Escherichia coli	17	$10^{4.1}$
Obligate anaerobes		
Prevotella bivia	61	$10^{4.1}$
Prevotella species	14	$10^{3.4}$
Porphyromonas asaccharolytica	31	$10^{3.0}$
Bacteroides ureolyticus	36	$10^{3.0}$
Bacteroides fragilis group	9	$10^{3.5}$
Fusobacterium nucleatum	8	$10^{3.3}$
Peptostreptococcus species	92	$10^{4.2}$
Peptococcus niger	20	$10^{2.7}$
Genital mycoplasmas		
Ureaplasma urealyticum	78	$10^{5.0}$
Mycoplasma hominis	15	$10^{3.5}$
Yeast		
Candida albicans	31	ND[b]

[a] Modified from Hillier et al. (1993).
[b] ND, not determined.

ulation. In another study, which included pregnant Japanese and Thai women, similar results were obtained, with 87% of the women being colonized by H_2O_2-producing lactobacilli and 36% having *C. albicans* (Puapermpoonsiri et al., 1996).

These studies demonstrate that the vaginal ecosystem of pregnant women is complex and includes several microorganisms that are difficult to cultivate and identify and are therefore unfamiliar to many clinicians and microbiologists. Because of the increasingly recognized role of the endogenous flora in complications in pregnancy and infections of the upper genital tract, the importance of the composition and regulation of the vaginal ecosystem has been recognized. It has also become increasingly apparent that the concentration of the organisms present in the vagina plays an important role in the risk of adverse outcomes of pregnancy.

In the past, it was widely postulated that during pregnancy the vaginal flora changed to become more *Lactobacillus* predominant as the gestational age increased. In a cross-sectional study, women were evaluated at different points in pregnancy and postpartum (Goplerud et al., 1976). Different women were evaluated at each time point. The authors reported that 85% of women were positive for lactobacilli at 8 to 13 weeks gestation and 97% were positive at 34 to 40 weeks gestation, compared to only 64% at 6 weeks postpartum. However, since different groups of women were studied at each interval, the changes in *Lactobacillus* frequency over pregnancy may have reflected differences in the patient populations. More recent data derived from a cohort of pregnant women evaluated at three time points (23 to 26, 30 to 33, and 34 to 36 weeks gestation) have shown that the frequency of lactobacilli remains relatively constant over the second and third trimesters of pregnancy (Fig. 1) (Cotch et al., 1998).

Ethnicity has been reported to have an effect on the vaginal microflora of pregnant women. The vaginal microflora of women of different ethnic groups was evaluated in the Vaginal Infections and Prematurity Study of

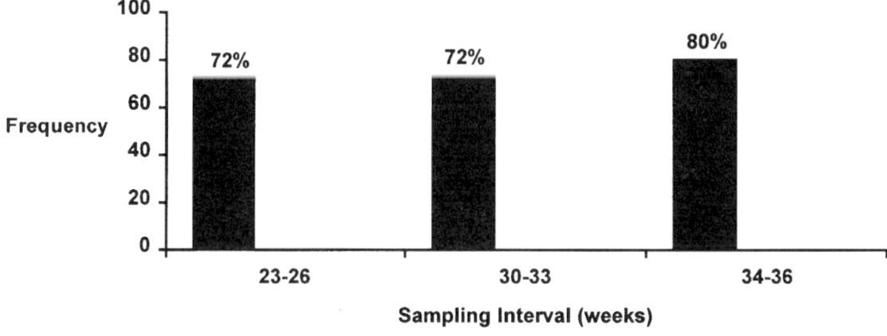

Figure 1 Prevalence of facultative lactobacilli at three sampling times during pregnancy. Modified from Cotch et al. (1998).

more than 13,000 women (Goldenberg et al., 1996). In that study, it was found that African American women were more likely to be colonized by group B *Streptococcus*, anaerobic gram-negative rods, *Mycoplasma hominis*, and *U. urealyticum* than were Caucasian or Hispanic women. African American women were also significantly more likely to have bacterial vaginosis, *T. vaginalis*, *C. trachomatis*, and *N. gonorrhoeae* than were Caucasian women. In contrast, Hispanic women were more likely than Caucasian women to be colonized by group B *Streptococcus* but were otherwise very similar to non-Hispanic Caucasian women with respect to the frequency of genital microorganisms. Asian women had comparatively lower frequency of all genital pathogens and had a statistically significant decrease in the frequency of *U. urealyticum* compared with Caucasian women (Table 2).

In a smaller study in Great Britain, African and Caribbean women were found to have higher levels of abnormal vaginal flora and bacterial vaginosis compared with Caucasian women, while Asian women were found to have lower frequencies of bacterial vaginosis and abnormal vaginal flora than did Caucasian women (Hay et al., 1994). It has been noted that when African American and Caucasian women of similar income levels are compared, there is still a twofold or greater discrepancy in the rate of preterm delivery (Goldenberg et al., 1996). Hispanic women, on the other hand, have one of the lowest rates of low-birth-weight infants even though the His-

Table 2 Frequency of genital microorganisms in women of different ethnic groups[a]

Organism or infection	Frequency (%) in ethnic group:			
	Caucasian (n = 4,049)	African American (n = 5,285)	Hispanic (n = 4,240)	Asian (n = 173)
Vaginal organisms				
Group B *Streptococcus*	14	24*	24*	13
Anaerobic gram-negative rods	14	25*	13	15
Mycoplasma hominis	27	46*	26	16
Ureaplasma urealyticum	73	85*	71	52*
Cervical organisms				
Chlamydia trachomatis	5	16*	6*	2
Neisseria gonorrhoeae	0.4	3*	0.6	0
Vaginal infections				
Bacterial vaginosis	9	23	16	6
Trichomoniasis	6	23	7	4

[a] Reprinted from Goldenberg et al. (1996) with permission.

[b] *, significantly different compared with Caucasian women ($P < 0.05$).

panic women included in studies have modest income levels. Some authors have postulated that the disproportionate burden of preterm low-birth-weight infants born to African American compared with Caucasian women may relate to the substantial differences in the rates of genital tract infections in those populations (Goldenberg et al., 1996).

Sexual behavior is thought to affect the vaginal ecosystem. Frequency of sexual intercourse during pregnancy was evaluated in the Vaginal Infections and Prematurity Study (Read and Klebanoff, 1993). Those investigators interviewed women at 23 to 26 weeks gestation, twice in the third trimester, and again at delivery. Not surprisingly, they found that 61% of the pregnant women reported having vaginal intercourse one or more times a week in the second trimester of pregnancy, while only 28% of women reported that frequency of intercourse in the last month of pregnancy. These authors reported that women who are colonized with *T. vaginalis* or *M. hominis* and who engaged in frequent sexual intercourse during pregnancy were at higher risk for preterm delivery than were women colonized by these organisms who did not have frequent intercourse. The authors speculated that frequent sexual intercourse may introduce organisms from the vagina into the cervix, which could begin the process of upper tract infection leading to preterm birth. What emerged from that study was that intercourse itself was not a risk factor for preterm birth but, rather, that it was frequent intercourse on the part of women who had certain lower genital tract infections.

CONSTITUENTS OF NORMAL FLORA AND ASSOCIATION WITH ADVERSE OUTCOMES OF PREGNANCY

Organisms Associated with Bacterial Vaginosis

Bacterial vaginosis is a condition in which high concentrations of vaginal lactobacilli are replaced by a mixed population of *Gardnerella vaginalis*, anaerobic gram-negative rods and cocci, and genital mycoplasmas. The anaerobic bacteria in the vagina of women with bacterial vaginosis that are thought to play the greatest role in virulence include *P. bivia* (formerly *Bacteroides bivius*) and the black-pigmented anaerobic gram-negative rods formerly referred to as *Bacteroides melaninogenicus*. As noted in Table 1, *U. urealyticum* is frequently found in the vagina of pregnant women without bacterial vaginosis. However, in women with bacterial vaginosis, *M. hominis* increases in concentration and frequency. *G. vaginalis*, the facultative gram-variable rod which has been most closely associated with bacterial vaginosis, is present in nearly 100% of women with this condition (Hillier et al., 1993). Some of the earliest studies evaluating the associations between bacterial vaginosis and adverse outcomes of pregnancy focused on individual organisms associated with bacterial vaginosis rather than the syndrome itself.

In 1984, Minkoff et al. published an elegant longitudinal study in which 233 women enrolled for prenatal care at 14 weeks gestation were observed through delivery. Vaginal cultures for anaerobic gram-negative rods (*Bacteroides* species) and *M. hominis* were performed. The presence of *Bacteroides* in the vagina was associated with preterm delivery (relative risk = 1.4, $P < 0.03$), premature rupture of membranes (relative risk = 2.8, $P = 0.03$), and delivery of an infant weighing less than 2,500 g (relative risk = 1.8, $P < 0.04$) in a stepwise logistical regression adjusting for maternal age, parity, previous preterm delivery, abortion, and other vaginal organisms. The Minkoff et al. (1984) study was the first to describe the association between vaginal anaerobic bacteria and complications of pregnancy.

Other studies also have examined the association between *M. hominis* and low birth weight. Berman et al. (1987) studied 12,024 Native American women enrolled at 8 to 24 weeks gestation and reported that colonization by *M. hominis* was significantly correlated with low birth weight (less than 2,500 g (relative risk = 1.4, $P < 0.05$). In a study in which 3,293 women were enrolled during prenatal care, colonization with *M. hominis* was associated with a 40% increased risk of low birth weight (relative risk = 1.4, $P < 0.05$) (Sweet et al., 1987). Another group of investigators also reported an association between colonization with *M. hominis* and preterm delivery (odds ratio = 2.0, 95% confidence interval) in a study of 801 women screened during prenatal care between 22 and 30 weeks gestation (Investigators of the Johns Hopkins Study of Cervicitis and Adverse Pregnancy Outcome, 1989).

Three more recent studies have confirmed the original observation by Minkoff et al. (1984) that high-density vaginal colonization by anaerobic gram-negative rods (*Bacteroides* species) is associated with preterm or low-birth-weight delivery or both. Krohn et al. (1991) reported that women with vaginal *B. bivius* (now known as *Prevotella bivia*) or *B. fragilis* had an increased rate of preterm delivery at less than 34 weeks gestation (relative risk = 2.0, $P < 0.05$). In a similar study performed in Australia, vaginal colonization by anaerobic gram-negative rods was related to a 60% increased risk of delivery at less than 34 weeks gestation (McDonald et al., 1991). In the Vaginal Infections and Prematurity Study, the role of *Bacteroides* and *M. hominis* was evaluated in the presence or absence of concurrent bacterial vaginosis (Hillier et al., 1995a). Women vaginally colonized by both *Bacteroides* and *M. hominis* in the absence of bacterial vaginosis still had a 50% increased risk of giving birth to a preterm and low-birth-weight infant. In addition, women with bacterial vaginosis who were colonized vaginally by both *Bacteroides* and *M. hominis* had an increased risk for preterm low-birth-weight delivery compared with women who had bacterial vaginosis without those organisms. Taken together, these studies suggest that vaginal high-density colonization by anaerobic gram-negative rods and

M. hominis places women at increased risk for preterm delivery even after accounting for the presence of bacterial vaginosis.

The association between bacterial vaginosis-associated organisms and amniotic fluid infection has been evaluated in three studies. In the first study, women with an abnormal vaginal flora as assessed by Gram stain were shown to have an increased incidence of amniotic fluid infection (Silver et al., 1989) and were more likely to have *G. vaginalis* and *M. hominis* in their amniotic fluid. In the second study, the largest study done to date, the presence of several vaginal organisms in the second trimester of pregnancy was linked to the development of amniotic fluid infection as diagnosed by an oral temperature of greater than or equal to 38°C along with two or more signs of amniotic fluid infection including maternal or fetal tachycardia, uterine tenderness, purulent amniotic fluid, or increased maternal peripheral leukocyte count. Women having high-density vaginal colonization by *G. vaginalis, Bacteroides* species, and *M. hominis* had an increased risk for amniotic fluid infection after excluding women who had gonorrhea or chlamydial infection (Krohn et al., 1995). Women vaginally colonized by *G. vaginalis, Bacteroides* species, and *M. hominis* had more than a twofold increased risk for amniotic fluid infection compared with women not colonized by any of those organisms (Table 3). The third study investigated amniotic fluid infection in women in preterm labor who had intact fetal membranes (Hillier et al., 1995b). These authors reported that women with *Lactobacillus*-predominant vaginal flora were less likely to have bacteria in their amniotic fluid (Hillier et al., 1995b). Further, women with

Table 3 Relationship of *G. vaginalis, Bacteroides* species, and *M. hominis* with amniotic fluid infection[a,b]

Presence of:			% with amniotic fluid infection	Relative risk (95% confidence interval)[c]
G. vaginalis	*Bacteroides* species	*M. hominis*		
+	+	+	3.7	2.6 (1.7–3.9)
+	+	−	3.2	2.3 (1.3–4.0)
+	−	+	3.2	2.3 (1.6–3.2)
−	+	+	2.9	2.0 (0.5–8.0)
+	−	−	2.3	1.6 (1.1–2.3)
−	+	−	1.6	1.1 (0.4–3.1)
−	−	+	2.7	1.9 (0.9–3.6)
−	−	−	1.4	Reference

[a]From Krohn et al. (1995) with permission.
[b]Women whose specimens yielded *N. gonorrhoeae* or *C. trachomatis* were excluded.
[c]Test for trend, $P < 0.001$.

Fusobacterium nucleatum or *Bacteroides ureolyticus* in the vagina, two organisms found more frequently in those with bacterial vaginosis (Hillier et al., 1993), were more likely to develop amniotic fluid cultures positive for those organisms.

Group B *Streptococcus*

A number of studies have evaluated the association between genital or urinary tract colonization with group B streptococci and adverse outcomes of pregnancy. Urogenital colonization by group B streptococci has been associated with premature rupture of membranes in several studies (Alger et al., 1988; Moller et al., 1984; Newton and Clark, 1988; Regan et al., 1981) and with preterm labor and delivery in several others (McDonald et al., 1989; Regan et al., 1996; Sweet et al., 1987). In the Vaginal Infections and Prematurity Study, vaginal colonization by group B streptococci was characterized as light (growth of group B streptococci only in selective broth media) or heavy (growth on the nonselective agar plate) (Regan et al., 1996). For women who were heavily colonized by group B streptococci, the rate of preterm and low-birth-weight delivery was 7%, compared to 4.6% for women with no group B streptococci (odds ratio = 1.6; 95% confidence interval, 1.2 to 2.1). For women who were heavily colonized by group B streptococci and received antibiotics effective against group B streptococci, the incidence of preterm low-birth-weight delivery was identical to that for women who were not colonized by group B streptococci. A subset of 2,874 women had additional cultures obtained at the time of delivery. Heavy vaginal colonization by group B streptococci in the delivery culture also was significantly associated with preterm birth (odds ratio = 1.4; 95% confidence interval, 1.03 to 1.8), as well as with preterm premature rupture of membranes (odds ratio = 1.5; 95% confidence interval, 1.0 to 2.4). Light colonization by group B streptococci at 23 to 26 weeks gestation or at delivery was not associated with adverse outcomes of pregnancy.

The mechanism by which group B streptococci might cause preterm birth could be related to invasion of the chorioamnion. In one case-control study of placentas obtained from women delivered preterm or at term, it was found that chorioamnion invasion by group B streptococci was associated with both preterm birth and histologic chorioamnionitis (Hillier et al., 1991). Additional studies are needed to further clarify whether chorioamnion invasion by group B streptococci is also a risk factor for neonatal sepsis. However, data from one study indicate that high density vaginal colonization by group B streptococci may be a risk for amnionitis (Yancey et al., 1994). Furthermore, some women in preterm labor with intact fetal membranes have group B streptococci in the amniotic fluid, suggesting that this bacterium can cross intact membranes (Hillier et al., 1995b).

E. coli

Some strains of *E. coli* with particular capsule types have long been recognized as a cause of such neonatal diseases as sepsis and meningitis. Two published studies have reported an association between vaginal colonization by *E. coli* and preterm or low-birth-weight delivery or both. McDonald et al. (1991) performed a case-control study of 428 women in preterm labor compared to 568 women in labor at term in Adelaide, Australia. They reported that vaginal colonization by *E. coli* was more frequent in women delivered preterm than in those giving birth at term (odds ratio = 1.7; 95% confidence interval, 1.1 to 2.8). More recently, in a cross-sectional study of 2,646 women giving birth at the University of Washington Medical Center in Seattle, the recovery of *E. coli* from the vagina was characterized as high density (present in the third or fourth streak zone of the agar plate) or low density (present in only the first or second streak zone of the agar plate). High-density vaginal colonization with *E. coli* was associated with a significantly increased risk for preterm delivery and a 70% increased risk for delivery between 20 and 33 weeks gestation (relative risk = 1.7; 95% confidence interval, 1.3 to 2.3) (Krohn et al., 1997). High-density vaginal colonization with *E. coli* also was associated with a 90% increased risk of giving birth to an infant weighing between 500 and 1,499 g and a 50% increased risk of giving birth to an infant weighing between 1,500 and 2,499 g (Krohn et al., 1997).

To date, there are no longitudinal studies demonstrating that vaginal *E. coli* colonization earlier in pregnancy is a risk factor for preterm birth, nor are there studies demonstrating that treatment of vaginal *E. coli* can prevent preterm birth. However, numerous studies have demonstrated that bacteriuria early in pregnancy is associated with preterm birth and that the most common organism recovered from these women is *E. coli* (Romero et al., 1989). It is likely that the historical relationship between *E. coli*, bacteriuria, and preterm birth may be attributable more to the risks associated with invasion of the upper genital tract than to the risk associated with colonization of the urinary tract. It has been shown that chorioamnion invasion by *E. coli* is a risk factor for preterm birth and histologic chorioamnionitis (Hillier et al., 1991). Additional studies are urgently needed to clarify which strains of *E. coli* are associated with preterm birth and the relevance of screening for vaginal *E. coli* rather than bacteriuria as a marker for risk of preterm delivery.

Candida

Vaginal colonization by *Candida* species is known to occur in up to one-third of pregnant women, although most of these are asymptomatic. In one study of 2,929 women at several centers across the United States, yeast was detected by potassium hydroxide wet mount of the vaginal fluid in nearly

30% of the women at either 24 or 28 weeks gestation (Meis et al., 1995). Women found to be colonized by yeast were not at increased risk of delivering prior to 35 weeks gestation. An earlier study by Hardy et al. (1984) similarly found that there was no association between vaginal colonization by yeast and adverse pregnancy outcome for inner-city adolescents. Most recently, the Vaginal Infections and Prematurity Study evaluated 13,914 women between 23 and 26 weeks gestation (Cotch et al., 1998). These authors reported that high-density vaginal colonization by *Candida* (defined as growth in the third or fourth streak zone of the agar plate) was present in 10% of the women. They reported that 83% of the women colonized by yeast carried *C. albicans* and that *Candida* colonization was positively associated with colonization by *T. vaginalis*, group B streptococci, and aerobic *Lactobacillus*. However, high-density vaginal colonization by yeast was not associated with adverse outcomes of pregnancy.

Lactobacilli

While many constituents of the normal flora have been linked with adverse outcomes of pregnancy, there is a substantial body of data which suggests that vaginal colonization by lactobacilli may protect against adverse outcomes of pregnancy. If lactobacilli protect against complications of pregnancy, the protection is probably related to the concentration of lactobacilli in the vagina and whether they are the predominant members of the vaginal microflora. It may also be related to hydrogen peroxide production by lactobacilli. In 1988, Martius et al. reported that women having vaginal lactobacilli as detected by culture were less likely to give birth preterm than were women lacking vaginal lactobacilli. In 1991, Krohn et al. published a study of 211 women who were seen during preterm labor occurring before 34 weeks gestation. Quantitative vaginal cultures were performed on samples from the women. The rate of preterm birth was 40% lower in women having greater than 10^7 CFU of facultative *Lactobacillus* per g of vaginal fluid (rate ratio = 0.6; 95% confidence interval, 0.4 to 0.9). Holst et al. (1994) performed a small case-control study of 87 women in which they reported that only 18% of women giving birth preterm were vaginally colonized by hydrogen peroxide-producing lactobacilli, compared to 78% of women giving birth at term ($P < 0.001$). By contrast, lactobacilli that did not produce hydrogen peroxide were recovered equally often from those delivering preterm and at term, suggesting that hydrogen peroxide-producing lactobacilli were more protective against pregnancy complications than were strains that were negative for hydrogen peroxide.

In some cases, detection of lactobacilli in the vagina is performed by direct examination of a Gram-stained vaginal smear rather than by culture of vaginal fluid. In those cases, the *Lactobacillus* morphotypes are visualized and their relative quantity is compared with that of small gram-negative or gram-variable rods (Nugent et al., 1991). In one such study conducted in Great Britain, it was reported that women having *Lactobacillus*-predominant vaginal flora had a rate of pregnancy loss at 16 to 24 weeks gestation of only 1%, compared to 5% for those with reduced numbers of lactobacilli and 7% for those lacking vaginal lactobacilli (Hay et al., 1994). These authors reported a decreased incidence of preterm birth in women having vaginal lactobacilli compared with those from whom vaginal lactobacilli were absent. In the Vaginal Infections and Prematurity Study, women with *Lactobacillus* detected by culture or by vaginal Gram stain were significantly less likely to give birth to preterm and low-birth-weight infants (Hillier et al., 1995a). Women having vaginal *Lactobacillus* also were less likely to have intrauterine growth retardation in the study by Germain et al. (1994).

The mechanism by which lactobacilli could protect against adverse outcomes of pregnancy probably relates to their effect on other genital pathogens, including those associated with bacterial vaginosis. It is clear that many women treated for bacterial vaginosis do not become recolonized with *Lactobacillus* that produce hydrogen peroxide (Agnew and Hillier, 1995). Thus, additional strategies for reconstituting the vaginal microflora of women after treatment of bacterial vaginosis may be needed to prevent these adverse outcomes of pregnancy.

While lactobacilli appear to be protective against bacterial vaginosis, some cross-sectional studies also have shown that pregnant women who have *Lactobacillus*-predominant flora as assessed by vaginal Gram stain are less likely to be infected with sexually transmitted pathogens, including *N. gonorrhoeae*, *C. trachomatis*, and *T. vaginalis*. In one study of over 7,000 women assessed during the second trimester of pregnancy, it was shown that women having *Lactobacillus*-predominant flora were less likely to have all of these agents of sexually transmitted disease while women having reduced lactobacilli but not bacterial vaginosis still had an increased risk of sexually transmitted disease (Hillier et al., 1992a). Other studies in which the lactobacilli were tested for H_2O_2 production have similarly shown a decreased prevalence of bacterial vaginosis among women with H_2O_2-producing lactobacilli (Hillier et al., 1992b; Puapermpoonsiri et al., 1996). These data suggest that a *Lactobacillus*-predominant flora may also affect the susceptibility of a pregnant woman to genital tract infections.

ROLE OF MICROBIAL PRODUCTS IN INCREASING SUSCEPTIBILITY TO ADVERSE OUTCOMES OF PREGNANCY

The vaginal fluid of women contains not only the organisms present in the ecosystem but also the products of those organisms. While invasion of the organisms themselves is required for an adverse pregnancy outcome in some cases, it is likely that the microbial by-products are important in pathogenesis in other cases. For example, recent studies have demonstrated that women who have bacterial vaginosis also have significantly increased levels of endotoxin in vaginal washes and cervical mucus (Platz-Christensen et al., 1993). The likely source of endotoxin in the vaginal fluid is the cell walls of such gram-negative bacteria as *Bacteroides* or *E. coli*. It is known that endotoxin is a potent stimulator of the cytokine response, and it is believed to play a role in the induction of cytokines and in preterm birth. McGregor et al. (1990) have evaluated a number of microbial by-products in the vaginal wash for their association with preterm labor. An elevated level of bacterial protease was associated with preterm labor; it was present in 50% of women with preterm premature rupture of membranes.

Sialidases or neuramidases are recognized as enzymes that can alter the host response to bacterial infections (McGregor et al., 1994). Bacterial sialidases have been demonstrated to decrease collagen synthesis, to stimulate lymphocytes directly, to inhibit macrophage inhibitory factor, and to modify polymorphonuclear cell oxidative bursts. Sialidases also can cleave sialic acid from bacterial and epithelial cell surfaces, thus altering cell attachment. The vaginal flora that can produce sialidase includes some strains of *G. vaginalis* and *P. bivia* (Briselden et al., 1992). Women with high levels of these strains of *G. vaginalis* or *P. bivia* in the vagina have increased levels of sialidase. In one case-control study of 142 pregnant women with bacterial vaginosis and 129 women without bacterial vaginosis, it was reported that sialidase activity was detected in 45% of those with and 12% of those without bacterial vaginosis ($P < 0.001$) (McGregor et al., 1994). In another study of pregnant Thai and Japanese women, sialidase was detected in the vaginal fluid of 69% of those with bacterial vaginosis, compared with 3% of those without that syndrome (Puapermpoonsiri et al., 1996).

Mucinases also are produced by several common vaginal bacteria and are found more frequently in women with bacterial vaginosis (McGregor et al., 1994). In a case-control study of pregnant women with bacterial vaginosis, McGregor et al. (1994) reported that mucinase was detected in 44% of women with and 27% of women without bacterial vaginosis ($P = 0.007$). The presence of mucinase activity in the vagina was associated with recovery of *G. vaginalis* or *M. hominis*, even in the absence of bacterial vaginosis. The production of mucolytic enzymes by the organisms associated with bacterial vaginosis may be a key in explaining the ability of those organisms to bypass the mucus barrier and invade the upper genital tract to cause chorioamnionic infection, amnionitis, and postpartum endometritis.

SUMMARY AND AREAS FOR FURTHER INVESTIGATION

The vaginal ecosystem is complex. Although many organisms such as *P. bivia*, *E. coli*, group B streptococci, and *M. hominis* are considered part of the normal vaginal ecosystem, high-density colonization with these organisms has been shown to be a risk factor for preterm birth. In contrast, vaginal colonization by *Lactobacillus* correlates with protection against infection by other organisms as well as against preterm birth and premature rupture of membranes. While routine genital cultures of pregnant women are not recommended, any studies which seek to evaluate the etiology of preterm birth must take into consideration the components of the vaginal ecosystem so that the individual contribution of each risk factor can be taken into account.

There are a number of areas suitable for further research in the area of vaginal ecology and pregnancy. It is unknown why some but not all women colonized by high concentrations of these organisms develop upper genital tract infections. There are some data suggesting that women having an abnormal vaginal microflora are at increased risk for early pregnancy loss owing to invasion of the upper tract by vaginal bacteria (Hay et al., 1994; McGregor et al., 1995). It is unknown whether these infections occur temporally near the time of the miscarriage or whether they exist from the time of conception. Little is known about the interactions between the biological and hormonal effects on the ecosystem, as distinguished from the changes in behavior that could also affect this body site. Further research is needed into the means by which constituents of the vaginal flora could alter the mucus plug in pregnancy and how the microbial products produced by members of the microflora could increase a woman's susceptibility to upper genital tract infection. Finally, it is very important to identify means by which the vaginal flora of pregnant women can be optimized so that women are more resistant to genital infection. That might be accomplished through the use of a vaginal suppository containing human strains of *Lactobacillus* which produce hydrogen peroxide.

REFERENCES

Agnew, K. J., and S. L. Hillier. 1995. The effect of treatment regimens for vaginitis and cervicitis on vaginal colonization by lactobacilli. *Sex. Transm. Dis.* **22:**269–273.

Alger, L. S., J. C. Lovshik, J. R. Blackmon, and M. C. Crenshaw. 1988. The association of *Chlamydia trachomatis, Neisseria gonorrhoeae,* and group B streptococci with preterm rupture of the membranes and pregnancy outcome. *Am. J. Obstet. Gynecol.* **159:**397–404.

Berman, S. M., H. R. Harrison, W. T. Boyce, W. J. J. Haffner, M. Lewis, and J. Barney. 1987. Low birth weight, prematurity, and postpartum endometritis. Association with prenatal cervical *Mycoplasma hominis* and *Chlamydia trachomatis* infection. *JAMA* **257:**1189–1194.

Briselden, A. M., B. J. Moncla, C. E. Stevens, and S. L. Hillier. 1992. Silidases (neuraminidases) in bacterial vaginosis and bacterial vaginosis-associated microflora. *J. Clin. Microbiol.* **30:**663–666.

Cotch, M. F., S. L. Hillier, R. S. Gibbs, and D. A. Eschenbach for the Vaginal Infections and Prematurity Study Group. 1998. Epidemiology and outcomes associated with moderate to heavy *Candida* colonization during pregnancy. *Am. J. Obstet. Gynecol.* **178:**374–380.

Germain, M., M. A. Krohn, S. L. Hillier, and D. A. Eschenbach. 1994. The genital flora in pregnancy and its association with intrauterine growth retardation. *J. Clin. Microbiol.* **32:**2162–2168.

Goldenberg, R. L., M. A. Klebanoff, R. Nugent, M. A. Krohn, S. L. Hillier, and W. W. Andrews for the Vaginal Infections and Prematurity Study Group. 1996. Bacterial colonization of the vagina during pregnancy in four ethnic groups. *Am. J. Obstet. Gynecol.* **174:**1618–1621.

Goplerud, C. P., M. J. Ohm, and R. P. Galask. 1976. Aerobic and anaerobic flora of the cervix during pregnancy and the puerperium. *Am. J. Obstet. Gynecol.* **126:**858–868.

Hardy, P. H., J. B. Hardy, E. E. Nell, D. A. Graham, M. R. Spence, and R. C. Rosenbaum. 1984. Prevalence of six sexually transmitted disease agents among pregnant inner-city adolescents and pregnancy outcome. *Lancet* **ii:**333–337.

Hay, P. E., R. F. Lamont, D. Taylor-Robinson, D. J. Morgan, C. Ison, and J. Pearson. 1994. Abnormal bacterial colonization of the genital tract and subsequent preterm delivery and late miscarriage. *Br. Med. J.* **308:**295–298.

Hillier, S. L., M. A. Krohn, N. B. Kiviat, D. H. Watts, and D. A. Eschenbach. 1991. Microbial etiology and neonatal outcomes associated with chorioamnion infection. *Am. J. Obstet. Gynecol.* **165:**955–960.

Hillier, S. L., M. A. Krohn, R. P. Nugent, and R. S. Gibbs. 1992a. Characteristics of three vaginal flora patterns assessed by Gram stain among pregnant women. *Am. J. Obstet. Gynecol.* **166:**938–944.

Hillier, S. L., M. A. Krohn, S. J. Klebanoff, and D. A. Eschenbach. 1992b. The relationship of hydrogen peroxide-producing lactobacilli to bacterial vaginosis and genital microflora in pregnant women. *Obstet. Gynecol.* **79:**369–373.

Hillier, S. L., M. A. Krohn, L. K. Rabe, S. J. Klebanoff, and D. A. Eschenbach. 1993. The normal vaginal flora, H_2O_2-producing lactobacilli, and bacterial vaginosis in pregnant women. *Clin. Infect. Dis.* **16**(Suppl. 4):S273–S281.

Hillier, S. L., R. P. Nugent, D. A. Eschenbach, M. A. Krohn, R. S. Gibbs, D. H. Martin, M. F. Cotch, R. Edelman, J. G. Pastorek, A. V. Rao, D. McNellis, J. A. Regan, J. C. Carey, and M. A. Klebanoff for the Vaginal Infections and Prematurity Study Group. 1995a. Association between bacterial vaginosis and preterm delivery of a low-birth-weight infant. *N. Engl. J. Med.* **333:**1737–1742.

Hillier, S. L., M. A. Krohn, E. Cassen, T. R. Easterling, L. K. Rabe, and D. A. Eschenbach. 1995b. The role of bacterial vaginosis and vaginal bacteria in amniotic fluid infection in women in preterm labor with intact fetal membranes. *Clin. Infect. Dis.* **20**(Suppl. 2):S276–S278.

Holst, E., A. Rossel Goffeng, and B. Andersch. 1994. Bacterial vaginosis and vaginal microorganisms in idiopathic premature labor and association with pregnancy outcome. *J. Clin. Microbiol.* **32:**176–186.

Investigators of the Johns Hopkins Study of Cervicitis and Adverse Pregnancy Outcome. 1989. Association of *Chlamydia trachomatis* and *Mycoplasma hominis* with intrauterine growth retardation and preterm delivery. *Am. J. Epidemiol.* **129:**1247–1257.

Krohn, M. A., S. L. Hillier, M. L. Lee, L. K. Rabe, and D. A. Eschenbach. 1991. Vaginal *Bacteroides* species are associated with an increased rate of preterm delivery among women in preterm labor. *J. Infect. Dis.* **164:**88–93.

Krohn, M. A., S. L. Hillier, R. P. Nugent, M. F. Cotch, J. C. Carey, R. S. Gibbs, and D. A. Eschenbach. 1995. The genital flora of women with intraamniotic infection. *J. Infect. Dis.* **171:**1475–1480.

Krohn, M. A., S. S. Thwin, L. K. Rabe, Z. Brown, and S. L. Hillier. 1997. Vaginal colonization by *Escherichia coli* as a risk factor for very low birth weight delivery and other perinatal complications. *J. Infect. Dis.* **175:**606–610.

Martius, J., M. A. Krohn, S. L. Hillier, W. E. Stamm, K. K. Holmes, and D. A. Eschenbach. 1988. Relationships of vaginal *Lactobacillus* species, cervical *Chlamydia trachomatis,* and bacterial vaginosis to preterm birth. *Obstet. Gynecol.* **71:**89–95.

McDonald, H., R. Vigneswaran, and J. A. O'Loughlin. 1989. Group B streptococcal colonization and preterm labour. *Aust. N. Z. J. Obstet. Gynaecol.* **29:**291–293.

McDonald, H. M., J. A. O'Loughlin, P. Jolley, R. Vigneswaran, and P. J. McDonald. 1991. Vaginal infection and preterm labour. *Br. J. Obstet. Gynecol.* **98:**427–435.

McGregor, J. A., J. I. French, R. Richter, A. Franco-Buff, A. Johnson, S. L. Hillier, F. N. Judson, and J. K. Todd. 1990. Antenatal microbiologic and maternal risk factors associated with prematurity. *Am. J. Obstet. Gynecol.* **163:**1465–1473.

McGregor, J. A., J. I. French, W. Jones, K. Milligan, P. J. McKinney, E. Patterson, and R. Parker. 1994. Bacterial vaginosis is associated with prematurity and vaginal fluid mucinase and sialidase: results of a controlled trial of topical clindamycin cream. *Am. J. Obstet. Gynecol.* **170:**1048–1060.

McGregor, J. A., J. I. French, R. Parker, D. Draper, E. Patterson, W. Jones, K. Thorsgard, and J. McFee. 1995. Prevention of premature birth by screening and treatment for common genital tract infections: results of a prospective controlled evaluation. *Am. J. Obstet. Gynecol.* **173:**157–167.

Meis, P. J., R. L. Goldenberg, B. Mercer, A. Moawad, A. Das, D. McNellis, F. Johnson, J. D. Iams, E. Thom, W. W. Andrews, and the National Institute of Child Health and Human Development Maternal-Fetal Medicine Units Network. 1995. The preterm prediction study: significance of vaginal infections. *Am. J. Obstet. Gynecol.* **173:**1231–1235.

Minkoff, H., A. Grunebaum, R. H. Schwartz, J. Feldman, M. Cummings, W. Crombleholme, L. Clark, G. Pringle, and W. M. McCormack. 1984. Risk factors for prematurity and premature rupture of membranes: a prospective study of the vaginal flora in pregnancy. *Am. J. Obstet. Gynecol.* **150:**965–972.

Moller, E. R., A. C. Thomsen, K. Borch, K. Dinesen, and M. Zdravkovic. 1984. Rupture of fetal membranes and premature delivery associated with group B streptococci in urine of pregnant women. *Lancet* **ii:**69–70.

Newton, E. R., and M. Clark. 1988. Group B *Streptococcus* and preterm rupture of membranes. *Obstet. Gynecol.* **72:**198–202.

Nugent, R. P., M. A. Krohn, and S. L. Hillier. 1991. Reliability of diagnosing bacterial vaginosis is improved by a standardized method of Gram stain interpretation. *J. Clin. Microbiol.* **29:**297–301.

Platz-Christensen, J. J., I. Mattsby-Blatzer, P. Thomsen, and N. Wiqvist. 1993. Endotoxin and interleukin-1 alpha in the cervical mucus and vaginal fluid of pregnant women with bacterial vaginosis. *Am. J. Obstet. Gynecol.* **169:**1161–1166.

Puapermpoonsiri, S., N. Kato, K. Watanabe, K. Ueno, C. Chongsomachai, and P. Lumbiganon. 1996. Vaginal microflora associated with bacterial vaginosis in Japanese and Thai pregnant women. *Clin. Infect. Dis.* **23:**748–752.

Read, J. S., and M. A. Klebanoff. 1993. Sexual intercourse during pregnancy and preterm delivery: effects of vaginal microorganisms. *Am. J. Obstet. Gynecol.* **186:** 514–519.

Regan, J. A., S. Chao, and L. S. James. 1981. Premature rupture of membranes, preterm delivery, and group B streptococcal colonization of mothers. *Am. J. Obstet. Gynecol.* **141:**184–186.

Regan, J. A., M. A. Klebanoff, R. P. Nugent, D. A. Eschenbach, W. C. Blackwelder, Y. Lou, G. S. Gibbs, P. J. Rettig, D. H. Matrin, and R. Edelman for the Vaginal Infections and Prematurity Study Group. 1996. Colonization with group B streptococci in pregnancy and adverse outcome. *Am. J. Obstet. Gynecol.* **174:**1354–1360.

Romero, R. E., M. Oyarzun, M. Mazor, M. Sirtori, J. C. Hobbins, and M. Bracken. 1989. Meta-analysis of the relationship between asymptomatic bacteriuria and preterm delivery/low birth weight. *Am. J. Obstet. Gynecol.* **73:**576–582.

Silver, H. M., R. S. Sperling, P. J. St. Clair, and R. S. Gibbs. 1989. Evidence relating bacterial vaginosis to intraamniotic infections. *Am. J. Obstet. Gynecol.* **161:**808–812.

Sweet, R. L., D. V. Landers, C. Walker, and J. Schachter. 1987. *Chlamydia trachomatis* infection and pregnancy outcome. *Am. J. Obstet. Gynecol.* **156:**824–833.

Yancey, M. K., P. Duff, P. Clark, T. Kurtzer, B. H. Frentzen, and P. Kubilis. 1994. Peripartum infection associated with vaginal group B streptococcal colonization. *Obstet. Gynecol.* **84:**816–819.

3
Immunology and Adverse Outcome of Pregnancy Related to Sexually Transmitted Diseases

Joseph A. Hill

Sexually transmitted diseases (STDs) pose a significant problem to maternal, fetal, and perinatal health. While many cases of adverse pregnancy outcome may have an infectious etiology, the precise organisms responsible are often not identifiable. Furthermore, not all infections are associated with adverse pregnancy outcome. It is clear that maternal and fetal immunologic factors must be involved. However, immune responses to STD pathogens in pregnancy, their relationship to colonization and infection patterns, and their effects on pregnancy have not been clearly elucidated.

Human pregnancy is a time of attenuated immunity. There is a significant reduction in the total lymphocyte number and concentration in the peripheral circulation; specifically $CD4^+$ helper/inducer immune cell populations are reduced in number. Systemic immunity within the peripheral circulation may also be affected by pregnancy (Table 1) (Johnstone et al., 1994). Diminished natural killer (NK) cell activity and antibody-dependent cellular cytotoxicity have been reported to occur in normal pregnancy (Hill et al., 1986). Immunosuppression, as indirectly measured by loss of systemic responsiveness to previously seen antigens, appears necessary for maintenance of early pregnancy (Bermas and Hill, 1997). The normal human decidua is replete with many immune and inflammatory cell populations (Bulmer and Sunderland, 1984; Kabawat et al., 1985; Kamat and Isaacson, 1985). The majority of these cells are NK cells (large granulated lymphocytes expressing the CD56, NK-cell phenotype) (Bulmer et al., 1987; Starkey et al., 1988). These cells, as well as trophoblast tissues, can secrete cytokines that may enhance or depress the immune response to pregnancy (Tabib-

Joseph A. Hill, Reproductive Medicine, Department of Obstetrics, Gynecology and Reproductive Biology, Brigham and Women's Hospital, Harvard Medical School, Boston, MA 02115.

Sexually Transmitted Diseases and Adverse Outcomes of Pregnancy
Edited by P. J. Hitchcock, H. T. MacKay, J. N. Wasserheit, and R. Binder
©1999 American Society for Microbiology, Washington, D.C.

Table 1 Lymphocyte subpopulation values within the same individual while nonpregnant and while pregnant[a]

Parameter	Nonpregnant	Pregnancy	P
Leukocyte count (mm^{-3})	6,034 ± 307	7,348 ± 382	0.002
Lymphocytes (%)	21 (17–28)	14 (12–20)	<0.0001
Lymphocytes (mm^{-3})	1.1 (0.8–1.6)	1.0 (0.7–1.3)	<0.0001
$CD4^+$ cells (% of lymphocytes)	45 (42–49)	42 (39–45)	0.004
No. of $CD4^+$ cells (mm^{-3})	483 (368–671)	444 (302–514)	0.006
$CD8^+$ cells (% of lymphocytes)	33 (30–38)	35 (31–39)	0.7
No. of CD8 cells (mm^{-3})	391 (299–564)	359 (270–483)	0.1
CD4/CD8 ratio	1.4 (1.1–1.5)	1.3 (1.0–1.4)	0.01
DR^+ T cells (% of lymphocytes)	6 (5–7)	6 (4–9)	0.6
No. of CR^+ T cells (mm^{-3})	68 (38–96)	60 (37–84)	0.1

[a]Reprinted from Johnstone et al. (1994) with permission.

zadeh, 1990; Johnson, 1993a; King et al., 1995; Jokhi et al., 1994; Wegmann, 1986). The decidua may constitute a distinct immunologic microenvironment with its own immune and anti-inflammatory cell populations and specific cytokines (Dudley et al., 1990). In addition, fetal trophoblast cells forming the lining of the placenta have specialized features that protect them from maternal immunological attack. Syncytiotrophoblast cells at the maternal-fetal interface do not express the antigens of self, derived from mother or father. Specifically, the unique major histocompatibility complex class I and class II antigens are not expressed, with one exception. Human leukocyte antigen (HLA) C is expressed during the first trimester of pregnancy (Faulk and Temple, 1976; King et al., 1996). It confers protection from maternal anti-paternal cellular immune responses; the negative aspect of this is that it also makes cells resistant to cellular immunity directed against intracellular pathogens. The significance of the recent discovery that nonvillous human trophoblast cells express HLA-G antigens (Kovats et al., 1990) is unknown (Table 2). Perhaps these antigens protect the placenta from NK-cell-mediated lysis (Pazmany et al., 1996) and thus play a significant role in placental immunology and in the maintenance of normal pregnancy (Carosella et al., 1996). The expression of complement-regulatory proteins (Table 3) (Johnson, 1993a, 1993b) by trophoblast cells is also a double-edged sword, possibly protecting the cells that have paternal markers from the mother's antibody responses but also inhibiting antibody-dependent killing of intracellular pathogens. A number of soluble immunoregulating factors that could attenuate local immune defense mechanisms also have been found in decidual and placental tissues (Table 4).

Decreased systemic NK-cell activity and decreased antibody-dependent cellular cytotoxicity during pregnancy (Hill et al., 1986) may

Table 2 Expression of human leukocyte antigens in human term placenta[a]

Antigen	Antigen expression in:			
	Nonvillous invasive cytotrophoblasts	Syncytiotrophoblasts	Cytotrophoblasts	Hofbauer cells (macrophages)
Class I MHC				
HLA-A, B, C	–	–	–	++
HLA-G	++	–	–	–
Class II MCH				
HLA-DR, DP, DQ	–	–	–	++

[a]Reprinted from Johnson (1993b) with permission.

Table 3 Expression of complement regulatory proteins in the human term placenta[a]

Protein	Protein expression in:			
	Nonvillous invasive cytotrophoblasts	Syncytiotrophoblasts	Cytotrophoblasts	Hofbauer cells (macrophages)
Membrane cofactor protein (MCP, CD46)	++	++	+	+
Decay-accelerating factor (DAF, CD55)	++	++	+	+
Membrane attack complex inhibitory protein (CD59)	+	+	++	

[a]Reprinted from Johnson (1993b) with permission.

Table 4 Potential immunoregulating factors during pregnancy

Progesterone
Pregnancy-associated alpha$_{\alpha}$-glycoprotein
Alpha-fetoprotein
Prolactin
Transforming growth factor β
T-helper 1 cytokines (TNF-α, IFN-γ, IL-2)
T-helper 2 cytokines (IL-4, IL-5, IL-10)
Other cytokines (IC-13, GM-CSF, CSF-1, TGF-β, LIF)[a]

[a] GM-CSF, granulocyte-macrophage colony-stimulating factor; TGF-β, transforming growth factor β; LIF, leukemia-inhibiting factor.

explain the increased susceptibility of pregnant women to viral illness and intracellular parasitic infection (Tables 5 and 6) (Weinberg, 1984). Pregnant women also have a high prevalence of STDs (Table 7) and may be at increased risk of acquiring and transmitting STD pathogens due to systemic and local attenuation of immunity. Maternally acquired infections during pregnancy can lead to multiple adverse outcomes (Table 8). However, not every pregnant woman with an infection develops an adverse pregnancy outcome (Table 9).

Table 5 Risk among pregnant women of acquiring infectious diseases compared with that among nonpregnant women of childbearing age in the same community[a]

Agent	Risk of:[b]		
	Reactivation of subclinical infection	Development of clinical disease	Maternal death caused by the disease
Poliomyelitis virus		2.5	
Hepatitis A virus		4	2.4
Influenza A virus			7.1
Variola virus		2	3.3
Epstein-Barr virus	2.4		
Papovavirus	1.5		
Plasmodium falciparum		7	
Entamoeba histolytica			4.7

[a] Reprinted from Weinberg (1984) with permission.
[b] Number of times risk in pregnant women exceeds risk in nonpregnant women.

Table 6 Percent distribution of various infectious-disease agents according to trimester of human pregnancy[a]

Agent	% of infected women in trimester:		
	I	II	III
Cytomegalovirus	6	31	63
Papovavirus	3	37	60
Poliomyelitis virus	4	40	26
Hepatitis A virus	7	15	70
Hepatitis B virus	4	23	73
Influenza A virus	17	36	47
Coccidioides immitis	32	24	44
Mycobacterium tuberculosis	11	66	23

[a]Reprinted from Weinberg (1984) with permission.

Recent attention has focused on immunologic cytokines as potential mediators of reproductive function and their involvement in normal and abnormal pregnancy. Cytokines are immunoregulatory proteins with many functions, ranging from proliferation to differentiation to inhibition. There are eight major groups of cytokines (Table 10), which may overlap in specific function. Following immunologic activation by antigen, $CD4^+$ T cells produce one of two distinctive cytokine profiles, leading to their classification as T-helper 1 (Th1) and T-helper 2 (Th2) cells (Mosmann et al., 1986; Cherwinski et al., 1987; Kurt-Jones et al., 1987). The different cytokines produced by these cells lead to differences in immune system function (Cher and Mosmann, 1987; Mosmann et al., 1986). Th1 cells primarily se-

Table 7 Prevalence of STDs in pregnant women in the United States

Infection	% of pregnant women infected
Gonorrhea	1
Syphilis	0.15
Chlamydia	3–5
Bacterial vaginosis	15
Trichomoniasis	2
Mycoplasma infection	25
Ureaplasma	70–80
Herpes	25
Cytomegalovirus infection	30
Human papillomavirus infection	40
HIV infection	0.12

Table 8 Adverse pregnancy outcomes with potential infectious etiologies

Implantation failure
Spontaneous abortion
Chorioamnionitis
Intrauterine fetal demise
Premature rupture of placental membranes
Premature labor
Intrauterine growth retardation
Stillbirth
Postpartum endometritis
Septic shock
Neonatal infection

crete gamma interferon (IFN-γ) but also secrete interleukin-2 (IL-2) and tumor necrosis factor beta (TNF-β) and induce cellular immunity. Th2 cells primarily secrete IL-4 but also secrete IL-5 and IL-10 and down-regulate cellular immunity while playing a major role in the induction of antibody responses mediated by plasma cells. The cytokine TNF-α can be produced during both Th1 and Th2 immune responses, although levels are higher in Th1 responses and this cytokine is known for cytolytic effects that contribute to the efficacy of cellular immunity (Mosmann and Coffman, 1989a, 1989b; Romagnani, 1992).

Lymphocytes from a subgroup of women with unexplained recurrent spontaneous abortion respond to sperm and trophoblast antigen extracts in vitro by proliferating and secreting Th1-type soluble cytokines that adversely affect embryo and trophoblast viability (Hill et al., 1992). Lympho-

Table 9 Percentage of pregnant women with an STD experiencing an adverse pregnancy outcome

Infection	% of infected women experiencing:		
	Fetal loss	Premature delivery	Perinatal infection
Gonorrhea	Rare	11–25	30–60
Syphilis	20–25	15–50	40–80
Chlamydia	Rare	10–30	40–70
Genital herpes			
Primary	7–54	30–35	30–50
Recurrent	Rare	Rare	0.4–8
Bacterial vaginosis	Rare	10–25	Rare
Trichomoniasis	Rare	11–15	Rare

Table 10 Cytokine families

Antiviral agents
Interferons (IFN-α, β, γ [τ?])
Colony-stimulating factors (CSF)
CSF-1 or macrophage (M-CSF)
Granulocyte-macrophage (GM-CSF)
Granulocyte (G-CSF)
IL-3
Stem cell factors (SCF)
Erythropoietin
Thrombopoietin
Lymphoid growth factors
Interleukin-α, β
Interleukins-2 to -15 (IL-2–IL-15)
Growth promoters
Bone morphogeneic protein
Ciliary neurotrophic factors
Epidermal growth factor (EGF)
Fibroblast growth factors, acidic (aFGF-1), basic (bFGF-2)
Hepatocyte growth factors
Heregulin
Glial growth factors (neuregulins)
Insulin-like growth factors (IGF) I, II
Nerve growth factors
Platelet-derived growth factor (PDGF)
Transforming growth factor (TGF) α, β_{1-5}
Vascular endothelial cell growth factor (VEGF)
Growth inhibitors
Leukemia-inhibiting factor (LIF)
Oncostatin M
Mullerian inhibiting substance (MIS)
Transforming growth factor (TGF) α, β_{1-5}
Tumor necrosis factor α, β (TNF-α, -β)
Gamma interferon (IFN-γ)
Chemotatic factors
IL-8
Complement (C3)
Monocyte chemotactic protein 1 (MCP-1)
Macrophage inflammatory protein α, β (MIP-1α, β)
Macrophage migration inhibitory factory (MIF)
Regulated on activation, normal T-cell, expressed and secreted (RANTES)

cytes from parous women with a history of normal pregnancies do not show this response (Hill et al., 1992, 1995). The origin of this immune system sensitivity is unknown. One possibility is that previous infection of the reproductive tract serves as an adjuvant that promotes Th1-type sensitivity to normally nonimmunogenic reproductive antigens. Alternatively, Th1-type cytokines may have a direct adverse effect on pregnancy outcome. As evidence for the latter possibility, studies have demonstrated that Th1-type cytokines, especially IFN-γ and TNF-α, impair early embryo development (Hill et al., 1987) and trophoblast growth and function in vitro (Haimovici et al., 1991; Berkowitz et al., 1988) and cause abortion in mice (Chaouat et al., 1990). Since the human endometrium and decidua contain immune and inflammatory cells that are capable of secreting cytokines (Bulmer and Sunderland, 1984; Kabawat et al., 1985; Kamat and Isaacson, 1985; Bulmer et al., 1987; Starkey et al., 1988; Tabibzadeh, 1990; Johnson, 1993a, 1993b; Bulmer and Johnson, 1985; Bulmer, 1988), we have hypothesized that immune-cell activation by trophoblast, sperm, or microbial antigens leading to the release of Th1-type cytokines may be a mechanism for human recurrent spontaneous abortion (Yamada et al., 1994; Hill et al., 1995; Hill and Anderson, 1988). In contrast, Th2-type cytokines are secreted at the maternal-fetal interface during normal pregnancy in the mouse and have been proposed to play a role in normal pregnancy by suppressing cellular immune responses that could endanger the fetus while maintaining the humoral immunity vital for maternal defense against disease (Lin et al., 1993). Since Th1-type cytokines have been found in the decidua of aborting mice (Tangri et al., 1994), it appears reasonable to propose that reproductive success may depend on coordinated cytokine regulation during pregnancy.

A large body of literature concerning the association of STDs and adverse pregnancy outcome has accumulated (Handsfield et al., 1973; Edwards et al., 1978; Charles and Larsen, 1986; Sweet et al., 1987; McDonald et al., 1991; Fowler et al., 1992; Romero et al., 1992a, 1992b, 1992c; Gibbs et al., 1992; Kurki et al., 1992; Watts et al., 1992; Prober et al., 1992; Cassell et al., 1993; Read and Klebono, 1993; Towers et al., 1993). The immunologic consequences of STDs and their potential contribution to adverse pregnancy outcome are not well characterized. However, inflammatory cytokines whose level is elevated in the amniotic fluid of women in preterm labor, including IL-1, IL-6, IL-8, and TNF-α, have been proposed to be involved in pathogenesis of preterm labor and premature rupture of membranes. These cytokines stimulate prostaglandin E_2 and $F_{2\alpha}$ production by amnion and by decidual macrophages, respectively (Romero et al., 1989a, 1989b, 1992, 1993; Mitchell et al., 1991; Bry and Hallman, 1992; Norwitz et al., 1992; Creig et al., 1993; Hillier et al., 1993; Cox et al., 1993; Opsjon et al., 1993; Inglis et al., 1994). Surprisingly, the level of IL-4 is also elevated in amniotic fluid in women in preterm labor, particularly in association with chorioamnionitis. Although IL-4 is considered to be an anti-inflammatory molecule, it may play a paradoxical proinflammatory role in the pathogenesis of infection-associated preterm labor (Dudley et al., 1996a, 1996b). The mechanisms used to fight infection in the decidua and fetal-placental membranes are unknown, although chemokine production by the human chorion can be induced by group B streptococci (Dudley et al., 1996a, 1996b). Immune-cell activation in the decidua in response to maternal infection may result in myometrial contractions due to prostaglandin $F_{2\alpha}$ release by decidual macrophages. Ascending infection of the membranes may be less likely to stimulate prostaglandin E_2 production and therefore is less likely to cause contractions. However, spontaneous rupture of membranes may be more likely to occur in response to ascending infection than to blood-borne decidual infection. The contributions of the maternal, fetal, and placental-decidual inflammatory responses to specific infections are unknown. The concentrations of endotoxin and IL-1α have been reported to be significantly higher in the cervical-vaginal fluid of pregnant women with bacterial vaginosis than in pregnant women without bacterial vaginosis (Platz-Christensen et al., 1993), and bacterial vaginosis is associated with prematurity (McGregor et al., 1994) and premature rupture of membranes (McGregor et al., 1993). Neutrophil-attractant agents, and other chemotaxis agents including IL-8, have been found in response to infection in pregnant women and have been correlated with adverse outcomes including chorioamnionitis and preterm labor (Cherouny et al., 1992, 1993; Barclay et al., 1993). Immunologic cytokines including TNF-α, IL-6, and IL-10 also have been implicated in low birth weight and fetal wasting (Heyborne et al., 1992, 1994; Silver et al., 1993). Whether infectious agents are responsible for immune-cell activation resulting in the release of potentially growth-restricting cytokines remains to be elucidated. IL-8 may also play a fundamental role in cervical maturation in both normal and pathologic pregnancy (Maradny et al., 1994).

Immunologic cytokines may facilitate or hinder pregnancy depending on the type of cytokines present, their concentrations and route of administration, and the timing of their secretion relative to gestational age. Understanding host defense mechanisms including cytokine regulation in response to infectious organisms acquired or reactivated during pregnancy will enable the development of cost-effective intervention strategies to prevent adverse outcomes of pregnancy. Many questions need to be answered before host-pathogen interactions are identified and understood (Table 11). Multidisciplinary collaborative approaches combining both basic biomedical and clinical research will be required to formulate and implement effective investigative strategies to answer these fundamentally important questions.

Table 11 Research agenda questions for immunology and adverse pregnancy outcome related to STDs

Maternal
What is the immunology of the genital tract?
Where do immunologic responses occur within reproductive tissues?
When does systemic and mucosal immunity mature?
How does immunity occur within reproductive tissues, and what are the consequences?
Fetal
What is the immunology of the fetus and fetal membranes?
Where do immunologic responses occur within the fetus and fetal membranes?
When do immunologic responses occur (ontogeny)?
How does immunity occur within the fetus and fetal membranes, and what are the consequences?
Maternofetal interface
What is the immunology of the maternofetal interface?
Where do immunologic responses occur within the maternofetal interface?
When do immunologic responses occur?
How does immunity occur within the maternofetal interface, and what are the consequences?
Pathogens
What, where, when, and how are maternal and fetal immunologic responses affected by individual pathogens, including the ontogeny of the immune response to specific pathogens?
What, where, when, and how are individual pathogens affected by maternal and fetal immunity?

REFERENCES

Barclay, C. G., J. E. Brannand, R. W. Kelly, and A. A. Calder. 1993. Interleukin-8 production by the human cervix. *Am. J. Obstet. Gynecol.* **169:**625–632.

Berkowitz, R. S., J. A. Hill, C. B. Kurtz, and D. J. Anderson. 1988. Effects of products of activated leukocytes (lymphokines and monokines) on the growth of malignant trophoblast cells *in vitro*. *Am. J. Obstet. Gynecol.* **158:**199–203.

Bermas, B. L., and J. A. Hill. 1997. Proliferative responsiveness to recall antigens are associated with pregnancy outcome in women with a history of recurrent spontaneous abortion. *J. Clin. Invest.* **6:**15.

Bry, K., and M. Hallman. 1992. Transforming growth factor-β opposes the stimulatory effects of interleukin-1 and tumor necrosis factor on amnion cell prostaglandin E_2 production: implications for preterm labor. *Am. J. Obstet. Gynecol.* **167:** 222–226.

Bulmer, J. N. 1988. Immunopathology of pregnancy. *Bailliere's Clin. Immunol. Allergy* **2:**697–734.

Bulmer, J. N., and P. M. Johnson. 1985. Immunohistological characterization of the decidual leukocyte infiltrate related to endometrial gland epithelium in early human pregnancy. *Immunology* **5:**35.

Bulmer, J. N., and C. A. Sunderland. 1984. Immunohistological characterization of lymphoid cell populations in the early human placental bed. *Immunology* **52:**349–357.

Bulmer, J. N., D. Hollings, and A. Ritson. 1987. Immunocytochemical evidence that endometrial stromal granulocytes are granulated lymphocytes. *J. Pathol.* **153:**281–287.

Carosella, E. D., J. Dousset, and M. Kirszenbaum. 1996. HLA-G revisited. *Immunol. Today* **17:**407–409.

Cassell, L. H., K. B. Waites, H. L. Watson, D. T. Crouse, and R. Harasawa. 1993. *Ureaplasma urealyticum* intrauterine infection: role in prematurity and disease in newborns. *Clin. Microbiol. Rev.* **6:**69–87.

Chaouat, G., E. Mena, D. Clark, M. Dy, M. Minkowski, and T. G. Wegmann. 1990. Control of fetal survival in CBAxDBA/2 mice by lymphokine therapy. *J. Reprod. Fertil.* **89:**447.

Charles, D., and B. Larsen. 1986. Streptococcal puerperal sepsis and obstetric infections: a historical perspective. *Rev. Infect. Dis.* **8:**411–422.

Cher, D. J., and T. R. Mosmann. 1987. Two types of murine helper T cell clones. II. Delayed-type hypersensitivity is mediated by TH1 clones. *J. Immunol.* **138:**3688–3694.

Cherouny, P. H., G. A. Pankuch, J. J. Botti, and P. C. Appelbaum. 1992. The presence of amniotic fluid leukoattractants accurately identifies histologic chorioamnionitis and predicts tocolytic efficacy in patients with idiopathic preterm labor. *Am. J. Obstet. Gynecol.* **167:**683–688.

Cherouny, P. H., G. A. Pankuch, R. Romero, J. J. Botti, D. C. Kuhn, L. M. Demers, and P. C. Appelbaum. 1993. Neutrophil attractant/activating peptide-1/interleukin-8: association with histologic chorioamnionitis, preterm delivery, and bioactive amniotic fluid leukoattractants. *Am. J. Obstet. Gynecol.* **169:**1299–1303.

Cherwinski, H. M., J. H. Schumacker, K. D. Brown, and T. R. Mosmann. 1987. Two types of mouse helper T cell clones. III. Further differences in lymphokine synthesis between TH1 and TH2 clones revealed by RMA hybridization, functionally monospecific bioassays and monoclonal antibodies. *J. Exp. Med.* **166:**1229–1244.

Cox, S. M., M. R. King, L. Casey, and P. C. MacDonald. 1993. Interleukin-1β, -1a and -6 and prostaglandin in vaginal/cervical fluids of pregnant women before and during labor. *J. Clin. Endocrinol. Metab.* **77:**805–815.

Creig, P. C., J. M. Ernest, L. Teot, M. Erikson, and R. Talley. 1993. Amniotic fluid interleukin-6 levels correlate with histologic chorioamnionitis and amniotic fluid cultures in patients in premature labor with intact membranes. *Am. J. Obstet. Gynecol.* **169:**1035–1044.

Dudley, D. J., M. D. Mitchell, K. Creighton, and D. W. Branch. 1990. Lymphokine production during term human pregnancy: differences between peripheral leukocytes and decidual cells. *Am. J. Obstet. Gynecol.* **163:**1890–1893.

Dudley, D. J., S. S. Edwin, A. Gangerfield, J. Von Waggoner, and M. D. Mitchell. 1996a. Regulation of cultured human chorion cell chemokine production by group B streptococci and purified bacterial products. *Am. J. Reprod. Immunol.* **36:**264–268.

Dudley, D. J., C. Hunter, M. W. Varner, and M. D. Mitchell. 1996b. Elevation of amniotic fluid interleukin-4 concentrations in women with preterm labor and chorioamnionitis. *Am. J. Perinatal.* **13:**443–447.

Ecker, J. L., M. R. Laufer, and J. A. Hill. 1993. Measurement of embryotoxic factors is predictive of pregnancy outcome in women with history of recurrent abortion. *Obstet. Gynecol.* **81:**84–87.

Edwards, L. E., M. I. Barrada, A. A. Hamann, and E. Y. Hakanson. 1978. Gonorrhea in pregnancy. *Am. J. Obstet. Gynecol.* **132:**637–641.

Faulk, W. P., and A. Temple. 1976. Distribution of beta 2 microglobulin and HLA in chorionic villi of human placentae. *Nature* **262:**799–802.

Fowler, K. B., S. Stagno, R. F. Pars, W. J. Britt, T. J. Boll, and C. A. Alford. 1992. The outcome of congenital cytomegalovirus infection in relation to maternal antibody status. *N. Engl. J. Med.* **326:**663–667.

Gibbs, R. S., R. Romero, S. L. Hillier, D. A. Eschenback, and R. L. Sweet. 1992. A review of premature birth and subclinical infection. *Am. J. Obstet. Gynecol.* **166:** 1515–1528.

Haimovici, F., J. A. Hill, and D. J. Anderson. 1991. The effects of soluble products of activated lymphocytes and macrophages on blastocyst implantation events *in vitro*. *Biol. Reprod.* **44:**69–75.

Handsfield, H. H., A. Hudson, and K. K. Holmes. 1973. Neonatal gonococcal infection. I. Orogastric contamination with *Neisseria gonorrhoeae*. *JAMA* **225:**697–701.

Heyborne, K. D., S. S. Witkin, and J. A. McGregor. 1992. Tumor necrosis factor-a in mid trimester amniotic fluid is associated with impaired intrauterine fetal growth. *Am. J. Obstet. Gynecol.* **167:**920–925.

Heyborne, K. D., J. A. McGregor, G. Henry, S. S. Witkin, and J. S. Abranson. 1994. Interleukin-10 in amniotic fluid at midtrimester: immune activation and suppression in relation to fetal growth. *Am. J. Obstet. Gynecol.* **171:**55–59.

Hill, J. A. 1991. Implications of cytokines in male and female sterility, p. 269–275. *In* G. A. Chaouct and J. F. Mowbray (ed.), *Cellular and Molecular Biology of the Maternal-Fetal Relationship.* INSERM/John Libbey Eurotext, Paris, France.

Hill, J. A., and D. J. Anderson. 1988. Cell mediated immune mechanisms in recurrent spontaneous abortion, p. 171–179. *In* G. P. Talwar (ed.), *Contraceptive Research for Today and the Ninety's.* Springer-Verlag, New York, N.Y.

Hill, J. A., S. Hsia, D. W. Duran, and C. I. Bryans. 1986. Natural killer cell activity and antibody dependent cell-mediated cytotoxicity in pre-eclampsia. *J. Reprod. Immunol.* **9:**205–212.

Hill, J. A., F. Haimovici, and D. J. Anderson. 1987. Products of activated lymphocytes and macrophages inhibit mouse embryo development *in vitro*. *J. Immunol.* **139:**2250–2254.

Hill, J. A., K. Polgar, B. L. Harlow, and D. J. Anderson. 1992. Evidence of embryo and trophoblast toxic cellular immune response(s) in women with recurrent spontaneous abortion. *Am. J. Obstet. Gynecol.* **166:**1044–1052.

Hill, J. A., K. Polgar, and D. J. Anderson. 1995. T-helper I type cellular immunity to trophoblast antigens in women with recurrent spontaneous abortion. *JAMA* **273:**1933–1936.

Hillier, S. L., S. S. Witkin, M. A. Krohn, D. H. Watts, N. B. Kiviat, and D. A. Eschenback. 1993. The relationship of amniotic fluid cytokines and preterm delivery amniotic fluid infections, histologic chorioamnionitis and chorioamnion infection. *Obstet. Gynecol.* **81:**841–948.

Inglis, S. R., J. Jermias, K. Kuno, K. Lescale, Q. Peeper, F. A. Chervenok, and S. S. Witkin. 1994. Detection of tumor necrosis factor-a, interleukin-6, and fetal fibronectin in the lower genital tract during pregnancy. Relation to outcome. *Am. J. Obstet. Gynecol.* **121:**5–10.

Johnson, P. M. 1993a. Immunobiological characterization of the trophoblast-decidual interface in human pregnancy, p. 3–13. *In* T. G. Wegmann and T. Gill (ed.), *Immunobiology of Reproduction.* Springer Verlag, Boston, Mass.

Johnson, P. M. 1993b. Reproductive and maternofetal relations. *In* P. J. Lachman, D. K. Peters, F. S. Rosen, and M. J. Walport (ed.), *Clinical Aspects of Immunology,* 5th ed. Blackwell Scientific Publications, Oxford, United Kingdom.

Johnstone, F. D., K. J. Thong, A. G. Bird, and J. Whitlaw. 1994. Lymphocyte subpopulations in early human pregnancy. *Obstet. Gynecol.* **83:**941–946.

Jokhi, P. P., A. King, A. M. Sharkey, A. M. Sharkey, S. K. Smith, and Y. W. Loke. 1994. Screening for cytokine messenger ribonucleic acids in purified human decidual lymphocyte populations by the reverse-transcriptive polymerase chain reaction. *J. Immunol.* **153:**4427–4435.

Kabawat, S. E., M. Mostenfi-Zadeh, S. G. Driscol, and A. K. Bhan. 1985. Implantation site in normal pregnancy: a study with monoclonal antibodies. *Am. J. Pathol.* **118:**76–84.

Kamat, B. R., and P. G. Isaacson. 1985. The immunocytochemical distribution of leukocytoxic subpopulations in human endometrium. *Am. J. Pathol.* **127:**66–73.

King, A., P. P. Jokhi, S. K. Smith, A. M. Sharkey, and Y. W. Loke. 1995. Screening for cytokine mRNA in human villous and extravillous trophoblast, using the reverse transcription polymerase chain reaction (RT-PCR). *Cytokine* **7:**364–371.

King, A., C. Boocock, A. M. Charley, L. Gardner, A. Beretta, and A. G. Siccardi. 1996. Evidence for the expression of HLA-A-C class I mRNA and protein by human first trimester trophoblast. *J. Immunol.* **156:**2068–2076.

Kovats, S., E. K. Main, C. Kibrach, M. Stubbleline, S. J. Fisher, and R. DeMars. 1990. A class I antigen, L-HLA-G, expressed in human trophoblasts. *Science* **248:** 220–223.

Kurki, T., A. Sivonen, O. V. Renkonen, E. Savia, and O. Ylikerkala. 1992. Bacterial vaginosis in early pregnancy and pregnancy outcome. *Obstet. Gynecol.* **80:**173–177.

Kurt-Jones, E. A., S. Hamberg, J. Ohara, W. E. Paul, and A. K. Abbas. 1987. Heterogeneity of helper/inducer T-lymphocytes. I. Lymphokine production and lymphokine responsiveness. *J. Exp. Med.* **166:**1774–1787.

Lin, H., T. R. Mosmann, L. Guilbert, S. Tuntipopipat, and T. G. Wegmann. 1993. Synthesis of T-helper 2-type cytokines at the maternal-fetal interface. *J. Immunol.* **151:**4562–4573.

Maradny, E. E., N. Kanayama, A. Halim, K. Maehara, K. Sumimoto, and T. Tevao. 1994. Interleukin-8 induces cervical ripening in rabbits. *Am. J. Obstet. Gynecol.* **171:** 77–83.

McDonald, H. M., J. A. O'Loughlin, P. Jolley, R. Vignerswaran, and P. J. McDonald. 1991. Vaginal infection and preterm labor. *Br. J. Obstet. Gynecol.* **98:**427–435.

McGregor, J. A., J. I. French, and K. Seo. 1993. Premature rupture of membranes and bacterial vaginosis. *Am. J. Obstet. Gynecol.* **169:**463–466.

McGregor, J. A., J. I. French, W. Jones, K. Milligan, P. J. McKinney, E. Patterson, and R. Parker. 1994. Bacterial vaginosis is associated with prematurity and vaginal fluid mucinase and sialidase: results of a controlled trial of topical clindamycin cream. *Am. J. Obstet. Gynecol.* **170:**1048–1059.

Mitchell, M. D., D. W. Branch, S. Lardin-Schiller, R. J. Romero, R. A. Daynes, and D. J. Dudley. 1991. Immunologic aspects of preterm labor. *Semin. Perinatol.* **15:** 210–224.

Mosmann, T. R., and R. L. Coffmann. 1989a. Heterogeneity of cytokine secretion patterns and functions of helper T cells. *Adv. Immunol.* **46:**11.

Mosmann, T. R., and R. L. Coffmann. 1989b. TH1 and TH2 cells: different patterns of lymphokine secretion lead to different functional properties. *Am. Rev. Immunol.* **7:**145–173.

Mosmann, T. R., H. M. Cherwinski, M. W. Bord, M. A. Giedlin, and R. L. Coffman. 1986. Two types of murine helper T cell clones. I. Definition according to profiles of lymphokine activities and secreted proteins. *J. Immunol.* **136:**2348–2357.

Nolling, J., T. D. Pihl, A. Vriesema, and J. N. Reeve. 1995. Organization and growth phase-dependent transcription of methane genes in two regions of the *Methanobacterium thermoautotrophicum* genome. *J. Bacteriol.* **177:**2460–2468.

Norwitz, E. R., A. L. Bernard, and P. M. Starkey. 1992. Tumor necrosis factor-a selectively stimulates prostaglandin $F_{2\alpha}$ production by macrophages in human term decidua. *Am. J. Obstet. Gynecol.* **167:**815–820.

Opsjon, S. L., N. C. Wathen, S. Tingulstad, G. Wiedwang, A. Sundan, A. Wange, and R. Austgulen. 1993. Tumor necrosis factor, interleukin-1 and interleukin-6 in normal human pregnancy. *Am. J. Obstet. Gynecol.* **169:**397–404.

Pazmany, L., O. Mandelboim, M. Vales-Gomez, D. M. Davis, H. T. Reyburn, and J. L. Strominger. 1996. Protection from natural killer cell-mediated lysis by HLA-G expression in target cells. *Science* **274:**792–795.

Platz-Christensen, J. J., I. Mattsby-Baltzer, P. Thomsen, and N. Wiqvist. 1993. Endotoxin and interleukin-1a in the cervical mucus and vaginal fluid of pregnant women with bacterial vaginosis. *Am. J. Obstet. Gynecol.* **169:**1161–1166.

Prober, C. G., L. Carey, Z. A. Brown, P. A. Hensleitgh, L. M. Frenhel, Y. J. Gryson, J. R. Whitley, and A. M. Avvin. 1992. The management of pregnancies complicated by genital infections with herpes simplex virus. *Clin. Infect. Dis.* **15:**1031–1038.

Read, J. S., and F. F. Klebono. 1993. MA for the vaginal infections and prematurity study groups. Sexual intercourse during pregnancy and preterm delivery: effects of vaginal microorganisms. *Am. J. Obstet. Gynecol.* **168:**514–519.

Romagnani, S. 1992. Human TH1 and TH2 subsets: regulation of differentiation and role in protection and immunopathology. *Int. Arch. Allergy Immunol.* **4:**279–285.

Romero, R., S. Durum, C. Dinarello, E. Oyarzun, J. C. Hobbins, and M. D. Mitchell. 1989a. Interleukin-1 stimulates prostaglandin biosynthesis by human amnion. *Prostaglandin* **37:**13–22.

Romero, R., D. T. Brody, E. Oyarzun, M. Mazor, Y. K. Wu, J. C. Hobbins, and S. K. Durum. 1989b. Infection and labor. III. Interleukin 1: a signal for the onset of parturition. *Am. J. Obstet. Gynecol.* **160:**1117–1123.

Romero, R., M. Mazor, W. Sepulveda, C. Avila, D. Copeland, and J. Williams. 1992a. Tumor necrosis factor in preterm and term labor. *Am. J. Obstet. Gynecol.* **166:**1576–1587.

Romero, R., M. McZor, R. Morrotti, C. Avila, E. Oyarzun, A. Insunza, M. Parra, E. Bhenke, F. Montiel, and G. H. Carsell. 1992b. Infection and labor. VII. Microbial invasion of the amniotic cavity in spontaneous rupture of membranes at term. *Am. J. Obstet. Gynecol.* **166:**129–133.

Romero, R., W. Sepulveda, M. Mazor, F. Brandt, D. B. Cotton, C. A. Dinarello, and M. D. Mitchell. 1992c. The natural interleukin-1 receptor antagonist in term and preterm parturition. *Am. J. Obstet. Gynecol.* **167:**863–872.

Romero, R., B. H. Yoon, M. Mazor, R. Gomez, M. P. Diamond, J. S. Kenney, M. Ramirez, P. L. Fidel, Y. Sorokin, D. Cotton, and P. Sehgal. 1993. The diagnostic and prognostic value of amniotic fluid white blood cell counts, glucose, interleukin-6, and gram stain in patients with preterm labor and intact membranes. *Am. J. Obstet. Gynecol.* **169:**805–816.

Silver, R. M., B. Schwinzer, and J. A. McGregor. 1993. Interleukin-6 levels in amniotic fluid in normal and abnormal pregnancies: preeclampsia, small-for-gestational-age fetus, and premature labor. *Am. J. Obstet. Gynecol.* **169:**1101–1105.

Starkey, P. M., I. L. Sargent, and C. W. G. Redman. 1988. Cell populations in early pregnancy decidua: characterization and isolation of large granular lymphocytes by flow cytometry. *Immunology* **64:**129.

Sweet, R. L., D. V. Landers, C. Walker, and J. Schachter. 1987. Chlamydia trachomatis infection and pregnancy outcome. *Am. J. Obstet. Gynecol.* **156:**824–833.

Tabibzadeh, S. 1990. Evidence of T-cell activation and potential cytokine action in human endometrium. *J. Clin. Endocrinol. Metab.* **71:**645–649.

Tangri, S., T. G. Wegmann, H. Lin, and R. Raghupathy. 1994. Maternal fetal placental reactivity in natural immunologically mediated fetal resorptions. *J. Immunol.* **152:**4903–4911.

Towers, C. V., D. F. Lewis, T. Asrat, K. Gardner, and J. H. Perlow. 1993. The effect of colonization with group B streptococci on the latency phase of patients with preterm premature rupture of membranes. *Am. J. Obstet. Gynecol.* **169:**1139–1143.

Walsh, T. J., T. G. Mitchell, and D. H. Larone. 1995. *Histoplasma, Blastomyces, Coccidioides,* and other dimorphic fungi causing systemic mycoses, p. 749–764. *In* P. R. Murray, E. J. Baron, M. A. Pfaller, F. C. Tenover, and R. H. Yolken (ed.), *Manual of Clinical Microbiology,* 6th ed. American Society for Microbiology, Washington, D.C.

Watts, D. H., M. A. Krohn, S. L. Hillier, and D. A. Eschenbach. 1992. The association of occult amniotic fluid infection with gestational age and neonatal outcome among women in preterm labor. *Obstet. Gynecol.* **79:**351–357.

Weinberg, E. D. 1984. Pregnancy-associated depression of cell-mediated immunity. *Rev. Infect. Dis.* **6:**814–831.

Wegmann, T. G. 1986. Placental immunotrophism: maternal T cells enhance placental growth and function. *Am. J. Reprod. Immunol.* **15:**67–69.

Yamada, H., K. Polgar, and J. A. Hill. 1994. Evidence of cell-mediated immunity to trophoblast antigens in women with recurrent spontaneous abortion. *Am. J. Obstet. Gynecol.* **170:**1339–1344.

CLINICAL OUTCOMES AND METHODS

4
Prematurity: Premature Rupture of the Membranes and Preterm Labor

Ronald S. Gibbs

Premature birth and low birth weight are the leading perinatal problems in the Western world. In the United States, 6% of infants have low birth weight, but these infants account for approximately 75% of all perinatal deaths (Gibbs et al., 1992). Current strategies, which are aimed at identifying clinically evident risk factors, and use of marginally effective tocolytic drugs (which arrest uterine contractions) have had no effect on low-birth-weight rates in the United States. For over 50 years, it has been recognized that clinical infections such as sexually transmitted diseases, bacterial vaginosis, pneumonia, pyelonephritis, and even typhoid fever have been associated with premature labor and premature birth. Within the past few years, exciting information has been gathered to suggest that subclinical infection may be an important—and reversible—cause of premature birth. This chapter reviews the evidence supporting a linkage of subclinical infection and inflammation with preterm birth.

The hypothesis is that microbes or microbial toxins arrive in the uterine cavity either by the ascending route from the lower genital tract or by the blood-borne route from a remote focus. Once in the cavity, these microbes, probably acting at the level of the decidua or possibly the membranes, activate the decidua and the cytokine cascade, leading to prostaglandin synthesis. Prostaglandins, in turn, cause uterine contractions, which themselves lead to further cervical dilatation, more membrane exposure, and entry of more bacteria into the uterine cavity. Thus, a vicious cycle ensues.

Histologic chorioamnionitis is consistently associated with preterm birth. Examination of tissue reveals that for newborns greater than 2,500 g,

Ronald S. Gibbs, Department of Obstetrics and Gynecology, University of Colorado Health Sciences Center, 4200 E. 9th Ave., Box 198, Denver, CO 80262.

Sexually Transmitted Diseases and Adverse Outcomes of Pregnancy
Edited by P. J. Hitchcock, H. T. MacKay, J. N. Wasserheit, and R. Binder
©1999 American Society for Microbiology, Washington, D.C.

approximately 20% of placentas had histologic lesions of chorioamnionitis, but for newborns less than 1,000 g, over 70% of placentas had chorioamnionitis (Hillier et al., 1988).

For births of premature infants, clinically evident infection in infants and mothers is increased. This has been a consistent observation. Seo et al. (1992) found that only 0.5% of babies delivered at term with intact membranes were infected (with culture confirmation) but that 19% of babies born earlier than 28 weeks with intact membranes were infected. For pregnancies ending with premature rupture of membranes, the rates were approximately two to three times greater for all gestational ages (Seo et al., 1992) (Table 1).

For both the above observations, however, the etiologic agents are often undocumented. Histologic chorioamnionitis is probably a response to infection, and infection in preterm newborns could also reflect invasive procedures or longer stays in the nursery.

Associations have been made between some organisms or infections and subsequent preterm birth. For sexually transmitted organisms such as *Ureaplasma urealyticum*, *Trichomonas vaginalis*, and *Chlamydia trachomatis*, such associations have been rather inconsistently reported (Gibbs et al., 1992; Ryan et al., 1990). However, for women who have *C. trachomatis* infection and who have chlamydia-specific immunoglobulin M antibodies in the serum, two studies have shown associations with preterm birth (Sweet et al., 1987). In addition, bacterial vaginosis has been shown to be associated with preterm birth. The relationship between sexually transmitted organisms and preterm birth is addressed in chapter 5.

The rate of positive cultures of amniotic fluid from otherwise asymptomatic women in premature labor has varied from as low as 3% to as high as 24%. This variation is not surprising in view of the different culture techniques used and the vagaries of diagnosis of premature labor itself. In the largest study, Romero et al. (1989) defined a subgroup of patients in preterm labor who gave birth within 48 h (Fig. 1). In this group of 111

Table 1 Preterm birth and neonatal infection based on diagnosis by culture[a]

Time of gestation (wk)	% of premature babies infected after delivery with:	
	Ruptured membranes	Intact membranes
<28	39.1	19.0
28–30	17.1	6.1
31–33	5.4	2.0
34–36	3.0	1.8
>37	1.2	0.5

[a]Reprinted from Seo et al. (1992) with permission.

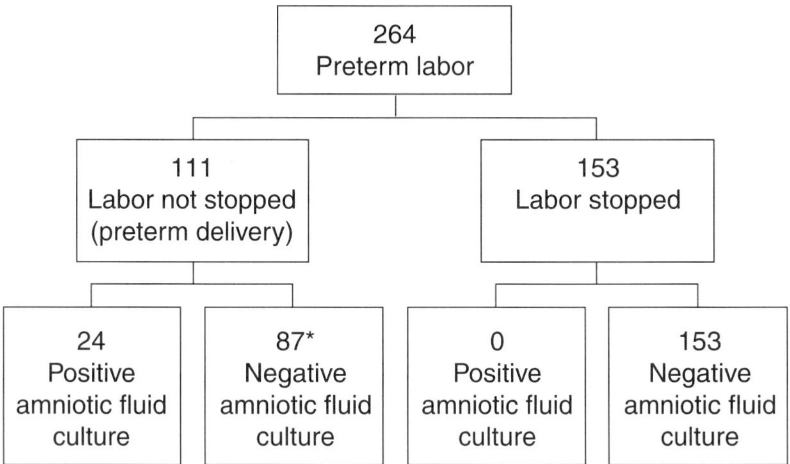

Figure 1 Amniotic fluid cultures in patients in preterm labor. The asterisk indicates that although amniotic fluid cultures were negative, three neonates had evidence of infectious morbidity. Reprinted from Romero et al. (1989) with permission.

patients, the likelihood of a positive culture, by using careful microbiological techniques, was 22.6%. Again, causality is uncertain with this observation, because the bacteria may enter the amniotic cavity as a consequence of premature labor. In such a case, it is likely that the amniotic fluid was colonized relatively late in the course of preterm labor. Accordingly, the study by Hillier et al. (1988) is of interest. In that study, very careful techniques were used to culture the chorioamnion of patients at varying stages of gestation. For women with newborns weighing more than 2,500 g, the likelihood of a positive culture was in the range of 20%, but for women with newborns weighing less than 1,500 g, the likelihood of a positive culture was 70 to 80%.

More recent reports, summarized by Gibbs et al. (1992), have shown that the biochemical consequences of infection or inflammation can lead to preterm birth. Prostaglandins are associated with the onset of both preterm and term labor, and it has been suggested that the cytokines that are released as the result of amnionitis or chorioamnionitis stimulate prostaglandin synthesis (Gibbs et al., 1992). This, in turn, stimulates the onset of labor. In women in preterm labor with evidence of infection or with poor response to tocolytic drugs, concentrations of prostaglandins and cytokines in amniotic fluid are elevated (Gibbs et al., 1992). In vitro, cytokines such as tumor necrosis factor and interleukin-1 stimulate gestational tissues to produce prostaglandins. In vitro, interleukin-1 can also stimulate the contraction of uterine muscles. Bacterial products such as endotoxin can also stimulate uterine muscle contraction in vitro (Gibbs et al., 1992).

Bacteria or bacterial products have induced preterm birth in several animal models, including monkeys (see chapter 20), mice, and rabbits (McDuffie and Gibbs, 1994). In a series of experiments, our group has demonstrated that introduction of bacteria via a hysteroscope into the uterine cavity of rabbits regularly leads to preterm delivery at 70% of gestation, with histologic and microbiological evidence of infection. In saline-inoculated control animals, labor occurred infrequently and the fetuses remained alive in the vast majority of cases (Dombroski et al., 1990) (Table 2). When *Escherichia coli* or *Fusobacterium necrophorum* were inoculated, labor uniformly ensued, with delivery in approximately 26 to 32 h. The fetuses were nearly always born dead. When *Prevotella bivia* was inoculated, preterm labor occurred less commonly, delivery occurred after a longer interval, and fewer rabbit pups died. Inoculation with *E. coli* was also accompanied by rises in the levels of inflammatory cytokines in amniotic fluid (McDuffie et al., 1992).

Of greatest clinical interest are the antibiotic trials designed to prevent prematurity. These trials are of three different types, including trials conducted during prenatal care of women at high risk (generally greater than 10%) for preterm birth, trials involving women in preterm labor with intact membranes when the antibiotics are used concurrently with tocolytic drugs, and trials involving women with premature rupture of the membranes.

Early studies suggested that treatment with oral erythromycin in randomized trials decreased adverse outcomes of pregnancy (Kirschbaum, 1993; Gibbs and Eschenbach, 1997). In historically controlled trials, it was observed that the treatment of chlamydia infection in pregnancy also mitigated adverse outcomes. For example, Ryan and colleagues reported that premature rupture of membranes, low birth weight, and mortality of neo-

Table 2 Pregnancy outcome in a rabbit model[a]

Inoculum	No. of rabbits delivered/total no.	Time to delivery (h)	No. of rabbits with live fetuses/total no.
Saline	2/9	134	7/9
E. coli	16/16[b]	32	0/16
F. necrophorum	6/7[b]	28	0/7
P. bivia	8/32	90	28/32

[a] Reprinted from Dombroski et al. (1990) with permission.
[b] $P < 0.05$ versus saline group.

nates were all decreased in women who were successfully treated for *C. trachomatis* compared to untreated *C. trachomatis*-positive women (Ryan et al., 1990).

However, in the large Vaginal Infections and Prematurity study, co-sponsored by the National Institute of Child Health and Human Development and the National Institute of Allergy and Infectious Diseases, National Institutes of Health, results have not been so encouraging. For example, in the subgroup of women enrolled in the study because of lower genital tract colonization with *Ureaplasma urealyticum*, erythromycin treatment had no demonstrable benefit compared to placebo (Eschenbach et al., 1991). Similarly, in the subgroup of women with group B streptococcal colonization, erythromycin therapy had no effect compared to placebo in decreasing adverse outcomes (Regan et al., 1996; Klebanoff et al., 1995). Three prospective trials (two of which were randomized) demonstrated significant improvement in pregnancy outcome when women with a history of a premature birth and with bacterial vaginosis were treated as part of their prenatal care (Hauth et al., 1995; Morales et al., 1994; McGregor et al., 1995).

Randomized clinical trials of the second type (i.e., of women in preterm labor with intact membranes) have reported conflicting results regarding delays in delivery. In the largest trial reported to date, Romero et al. (1993) compared ampicillin (followed by amoxicillin) plus erythromycin to placebo. No demonstrable benefits were associated with antibiotic treatment. However, administration of antibiotic after the onset of labor may be too late with respect to the pathogenesis of infection-induced premature rupture of the membranes. A recent meta-analysis of seven studies concluded that there was no overall benefit of antibiotic therapy in this clinical situation (Egarter et al., 1996).

Most of the antibiotic trials involving patients with premature rupture of the membranes have demonstrated a significant delay in delivery (Gibbs and Eschenbach, 1997). Similarly, the Maternal Fetal Medicine Network masked trial showed significant prolongation of pregnancy complicated by premature rupture of membranes when ampicillin plus erythromycin was given compared to placebo. Other benefits observed in the group given antibiotics were reductions in a prospectively defined composite outcome (neonatal death, respiratory distress syndrome, grade 3 or 4 intraventricular hemorrhage, grade 2 or 3 necrotizing enterocolitis, or neonatal sepsis), respiratory distress syndrome, chorioamnionitis, neonatal sepsis, and neonatal pneumonia (Mercer et al., 1997). In addition, a meta-analysis concluded that use of antibiotics in patients with premature rupture of membranes prolonged pregnancy and led to a reduction in chorioamnionitis and in confirmed neonatal sepsis (Mercer and Arheart, 1995).

If we try to place these current data into a clinical context, recommendations would include screening for and treating bacteriuria, providing antibiotic prophylaxis against group B streptococci (to prevent neonatal sepsis), and screening for and treating *Neisseria gonorrhoeae* and *Chlamydia trachomatis* (to control STDs and to prevent neonatal infection). In addition, it may be appropriate to consider other practices (Gibbs and Eschenbach, 1997). There is good evidence to recommend treatment in women at high risk for preterm birth, not in all women. Specific risk factors for preterm birth in reported trials have included a history of a previous preterm delivery (Morales et al., 1994), low prepregnancy weight (Hauth et al., 1995), and attendance at an inner-city clinic with a high rate of premature delivery (McGregor et al., 1995). There is no evidence to recommend prenatal treatment of *U. urealyticum* or group B *Streptococcus* genital tract colonization. However, the presence of group B *Streptococcus* in the urine indicates bladder infection and should be treated.

In spite of considerable new data on the relationship between sexually transmitted infections and preterm labor and delivery, there are some important gaps in our knowledge. Because preterm birth may be multifactorial and the risk associated with infection is usually modest, it is difficult to design trials to test the hypothesis. The causal association between certain sexually transmitted diseases and preterm labor must be further elucidated by randomized trials in low-risk women before recommendations for screening and treatment can be developed. While there are data from in vitro studies linking amniotic fluid infection with cytokine production and subsequent release of prostaglandins, the precise timing of events through which infection results in preterm labor has yet to be elucidated. These data are necessary to develop recommendations for the timing of screening and treatment.

Specific research recommendations to address the gaps in our knowledge include developing better animal models to mimic human preterm labor and conducting more targeted antibiotic trials. Examples of such trials include prenatal treatment of *Trichomonas vaginalis* or treatment of low-risk patients with bacterial vaginosis. Such trials would have to be large enough to account for spontaneous resolution of these infections, the modest relative risk of adverse outcome associated with these infections, and recurrence after treatment of infection. Additional trials that monitor selected women in preterm labor with intact membranes also seem appropriate. However, such trials would need to enroll patients who have been identified as being at high risk for infection-related preterm labor.

REFERENCES

Dombroski, R. A., D. S. Woodard, M. J. K. Harper, and R. S. Gibbs. 1990. A rabbit model for bacteria induced preterm pregnancy loss. *Am. J. Obstet. Gynecol.* **163:** 1938–1943.

Egarter, C., H. Leitich, H. Karas, and F. Wieser. 1996. Antibiotic treatment in preterm premature rupture of membranes and neonatal morbidity: a meta-analysis. *Am. J. Obstet. Gynecol.* **174:**589–597.

Eschenbach, D. A., R. P. Nugent, and A. V. Rao. 1991. A randomized placebo-controlled trial of erythromycin for the treatment of *Ureaplasma urealyticum* to prevent premature delivery. *Am. J. Obstet. Gynecol.* **164:**734–742.

Gibbs, R. S., and D. A. Eschenbach. 1997. Use of antibiotics to prevent preterm birth. *Am. J. Obstet. Gynecol.* **177:**375–380.

Gibbs, R. S., R. Romero, S. L. Hillier, D. A. Eschenbach, and R. L. Sweet. 1992. A review of premature birth and subclinical infection. *Am. J. Obstet. Gynecol.* **166:** 1515–1528.

Hauth, J. C., R. L. Goldenberg, W. W. Andrews, M. B. DuBard, and R. L. Cooper. 1995. Reduced incidence of preterm delivery with metronidazole and erythromycin in women with bacterial vaginosis. *N. Engl. J. Med.* **333:**1732–1736.

Hillier, S. L., J. Martius, and M. A. Krohn. 1988. A case controlled study of chorioamnionitis infection and histologic chorioamnionitis. *N. Engl. J. Med.* **319:**1972–1978.

Kirschbaum, T. 1993. Antibiotics in the treatment of preterm labor. *Am. J. Obstet. Gynecol.* **168:**1239–1246.

Klebanoff, M. A., J. A. Regan, V. Rao, R. P. Nugent, W. C. Blackwelder, D. A. Eschenbach, J. G. Pastorek, S. Williams, and R. S. Gibbs. 1995. Outcome of the vaginal infections and prematurity study: results of a clinical trial of erythromycin among pregnant women colonized with group B streptococci. *Am. J. Obstet. Gynecol.* **172:**1540–1545.

McDuffie, R. S., and R. S. Gibbs. 1994. Animal models of ascending genital tract infection in pregnancy. *Infect. Dis. Obstet. Gynecol.* **2:**60–70.

McDuffie, R. S., M. P. Sherman, and R. S. Gibbs. 1992. Amniotic fluid tumor necrosis factor-α and interleukin-1 in a rabbit model of bacterially induced preterm pregnancy loss. *Am. J. Obstet. Gynecol.* **167:**1583–1588.

McGregor, J. A., J. I. French, R. Parker, D. Draper, and E. Patterson. 1995. Prevention of premature birth by screening and treatment for common genital tract infections: results of a prospective controlled evaluation. *Am. J. Obstet. Gynecol.* **173:** 157–167.

Mercer, B. M., and K. L. Arheart. 1995. Antimicrobial therapy in expectant management of preterm premature rupture of the membranes. *Lancet* **346:**1271–1279.

Mercer, B. M., M. Miodovnik, G. Thurnau, R. L. Goldenberg, A. Das, R. D. Ramsey, Y. A. Rabello, P. J. Meis, A. H. Moawad, J. D. Iams, J. P. Van Dorsten, R. H. Paul, S. F. Bottoms, G. Merenstein, E. A. Thom, J. M. Roberts, and D. McNellis. 1997. Antibiotic therapy for reduction of infant morbidity after preterm premature rupture of the membranes. *JAMA* **278:**989–995.

Morales, W. J., S. Schorr, and J. Albritton. 1994. Effect of metronidazole in patients with preterm birth in preceding pregnancy and bacterial vaginosis: a placebo-controlled, double-blind study. *Am. J. Obstet. Gynecol.* **171:**345–349.

Regan, J. A., M. A. Klebanoff, R. P. Nugent, D. A. Eschenbach, W. C. Blackwelder, Y. Lou, and R. S. Gibbs. 1996. Colonization with group B streptococci in pregnancy and adverse outcome. *Am. J. Obstet. Gynecol.* **174:**1354–1360.

Romero, R., M. Sirtori, E. Oyarzun, and C. Avila. 1989. Infection and labor. *Am. J. Obstet. Gynecol.* **161:**817–824.

Romero, R., B. Sibai, S. Caritis, R. Paul, and R. Depp. 1993. Antibiotic treatment of preterm labor with intact membranes: a multicenter, randomized, double-blinded, placebo-controlled trial. *Am. J. Obstet. Gynecol.* **169:**764–774.

Ryan, G. M., Jr., T. N. Abdella, S. G. McNelly, V. S. Baselski, and D. E. Drummond. 1990. Chlamydia trachomatis infection in pregnancy and effect of treatment on outcome. *Am. J. Obstet. Gynecol.* **162:**34–39.

Seo, K., J. A. McGregor, and J. I. French. 1992. Preterm birth is associated with increased risk of maternal and neonatal infection. *Am. J. Obstet. Gynecol.* **79:**75–80

Sweet, R. L., D. V. Londres, C. Walker, et al. 1987. *Chlamydia trachomatis* infection and pregnancy outcome. *Am. J. Obstet. Gynecol.* **156:**824.

5
Postpartum Endometritis

Richard L. Sweet

Despite the introduction of potent broad-spectrum antimicrobial agents for treatment of infection and the widespread use of perioperative antibiotics in patients undergoing cesarean section, postpartum (puerperal) infections remain common. Although the incidence of maternal deaths due to puerperal sepsis is low in industrialized countries, puerperal infection is a common cause of morbidity, an occasional cause of severe infectious complications, and accountable for approximately 15% of maternal mortality (Sweet and Gibbs, 1995; Monga and Oshiro, 1993; Gabel, 1987). In addition, postpartum endometritis may have an adverse effect on the future reproductive health of the mother (Hurry et al., 1984).

The definition of "standard puerperal morbidity" as suggested by the U.S. Joint Committee on Maternal Welfare is "a temperature of 100.4°F (38°C), the temperature to occur in any two of the first ten days postpartum, exclusive of the first 24 hours, and to be taken by mouth by a standard technique at four times daily." However, because of early-patient-discharge practices following delivery and early intervention with potent bactericidal antimicrobial agents, it is often difficult to monitor for these infections.

The most common site of postpartum infection is the upper genital tract (e.g., endometritis) (Sweet and Gibbs, 1995). Other important contributors to puerperal morbidity include urinary tract infection, wound or episiotomy infection, mastitis, pneumonia, septic pelvic thrombophlebitis, and pelvic abscess (Table 1). The remainder of this chapter focuses on postpartum endometritis, especially the role of sexually transmitted organisms or

Richard L. Sweet, Department of Obstetrics, Gynecology and Reproductive Sciences, University of Pittsburgh School of Medicine/Magee-Womens Hospital, Pittsburgh, PA 15213-3180.

Sexually Transmitted Diseases and Adverse Outcomes of Pregnancy
Edited by P. J. Hitchcock, H. T. MacKay, J. N. Wasserheit, and R. Binder
©1999 American Society for Microbiology, Washington, D.C.

Table 1 Causes of postpartum infection

Endomyometritis
Urinary tract infection
Wound or episiotomy infection
Mastitis
Pneumonia
Septic pelvic thrombophlebitis
Pelvic abscess

syndromes and the adverse effects of these infections on the reproductive health of young women.

Endometritis occurs in 1 to 3% of vaginal deliveries. Cesarean section is associated with a 10- to 30-fold-increased incidence of postpartum endometritis (Sweet and Gibbs, 1995; Gibbs, 1985; Gilstrap and Cunningham, 1979; Sweet and Ledger, 1973). Similarly, the incidence of bacteremia is higher among women delivering by cesarean section (8 to 20%) compared to vaginally (5%). Before the use of prophylactic antibiotics for cesarean section, the incidence of endometritis after cesarean section ranged from 10 to 86% with a mean of 35% (Sweet and Gibbs, 1995). Within the cesarean section group, the infection rate is generally higher for clinic patients (20 to 60%) than for private patients (10 to 25%). Even with the widespread introduction of prophylactic antibiotics immediately after cord clamping, significant rates of endometritis (1 to 31%) still occur in association with cesarean delivery (Swartz and Grolle, 1981). Chang and Newton (1992) have reported a study assessing predictors of antibiotic prophylactic failure and post-cesarean endometritis. Using multivariate analysis, these authors identified four predictors of prophylaxis failure: (i) parity, (ii) number of vaginal examinations, (iii) gestational age, and (iv) type of prophylaxis. Six or more vaginal examinations during labor was associated with a significant increased risk for failure, and the risk increased as the number of vaginal examinations increased. Regardless of other risk factors, nulliparity and more than six vaginal examinations were the two most important predictors of prophylaxis failure. The use of cefazolin rather than ampicillin for prophylaxis and gestational age less than 37 weeks were less powerful predictors of failure.

Rarely, serious infectious complications of endometritis occur. The incidence of these serious, life-threatening sequelae is as follows: bacteremia, 10% (range, 0 to 25%); septic shock, <1%; pelvic abscess, <1%; and septic pelvic thrombophlebitis, <1% (Table 2). Group B *Streptococcus* appears to have a unique propensity to cause bacteremia when associated with puerperal infection, especially after cesarean section (Table 3). Puerperal infec-

Table 2 Incidence of bacteremia in association with endometritis

Study	Location	% of patients with endometritis who develop bacteremia
Sweet and Ledger (1973)	University of Michigan	8
Gibbs and Blanco (1981)	San Antonio, Tex.	8
DiZerega et al. (1979)	Los Angeles, Calif.	25
Blanco et al. (1981)	San Antonio, Tex.	9.7
Gall and Hill (1980)	Durham, N.C.	4.7
Gilstrap and Cunningham (1979)	Dallas, Tex.	11.7
Duff (1980)	Washington, D.C.	0

tion with group B *Streptococcus* is characterized by rapid onset (<24 h), high fever (≥39°C), and lack of localizing signs. Nearly one-third of the cases of group B *Streptococcus* endometritis are complicated by bacteremia (Table 3). The incidence of group B *Streptococcus* puerperal sepsis ranges from 6.5 to 13 per 1,000 deliveries.

Not only are bacteremia and sepsis relatively uncommon in association with puerperal infections, but when they do occur, the risk of septic shock and mortality is significantly lower than for medical or surgical patients (Table 4). Bacteremia is complicated by septic shock in 20 to 50% of medical and surgical patients compared to 0 to 12% of obstetric patients. The mortality rate among endometritis patients with bacteremia ranges from 0 to 4.3%; if septic shock occurs, mortality ranges from 0 to 67%. This compares very favorably with the high mortality rates noted in medical and surgical patients. Two factors contribute to the better outcomes seen in endometritis patients. First, the mothers are generally young and healthy, have few chronic medical illnesses, and have intact immune systems. Second, if nec-

Table 3 Incidence of bacteremia in group B streptococcal puerperal infection

Study	No. of patients	No. (%) of cases of bacteremia	No. (%) of patients undergoing cesarean section	Incidence (%) of puerperal infection
Faro (1981)	40	14 (35)	38 (95)	13
Gibbs and Blanco (1981)	48	48 (100)	31 (68)	NS[a]
Pass et al. (1982)	68	21 (31)	38 (56)	6.5

[a] NS, not stated.

Table 4 Bacteremia, septic shock, and mortality in obstetrical and gynecologic infections

Study	No. of cases/1,000 deliveries	No. of patients with bacteremia	No. (%) of patients with septic shock	No. (%) of patients who died
Blanco et al. (1981)	7.5	176	0 (0)	0 (0)
Ledger et al. (1975)	5	139	6 (4)	4 (3)
Bryan et al. (1984)	2	92		4 (4.3)
Chow and Guze (1974)		32	4 (12)	0
Weinstein et al. (1983)	5.3 (obstetric) 4.6 (gynecologic)	38		1 (2.6)

essary, the infected tissue can be surgically removed. Thus, in a septic abortion, the infected uterine and placental tissue can be evacuated by performing dilation and curettage. If there is extensive endometritis, a hysterectomy, with or without removal of ovaries and tubes, can be performed.

Additional concern has recently been raised about whether postpartum infection, especially endometritis, leads to adverse effects on the future reproductive function of the mother as a result of tubal factor infertility and/or ectopic pregnancy. Initial studies by Hurry et al. (1984) and Valenzuala (1984) suggested that there was no such association. Hurry et al. reported that among 1,300 patients delivering by cesarean section, the following 5-year cumulative pregnancy rate was 88%. They noted no difference in infertility whether or not the patients developed a postpartum endometritis. However, if the infection spread beyond the uterus and involved the ovaries or tubes, especially with abscess formation, the pregnancy rate was only 43%. Similarly, Valenzuala (1984) noted that the number of pregnancies following cesarean section was similar whether or not postpartum infection occurred.

Toth et al. (1993) assessed the impact of previous pelvic infection on pregnancy outcome. Previous pelvic infection was defined as a diagnosis of pelvic inflammatory disease (PID), amnionitis, or postpartum or postabortion endometritis-salpingitis. The study included 183 women with such infections compared to randomly selected controls. Full-term vaginal delivery occurred in only 14.2% of women with a history of pregnancy-associated infection versus 56% of the controls ($P < 0.001$). Women with a history of PID were significantly more likely to have a spontaneous abortion in a subsequent pregnancy (21.6 and 7.3%, respectively; $P = 0.013$) or to have preterm labor (10 and 0%, respectively). Those with amnionitis were at increased risk for preterm labor in subsequent pregnancies (25 and 0%, respectively). There was no increased prevalence of pregnancy complications among women with a history of postpartum endometritis. Unfortunately, this study design did not measure subsequent fertility. However, the rate of ectopic pregnancy was similar in the postpartum endometritis group and the control group. The most common antecedent risk factor for ectopic pregnancy was previous salpingitis. Thus, this study suggests that fertility may not be adversely affected by postpartum endometritis. On the other hand, as discussed later in this chapter, Plummer et al. (1987) have demonstrated that the sexually transmitted disease organisms *Neisseria gonorrhoeae* and *Chlamydia trachomatis* frequently cause postpartum endometritis that involves the fallopian tubes and may cause subsequent tubal factor infertility.

RISK FACTORS

Numerous studies have attempted to define risk factors for the development of postpartum infections (Sweet and Gibbs, 1995; Monga and Oshiro, 1993; Gibbs, 1985; Gilstrap and Cunningham, 1979; Gibbs et al., 1978; D'Angelo and Sokol, 1980; Rehu and Nilsson, 1980; Hawrylyshyn et al., 1981; Hagglund et al., 1983; Hager, 1975; Gassner and Ledger, 1976). The process of risk assessment has been difficult because of the complex interaction of underlying factors such as socioeconomic status, status of the immune system, antibacterial activity of amniotic fluid, and differences in vaginal microfloras. A large number of risk factors for postpartum endometritis, including labor, rupture of membranes, number of vaginal examinations, use of an internal fetal monitor, low parity, general anesthesia, skill of the surgeons, duration of surgery (>60 min), estimated blood loss (>500 ml), postoperative anemia, positive amniotic fluid culture, vaginal or cervical colonization with a variety of microorganisms including sexually transmitted organisms, absence of amniotic fluid-inhibiting factor(s), failure for labor to progress, and delivery by cesarean section, have been evaluated. Table 5 lists the generally accepted risk factors for puerperal endometritis.

Cesarean section is the major predisposing factor for both frequency and severity of pelvic infection in the postpartum period. Cesarean section is associated with a 5- to 30-fold increase in the risk of postpartum infection compared to that for patients delivered vaginally (Sweet and Gibbs, 1995; Monga and Oshiro, 1993; Gibbs, 1985; Gilstrap and Cunningham, 1979). The increased risk for developing endometritis following cesarean section is due to a combination of factors including trauma and tissue death associated

Table 5 Risk factors for postpartum endomyometritis

Cesarean section
Ruptured membranes
Labor
Low socioeconomic status
Vaginal examinations
Internal fetal monitoring
Presence of high-virulence bacteria or *Mycoplasma hominis* in amniotic fluid
Bacterial vaginosis
Group B *Streptococcus* colonization

with the surgical site, contamination with bacteria from the lower genital tract, and postoperative collection of fluid at the surgical site. Attempts to correlate postoperative infection after cesarean section with results of culture of the amniotic fluid obtained at the time of the cesarean section have not been useful. In particular, qualitative cultures do not predict outcome, since patients with positive culture do not develop infection and those with sterile amniotic fluid may subsequently develop postpartum endometritis. Gibbs (1985) has suggested that a better correlation can be obtained by performing quantitative cultures and microbiological evaluations. Placental and uterine biopsies have also been attempted as a tool for identifying patients at risk for postpartum infection. To date, evaluation of these tissues has not proven clinically useful. Clearly, the most significant risk factor for the development of post-cesarean endometritis is the duration of labor. When labor continued for 8 h or more, a fourfold increase in the incidence of post-cesarean endometritis occurred (Gibbs et al., 1978). The duration of ruptured membranes is an additional, very significant risk factor for the development of postpartum endometritis (Gibbs et al., 1978; D'Angelo and Sokol, 1980; Hagglund et al., 1983; Gilstrap and Cunningham, 1979). For example, Gilstrap and Cunningham (1979) have demonstrated that 100% of amniocentesis specimens from women of low socioeconomic levels who had membrane rupture more than 6 h prior to delivery were culture positive; 95% of these women subsequently developed post-cesarean endometritis.

The use of internal fetal monitoring has been accompanied by concerns about increased intrauterine infection both pre- and postdelivery. In the past, it has been difficult to separate the role of internal fetal monitoring from other covariables such as prolonged labor, premature rupture of membranes, and complicated medical situations during pregnancy. While initial studies (Gibbs et al., 1978) concluded that fetal monitoring played little or no role as a risk factor, more recent studies have demonstrated that it is a significant factor (Monga and Oshiro, 1993).

Socioeconomic status has been demonstrated to significantly influence the rate of postpartum infection. Most studies demonstrate that indigent patients, regardless of race, have significantly higher postpartum infection rates than do patients of middle to upper middle class socioeconomic status. Commonly cited explanations for this phenomenon include differences in vaginal flora, hygiene practices (douching), presence or absence of bacterial inhibiting factors in amniotic fluid, and nutritional status. It has also been suggested that indigent patients on clinic services staffed by residents may have many more vaginal examinations during labor and longer labor than patients in a private setting.

More than two decades ago, recommendations were made based on the belief that vaginal examinations in labor carried no greater risk for infection than did rectal examinations. Subsequently, vaginal examination became the standard approach for the assessment of labor. However, several studies using newer methods of statistical analysis, including multivariate analysis, have refuted this notion and documented that an increased number of vaginal examinations is associated with a greater risk for infection. Using multivariate analysis, Gibbs et al. (1978) found that the number of examinations was a definite risk factor for puerperal infection following cesarean section. Chang and Newton (1992) confirmed this finding and showed that a larger number of vaginal examinations (six or more) was a significant risk factor in women who were not protected with prophylactic antibiotics and developed post-cesarean endometritis. It is believed that with an increasing number of vaginal examinations a higher bacterial inoculum is introduced into the upper genital tract and causes this increased risk for infection.

The presence of virulent bacteria, including genital mycoplasmas, in the amniotic fluid is a significant risk factor for the development of postpartum endometritis, especially post-cesarean section (Rosene et al., 1986; Williams et al., 1987). These studies concluded that post-cesarean section endometritis was significantly associated with the presence of virulent bacteria (predominantly coliforms, streptococci, anaerobic cocci, and *Bacteroides* spp.) or *Ureaplasma urealyticum*. For the patients developing post-cesarean section endometritis, 35 to 60% of intraoperative cultures obtained from the amniotic fluid or the lower uterine segment contained virulent bacteria, compared to 10 to 24% of cultures for noninfected patients. The recovery rate of ureaplasma was 15 to 42% in the infected women compared to 0 to 10% in uninfected women. More recently, Newton et al. (1990) evaluated clinical and microbiologic risk factors for postpartum endometritis in over 600 asymptomatic women in labor, of whom 100 subsequently developed postpartum endometritis. Multivariate analysis demonstrated that the presence of virulent bacteria or *Mycoplasma hominis* in the amniotic fluid increased the risk of infection, with a relative risk of 1.4 ($P < 0.01$). In patients undergoing vaginal delivery, organisms associated with bacterial vaginosis (anaerobes, *Gardnerella vaginalis*, or *M. hominis*) were significant risk factors for the development of endometritis, with a relative risk of 14.2 ($P < 0.001$). In addition, aerobic gram-negative rods in the amniotic fluid significantly increased the risk (relative risk, 4.2; $P < 0.01$). In this study, although clinical variables such as duration of labor, duration of ruptured membranes, and internal fetal monitoring were significantly associated with endometritis on univariate analysis, these risk factors were not shown to be significant on multivariate analysis. Rather, it was concluded that these clinical variables facilitated infection by bacterial vaginosis-related organisms.

Subsequent studies have continued to demonstrate the important role of bacterial vaginosis in the etiology of postpartum endometritis. Clearly, the organisms which have been recovered from the upper genital tract of patients with postpartum endometritis over the last two decades have been organisms associated with bacterial vaginosis. These include anaerobes such as *Peptostreptococcus* and *Prevotella*, aerobic streptococci, and *M. hominis*. Watts et al. reported that the odds ratio for development of postpartum endometritis associated with bacterial vaginosis was 6.1 (95% confidence interval, 3.3 to 15.9) after adjusting for age, duration of labor, and duration of membrane rupture (Watts et al., 1990).

While most attention has focused on vaginal colonization by group B *Streptococcus* and its role in early-onset neonatal sepsis and mortality, this condition is also a predictor of women at increased risk for postpartum endometritis. Particularly characteristic of group B streptococcal infection is a very rapid onset, post-cesarean section high fever and lack of localizing signs despite a high incidence of bacteremia (Gibbs and Blanco, 1981; Faro, 1981; Pass et al., 1982). Studies have demonstrated that universal screening and selective intrapartum prophylaxis can prevent post-delivery group B streptococcal infections of the upper genital tract as well as neonatal mortality and morbidity.

MICROBIOLOGY

Postpartum endometritis, like other upper genital tract infections in the female, can be caused by a wide variety of anaerobic and facultative bacteria. The role of sexually transmitted organisms such as *C. trachomatis*, *N. gonorrhoeae*, and the genital mycoplasmas has been controversial. Elucidation of the microbiological etiology of postpartum endometritis is complicated by the need to obtain specimens from the endometrial cavity that have not been contaminated by the normal flora of the vagina and cervix. Sophisticated tools including double-lumen swabs, brushes and lavage techniques, and triple-lumen aspiration catheters have been developed to overcome the problems of contamination (Rosene et al., 1986; Knuppel et al., 1981; Duff et al., 1983; Eschenbach et al., 1986).

The microorganisms commonly recovered from the endometrial cavity of patients with postpartum endometritis are listed in Table 6. In general, studies have demonstrated that the anaerobic gram-negative bacilli are present in 40 to 50% of patients with postpartum endometritis. The following microorganisms have also been recovered from these patients: facultative gram-negative bacilli in 10 to 20%, peptostreptococci in 45 to 55%, enterococci in 5 to 10%, and group B streptococci in 10 to 20%. On the average, two or three different microorganisms can be recovered from the endometrial cavity in women with postpartum endometritis, but up to eight organisms are isolated in some patients. Aerobic or facultative bacteria are recovered from approximately 70% of the upper genital tract cultures. In the past, it was believed that *Escherichia coli* was the most common of the gram-negative bacilli. However, with use of selective media, it has more recently been demonstrated that *G. vaginalis* is the most common of these gram-negative bacilli (Rosene et al., 1986). The streptococci are the most frequently isolated aerobic pathogens in women with postpartum endometritis. Of these gram-positive isolates, group B *Streptococcus* is the most common, being recovered from 10 to 20% of patients. The enterococci are reportedly recovered from 5 to 10% of patients, but their role as pathogens is controversial. Several studies have demonstrated that the enterococci may be a particular concern in instances where the vaginal flora has been altered by prophylactic antibiotics, especially broad-spectrum cephalosporins (Chang and Newton, 1992). Fortunately, organisms such as *Staphylococcus aureus* and *Pseudomonas aeruginosa* are rare in patients with postpartum endometritis.

Anaerobic bacteria can be recovered in 40 to 60% of patients with postpartum endometritis when appropriate anaerobic microbiologic collection

Table 6 Microbiology of postpartum endomyometritis

Facultative organisms		Anaerobic organisms		Sexually transmitted organisms
Gram positive	Gram negative	Gram positive	Gram negative	
Group B *Streptococcus*	*G. vaginalis*	Peptostreptococci	*Prevotella bivia*	*N. gonorrhoeae*
Enterococci	*E. coli*	Clostridia	*Prevotella disiens*	*C. trachomatis*
Nonhemolytic streptococci	*Klebsiella* spp.		Other *Prevotella* spp.	*M. hominis*
S. aureus	*Proteus mirabilis*		*Porphyromonas* spp.	*U. urealyticum*
	Enterobacter spp.		*Bacteroides fragilis*	

and processing techniques are used (Duff et al., 1983; Eschenbach et al., 1986; Watts et al., 1990). The most common organisms among the anaerobic bacteria are the *Prevotella* organisms (formerly known as *Bacteroides*); in particular, *Prevotella bivia* and *Prevotella disiens* are the most important in this group. *Bacteroides fragilis*, while responsible for less than 5% of cases of postpartum endometritis, is a virulent pathogen and has been associated with severe infections such as abscess formation and septic pelvic thrombophlebitis. The other common anaerobic isolates are members of the *Peptostreptococcus* group. In addition, *Fusobacterium* and *Clostridium* spp. have been associated with postpartum endometritis. It should be noted that patients are rarely infected with *Clostridium perfringens*; these infected women generally do well with antimicrobial therapy alone and do not require extensive tissue debridement or removal of reproductive organs. Such aggressive surgical intervention should be reserved for patients with definite evidence of muscle necrosis. Even with bacteremia due to *Clostridium* spp., patients usually respond to antimicrobial therapy if the muscle of the uterus is not infected.

While it has generally been accepted that the presence of *N. gonorrhoeae* at the time of delivery is associated with an increased risk for postpartum endometritis, this belief is based on studies conducted nearly 30 years ago. These studies did not control for the presence of other organisms such as *C. trachomatis*, genital tract mycoplasmas, or bacterial vaginosis-associated organisms. The role of other sexually transmitted disease organisms or syndromes has been the focus of much recent interest and investigation. The role of *C. trachomatis*, *M. hominis*, *U. urealyticum*, and bacterial vaginosis-associated organisms in the etiology of postpartum endometritis is discussed below. Unfortunately, the vast majority of studies of gonorrhea did not attempt to recover anaerobes, facultative bacteria, *C. trachomatis*, *M. hominis*, or *U. urealyticum*. Rosene et al. (1986), using a protected-lumen transcervical culture method, attempted to recover anaerobic, aerobic, and facultative bacteria, genital mycoplasmas, and *C. trachomatis* from the endometrial cavity of women with early postpartum endometritis. Table 7 is a summary of the endometrial isolates reported in that paper. At least one facultative and one anaerobic species of bacteria were recovered from 82% of the patients, and genital mycoplasmas were recovered from 76% of the women with endometritis. Bacteria and genital mycoplasmas were present in 61% of the women. Bacteria without mycoplasma were present in 20%, genital mycoplasmas alone were present in 16%, and *C. trachomatis* was present in 2%. The most common organisms included *G. vaginalis*, *Peptostreptococcus* species, *Prevotella* species, group B *Streptococcus*, and *U. urealyticum*.

TREATMENT

The majority of patients with postpartum endometritis respond clinically to appropriate antibiotics within a few days. Among patients with endo-

Table 7 Isolates obtained from the endometrial cavity with a triple-lumen catheter in 51 patients with postpartum endometritis[a]

Microorganism	No. (%) of isolates
Facultative gram-positive bacteria	51 (40)
Group B streptococci	8 (6)
Enterococci	7 (5)
S. aureus	1 (1)
Facultative gram-negative bacteria	28 (22)
G. vaginalis	15 (12)
E. coli	6 (5)
Enterobacterium spp.	2 (2)
Proteus mirabilis	2 (2)
Anaerobic bacteria	49 (38)
Prevotella bivia	11 (9)
Other *Prevotella* spp.	9 (7)
Peptostreptococci	22 (17)
Mycoplasmas	
M. hominis	11 (9)
U. urealyticum	39 (30)
C. trachomatis	2 (2)

[a]Adapted from Rosene et al. (1986).

metritis following vaginal delivery, the recovery rate is very high (>95%), even with therapy that does not specifically target the anaerobic bacteria. On the other hand, in patients with post-cesarean section endometritis, the response to antibiotics is less dramatic; effective treatment must include antibiotics active against bacterial vaginosis organisms including *B. fragilis* and the *Prevotella* spp. (Sweet, 1981; Sweet and Ledger, 1979). The landmark study of DiZerega et al. (1979) demonstrated that early treatment with antimicrobial agents with a spectrum of activity that includes *B. fragilis*, *P. bivia*, and other *Prevotella* species results in significantly higher cure rates and lower incidences of severe infection such as pelvic abscesses, bacteremia, and septic thrombophlebitis. Combinations of antibiotics such as clindamycin plus gentamicin or metronidizole plus gentamicin or broad-spectrum drugs such as cephalosporin that are effective against the gram-negative anaerobic bacilli can be used. Although organisms such as *M. hominis* and *U. urealyticum* have been commonly isolated from patients with postpartum endometritis, these patients respond to antibiotics that are not effective against these organisms. Thus, their role in postpartum infections remains unclear. Similarly, the role of *C. trachomatis* in the pathogenesis of postpartum endometritis remains controversial. Here again, while the organism may be recovered, treatment with antibiotics thought to be inactive against it results in clinical response.

The use of antibiotic prophylaxis immediately after cord clamping has been demonstrated to dramatically reduce the incidence of postpartum endometritis following cesarean section. Chang and Newton (1992) attempted to identify predictors of antibiotic prophylactic failure in post-cesarean endometritis. They were able to demonstrate that patients receiving a cephalosporin agent (cefazolin), as opposed to ampicillin, were more likely to fail to respond to prophylaxis. It is believed that this may be due to selective overgrowth by *Enterococcus* in these patients. Similarly, studies by Walmer et al. (1988) demonstrated an increase in enterococcal infections following cephalosporin prophylaxis.

SEXUALLY TRANSMITTED ORGANISMS

During pregnancy, vertical transmission of *N. gonorrhoeae* has been associated with neonatal ophthalmia neonatorum and with adverse pregnancy outcomes such as preterm labor and delivery, premature rupture of membranes, low-birth-weight babies, and intrauterine growth retardation (Sweet and Gibbs, 1995). In the United States, high-risk populations are routinely screened and treated for gonorrhea at the first prenatal visit and again in the third trimester. Because of this clinical practice, gonorrhea does not appear to play a major role in postpartum endometritis (Sweet and Gibbs, 1995). However, other high-risk populations are not so fortunate. Plummer et al. (1987) investigated the frequency of upper genital tract infection and its relationship to sexually transmitted diseases and other risk factors in over 1,000 women in a maternity hospital in Nairobi, Kenya. This was an extremely high-risk population with a prevalence of *N. gonorrhoeae* and *C. trachomatis* infections of 6.7 and 20.8%, respectively. Over 20% of the patients developed a postpartum genital tract infection. In this study, the development of postpartum upper genital tract infection was significantly associated with gonococcal infection (odds ratio, 4.4; $P < 0.0001$), chlamydial infection (odds ratio, 1.7; $P < 0.02$), presence of ophthalmia neonatorum (odds ratio, 2.6; $P < 0.0001$), and labor longer than 12 h (odds ratio, 1.8; $P < 0.01$). By univariate analysis, the development of upper genital tract infection was significantly correlated with maternal gonococcal infection. This significant association remained with a multivariate analysis. The presence of gonococcal infection of the cervix was significantly associated with the development of salpingitis postpartum (Table 8). As discussed above, when gonococcal postpartum endometritis spreads to involve the fallopian tube, the patients were at significant risk for tubal factor infertility. The odds ratio with gonococcal infection alone was nearly 13 for the development of salpingitis (Table 8).

Table 8 Risk of postpartum upper genital tract infection in women with gonococcal and/or chlamydial infection of the cervix[a]

Upper genital tract disease	No. of patients	Alone	Odds ratio (*P*)	All	Odds ratio (*P*)
Gonococcal infection					
None	394	17		26	
Endometritis	25	3	2.8 (NS)[b]	4	2.4 (NS)
Salpingitis	9		12.9 (<0.0001)	6	10.1 (<0.0001)
Salpingitis and endometritis	41	7	4.0 (<0.01)	14	5.17 (<0.0001)
Chlamydia infection					
None	394	111		120	
Endometritis	25	7	1.0 (NS)	8	1.0 (NS)
Salpingitis	9	9	3.6 (<0.05)	10	3.6 (<0.01)
Salpingitis and endometritis	41	19	1.64 (NS)	44	1.9 (<.0.01)

[a]Reprinted from Plummer et al. (1987) with permission. Alone, gonococcal infection alone or chlamydia infection alone; All, all gonococcal infection or all chlamydial infection.
[b]NS, not significant.

C. trachomatis has also been associated with early postpartum fever and postpartum endometritis. Of mothers who had cervical chlamydial infections or infants with chlamydial conjunctivitis, 26 to 61% developed postpartum pelvic infections (Thygeson and Stone, 1942; Mordhorst and Dawson, 1971; Wager et al., 1980; Harrison et al., 1983). In particular, postpartum chlamydial endometritis occurred predominantly among those undergoing vaginal deliveries (Wager et al., 1980). However, a number of studies have failed to confirm any association between *C. trachomatis* and postpartum endometritis (Harrison et al., 1983; Sweet et al., 1987; Heggie et al., 1981). Similar to the situation with *N. gonorrhoeae*, Plummer et al. (1987) have demonstrated that *C. trachomatis* is a significant risk factor for the development of postpartum upper genital tract infections (Table 8). The major concern is the association between chlamydial infection and the risk for salpingitis (odds ratio, 3.6; $P < 0.1$). While antibiotics which do not cover chlamydia have been demonstrated to be very effective in treating postpartum endometritis, this should not be taken as a sign that chlamydia is not involved in these infections. Clinical cure has been demonstrated in patients with chlamydial PID; however, the organism persists in the genital tract (Sweet et al., 1983). This is an important principle, because it is believed that persistent chlamydial organisms in the upper genital tract may cause tubal scarring, resulting in subsequent infertility and ectopic pregnancies (Patton et al., 1994; Morrison et al., 1989).

Even more controversial than the role of *C. trachomatis* in postpartum infections has been that of the genital mycoplasmas *M. hominis* and *U. urealyticum*. *M. hominis* and *U. urealyticum* are frequently found in specimens from the upper genital tract of women with postpartum endometritis when appropriate culture techniques are used. In addition, both of these organisms have, on occasion, been isolated from the blood of women with postpartum fever and infections. Evidence that genital mycoplasmas are involved in postpartum fever and/or postpartum infections includes the isolation of organisms from the blood of 4 to 13% of women with postpartum fever (Lamey et al., 1982; McCormack et al., 1973) and a fourfold antibody response to *M. hominis* in 50% of women with postpartum fever (Platt et al., 1980). Rosene et al. (1986) attempted to recover genital mycoplasmas simultaneously from the uterus and blood of women with postpartum endometritis. They isolated *U. urealyticum* alone or with *M. hominis* from 8 (16%) of 51 women with postpartum endometritis. The isolation of *U. urealyticum* from the blood in two of the six women with *U. urealyticum* alone in the endometrium suggests that the organism can cause postpartum infection. Overall, these authors recovered genital mycoplasmas from 76% of the women with endometritis. The genital mycoplasmas were recovered alone from 16% of the patients and in combination with bacteria from 61% of the patients. Similarly, Williams et al. (1987) were able to show that post-cesarean section endometritis was significantly associated with the presence of *U. urealyticum*. Of 20 women from whom *Ureaplasma* was isolated from the amniotic fluid, 5 went on to develop postpartum endometritis. By comparison, genital mycoplasmas were not isolated from the amniotic fluid in any of the patients who subsequently remained afebrile and without clinical infection. In the multivariate analysis, *U. urealyticum* in the amniotic fluid remained a significant factor associated with post-cesarean section endometritis ($P < 0.01$). These authors noted a very high degree of correlation between *U. urealyticum* and coisolation of virulent bacteria. This association of genital mycoplasmas and virulent bacteria in the amniotic fluid has also been observed by Blanco et al. (1983).

Bacterial vaginosis is a vaginal condition associated with increased concentrations of anaerobic bacteria and *G. vaginalis* (Eschenbach, 1993; Eschenbach et al., 1984). This condition has been associated with an ever-widening spectrum of female upper genital tract infections and undoubtedly plays a role in the etiology of postpartum endometritis, amnionitis, chorioamnionitis, post-hysterectomy pelvic infections, PID, postabortion PID, and preterm labor and delivery (Eschenbach, 1993). Watts et al. (1990)

demonstrated that women with bacterial vaginosis (diagnosed by Gram stain) were roughly six times more likely to develop postpartum endometritis after cesarean section than were women without this condition. In this population, bacterial vaginosis contributed to one-third of the cases of postpartum endometritis, despite the use of prophylactic antibiotics (Watts et al., 1990). This confirms previous work by Minkoff et al. (1982) that suggested antenatal colonization with the bacterial vaginosis-associated organisms was associated with adverse pregnancy outcomes.

FUTURE RESEARCH AREAS

Priorities in the area of postpartum endometritis include investigations of a role of *C. trachomatis* and genital mycoplasmas in the etiology of postpartum endometritis; development of diagnostic tests or algorithms that can identify patients who are likely to fail to respond to prophylaxis; evaluation of the risk for long-term sequelae (e.g., tubal infertility) after postpartum infection, including causal association with specific bacterial pathogens; evaluation of bacterial vaginosis screening and treatment interventions for prevention of postpartum endometritis; and evaluation of intervention strategies for prevention of maternal and neonatal group B *Streptococcus* sepsis.

REFERENCES

Blanco, J. D., R. S. Gibbs, and Y. S. Castaneda. 1981. Bacteremia in obstetrics clinical course. *Obstet. Gynecol.* **58:**621–625.

Blanco, J. D., R. S. Gibbs, and H. Malherber. 1983. A controlled study of genital mycoplasmas in amniotic fluid from patients with intra-amniotic infection. *J. Infect. Dis.* **147:**650–653.

Bryan, C. S., K. L. Reynolds, and E. E. Moore. 1984. Bacteremia in obstetrics and gynecology. *Obstet. Gynecol.* **64:**155–158.

Chang, P. L., and E. R. Newton. 1992. Predictors of antibiotic in post cesarean endometritis. *Obstet. Gynecol.* **80:**117–122.

Chow, A. W., and L. B. Guze. 1974. Bacteroidaceae bacteremia: clinical experience with 112 patients. *Medicine* **53:**93–99.

D'Angelo, L. J., and R. J. Sokol. 1980. Time-related peripartum determinants of postpartum morbidity. *Obstet. Gynecol.* **55:**319–323.

DiZerega, G., L. R. Yonekura, R. M. Nakamura, and W. J. Ledger. 1979. A comparison of clindamycin-gentamicin and penicillin-gentamicin in the treatment of post cesarean endometritis. *Am. J. Obstet. Gynecol.* **134:**238–242.

Duff, P. 1980. Pathophysiology and management of septic shock. *J. Reprod. Med.* **24:** 109–117.

Duff, P., R. Gibbs, J. Blanco, and P. J. St. Clair. 1983. Endometrial culture techniques in puerperal patients. *Obstet. Gynecol.* **61:**217–222.

Eschenbach, D. A. 1993. Bacterial vaginosis and anaerobes in obstetric-gynecologic infection. *Clin. Infect. Dis.* **16**(Suppl. 4):282–287.

Eschenbach, D. A., M. G. Gravett, and C. S. Chen. 1984. Bacterial vaginosis during pregnancy: an association with prematurity and postpartum complication. *Scand. J. Urol. Nephrol.* **86**(Suppl.):213–222.

Eschenbach, D. A., K. Rosene, L. S. Tompkins, H. Watkins, and M. G. Gravett. 1986. Endometrial cultures obtained by a triple-lumen method from afebrile and febrile postpartum women. *J. Infect. Dis.* **153:**1038–1045.

Faro, S. 1981. Group B beta hemolytic streptococci and puerperal infections. *Am. J. Obstet. Gynecol.* **139:**686–689.

Gabel, H. D. 1987. Maternal mortality in South Carolina from 1970 to 1984: an analysis. *Obstet. Gynecol.* **69:**307–311.

Gall, S. A., and G. B. Hill. 1980. High-dose cefamandole therapy in obstetric and gynecologic infections. *Am. J. Obstet. Gynecol.* **137:**914.

Gassner, C. B., and W. J. Ledger. 1976. The relationship of hospital-acquired maternal infection to invasive intrapartum monitoring techniques. *Am. J. Obstet. Gynecol.* **126:**33.

Gibbs, R. S. 1985. Infection after cesarean section. *Clin. Obstet. Gynecol.* **28:**697–707.

Gibbs, R. S., and J. D. Blanco. 1981. Streptococcal infections in pregnancy. A study of 48 bacteremias. *Am. J. Obstet. Gynecol.* **140:**405–411.

Gibbs, R. S., P. M. Jones, and C. J. Wilder. 1978. Antibiotic therapy of endometritis following cesarean section. *Obstet. Gynecol.* **52:**31–37.

Gilstrap, L. C., and F. G. Cunningham. 1979. The bacterial pathogenesis of infection following cesarean section. *Obstet. Gynecol.* **53:**545–549.

Hager, D. 1975. Maternal febrile morbidity associated with fetal monitoring and cesarean section. *Obstet. Gynecol.* **46:**260–262.

Hagglund, L. K., K. Christensen, P. Christensen, and C. Kamme. 1983. Risk factors in cesarean section infection. *Obstet. Gynecol.* **62:**145–150.

Harrison, H. R., E. R. Alexander, L. Weinstein, M. Lewis, M. Nash, and D. A. Sim. 1983. Cervical *Chlamydia trachomatis* and mycoplasma infection in pregnancy: epidemiology and outcome. *JAMA* **250:**1721–1727.

Hawrylyshyn, P. A., P. Bernstein, and F. R. Papsin. 1981. Risk factors associated with infection following cesarean section. *Am. J. Obstet. Gynecol.* **139:**294–297.

Heggie, A. D., C. G. Lumicao, L. A. Stuart, and M. T. Gyues. 1981. Chlamydia trachomatis infection in mothers and infants. A prospective study. *Am. J. Dis. Child.* **135:**507–511.

Hurry, D. J., B. Larsen, and D. Charles. 1984. Effects of post cesarean section febrile morbidity on subsequent fertility. *Obstet. Gynecol.* **64:**256–260.

Knuppel, R., J. Scerbo, and J. Dzink. 1981. Quantitative transcervical uterine cultures with a new device. *Obstet. Gynecol.* **57:**243–248.

Lamey, J. R., D. A. Eschenbach, S. H. Mitchell, J. M. Blumhagen, H. M. Foy, and G. E. Kenny. 1982. Isolation of mycoplasmas and bacteria from the blood of postpartum women. *Am. J. Obstet. Gynecol.* **143:**104–111.

Ledger, W. J., M. Norman, C. Gee, and W. Lewis. 1975. Bacteremia on an obstetric-gynecologic service. *Am. J. Obstet. Gynecol.* **121:**205–212.

McCormack, W. M., Y.-H. Lee, J.-S. L. Lin, and J. S. Rankin. 1973. Genital mycoplasmas in postpartum fever. *J. Infect. Dis.* **127:**193–196.

Minkoff, H. L., M. F. Sierra, G. F. Pringle, and R. H. Schwarz. 1982. Vaginal colonization with group B beta-hemolytic streptococcus as a risk factor for post cesarean section febrile morbidity. *Am. J. Obstet. Gynecol.* **142:**992–995.

Monga, M., and B. T. Oshiro. 1993. Puerperal infections. *Semin. Perinatol.* **17:**426–431.

Mordhorst, C. H., and C. Dawson. 1971. Sequelae of neonatal inclusion conjunctivitis and associated disease in parents. *Am. J. Ophthalmol.* **71:**861–867.

Morrison, R. P., R. J. Belland, K. Lyng, and H. D. Caldwell. 1989. Chlamydia disease pathogenesis. The 57 KD chlamydial hypersensitivity antigen is a stress response protein. *J. Exp. Med.* **170:**1271–1283.

Newton, E. R., T. J. Prihoda, and R. S. Gibbs. 1990. A clinical and microbiologic analysis of risk factors for puerperal endometritis. *Obstet. Gynecol.* **75:**402–406.

Pass, M. A., B. M. Gray, and H. C. Dillon, Jr. 1982. Puerperal and perinatal infections with Group B streptococci. *Am. J. Obstet. Gynecol.* **143:**147–152.

Patton, D. L., Y. T. C. Sweeney, and C.-C. Kuo. 1994. Demonstration of delayed hypersensitivity in *Chlamydia trachomatis* salpingitis in monkeys: a pathogenic mechanism of tubal damage. *J. Infect. Dis.* **169:**680–683.

Platt, R., J.-S. L. Lin, J. W. Warren, B. Rosner, K. C. Edelin, and W. M. McCormack. 1980. Infection with *Mycoplasma hominis* in postpartum fever. *Lancet* **ii:**1217–1221.

Plummer, F. A., M. Laga, R. C. Brunham, P. Piot, A. R. Ronald, V. Bhullar, J. Y. Mati, A. Ndinya, M. Cheang, and H. Nsanze. 1987. Postpartum upper genital tract infections in Nairobi, Kenya. Epidemiology, etiology and risk factors. *J. Infect. Dis.* **156:**92–97.

Rehu, M., and C. G. Nilsson. 1980. Risk factors for febrile morbidity associated with cesarean section. *Obstet. Gynecol.* **56:**269–273.

Rosene, K., D. A. Eschenbach, L. S. Tompkins, G. E. Kenny, and H. Watkins. 1986. Polymicrobial early postpartum endometritis with facultative and anaerobic bacteria, genital mycoplasmas and *Chlamydia trachomatis*: treatment with piperacillin or cefoxitin. *J. Infect. Dis.* **153:**1028–1037.

Swartz, W. H., and K. Grolle. 1981. The use of prophylactic antibiotics in cesarean section: a review of the literature. *J. Reprod. Med.* **26:**595–609.

Sweet, R. L. 1981. Treatment of mixed aerobic-anaerobic infections of the female genital tract. *J. Antimicrob. Chemother.* **8**(Suppl. D)**:**105–114.

Sweet, R. L., and R. L. Gibbs. 1995. *Infectious Diseases of the Female Genital Tract.* The Williams & Wilkins Co., Baltimore, Md.

Sweet, R. L., and W. J. Ledger. 1973. Puerperal infectious morbidity: a two year review. *Am. J. Obstet. Gynecol.* **117:**1093–1100.

Sweet, R. L., and W. J. Ledger. 1979. Cefoxitin: single-agent treatment of mixed aerobic-anaerobic pelvic infection. *Obstet. Gynecol.* **54:**193–198.

Sweet, R. L., J. Schachter, and M. O. Robbie. 1983. Failure of beta-lactam antibiotics to eradicate *Chlamydia trachomatis* from the endometrium in patients with acute salpingitis despite apparent clinical cure. *JAMA* **250:**2641–2645.

Sweet, R. L., D. V. Landers, C. Walker, and J. Schachter. 1987. *Chlamydia trachomatis* infection and pregnancy outcome. *Am. J. Obstet. Gynecol.* **156:**824–830.

Thygeson, P., and W. J. Stone. 1942. Epidemiology of inclusion conjunctivitis. *Arch. Ophthalmol.* **27:**91–122.

Toth, M., A. Chaudry, W. J. Ledger, and S. S. Witkin. 1993. Pregnancy outcome following pelvic infection. *Infect. Dis. Obstet. Gynecol.* **1:**12–15.

Valenzuala, G. 1984. Fertility following cesarean section endoparametritis. *Am. J. Obstet. Gynecol.* **149:**231–232.

Wager, G. P., D. H. Martin, L. Koutsky, D. A. Eschenbach, J. R. Daling, E. R. Alexander, and K. K. Holmes. 1980. Puerperal infectious morbidity relationship to route of delivery and to antepartum *Chlamydia trachomatis* infection. *Am. J. Obstet. Gynecol.* **138:**1028–1033.

Walmer, D., K. Walmer, and R. S. Gibbs. 1988. Enterococci in post cesarean endometritis. *Obstet. Gynecol.* **71:**159–161.

Watts, D. H., M. J. Krohn, S. L. Hillier, and D. A. Eschenbach. 1990. Bacterial vaginosis as a risk factor for post cesarean endometritis. *Obstet. Gynecol.* **75:**52–58.

Weinstein, M. P., J. R. Murphy, L. B. Reller, and K. A. Lichenstein. 1983. The clinical significance of positive blood cultures: a comprehensive analysis of 500 episodes of bacteremia and fungemia in adults. *Rev. Infect. Dis.* **5:**54–59.

Williams, C. M., D. M. Okada, J. R. Marshall, and A. W. Chow. 1987. Clinical and microbiologic risk evaluation for post cesarean section endometritis by multivariate discriminant analysis: role of intraoperative mycoplasma, aerobes, and anaerobes. *Am. J. Obstet. Gynecol.* **156:**967–974.

6
Methodologic Issues in Perinatal Research

Michael S. Kramer

This chapter presents an overview of the methods and study designs used to assess the possible association between sexually transmitted diseases (STDs) and adverse pregnancy outcomes. To be more specific, we are particularly interested in whether certain STDs can *cause* specific adverse outcomes, and if so, how often. The main question, from both a clinical and a public health perspective, is will prevention or treatment of the STD reduce the risk of the adverse pregnancy outcomes?

Satisfactory demonstration of a causal association requires that errors both random and systematic be minimized in the design and analysis of appropriate epidemiologic studies. This chapter will define what is meant by random and systematic error, explain how they relate to specific types of epidemiologic study designs, and suggest how errors can be minimized at both the design and analysis phases of investigation. The types of epidemiologic research designs and the quantitative estimates of effect that derive from such study designs will be reviewed. The importance of statistical power, and particularly adequate sample size, in minimizing random error will be considered. The various sources of systematic error (bias), with particular emphasis on how they relate to specific types of epidemiologic studies and how they can be reduced by appropriate design and analytic strategies, will be delineated. Randomized clinical trials and the design and analytic strategies used to minimize random and systematic error in the experimental setting will be discussed.

Michael S. Kramer, Department of Pediatrics and Department of Epidemiology and Biostatistics, McGill University Faculty of Medicine, Montreal, Quebec, Canada.

Sexually Transmitted Diseases and Adverse Outcomes of Pregnancy
Edited by P. J. Hitchcock, H. T. MacKay, J. N. Wasserheit, and R. Binder
©1999 American Society for Microbiology, Washington, D.C.

CHOOSING THE OUTCOME

Perinatal epidemiologic studies should focus on outcomes of major importance to the fetus, infant, or mother, including stillbirth, neonatal death, neonatal infant morbidity, major congenital malformations, and maternal mortality and morbidity.

These important adverse pregnancy outcomes are rare, however, and most epidemiologic studies are too small to detect all but the largest etiologic effects of potential risk factors. The exceptions are those risk factors reliably recorded on birth or death certificates, for which large sample sizes are quite feasible to obtain. Because STDs are not recorded on birth or death certificates, most epidemiologic studies depend on primary data collection and, owing to their consequently limited sample size, focus on surrogate adverse outcomes, such as preterm birth, intrauterine growth retardation, or low birth weight. It is known that these adverse outcomes increase the risk of fetal death and infant morbidity and mortality, but the link to STDs is unclear. Most growth-retarded infants are at low risk for mortality or major morbidity, except for those most severely affected (Kramer et al., 1990; Stein and Susser, 1984; Keirse, 1984). Preterm birth is of far greater import to infant health and survival (Hogue et al., 1987; Kessel et al., 1984; Kramer, 1990), although modern obstetric and neonatal care has reduced the risks for the majority of infants born over 32 weeks gestational age.

Low birth weight is a rather poor surrogate outcome. Although it too is statistically associated with fetal and infant morbidity and mortality, low-birthweight infants comprise both preterm and growth-retarded infants. Since preterm birth and intrauterine growth retardation have different etiologic determinants (Abrams and Newman, 1991; Barros et al., 1992; Kramer, 1987; Wen et al., 1990) and different prognostic implications (Hogue et al., 1987; Keirse, 1984; Kessel et al., 1984; Kramer, 1990; Kramer et al., 1990; Stein and Susser, 1984), the use of low birth weight as a study outcome can dilute or confuse the potential etiologic role of STDs.

For example, consider the data summarized in Table 1 (Abrams and Newman, 1991; Barros et al., 1992; Chomitz et al., 1992; Kramer, 1987; Kramer et al., 1992; Wen et al., 1990). Maternal short stature, low prepregnancy weight, and low rate of gestational weight gain are all important determinants of fetal growth and intrauterine growth retardation, but studies relating these outcomes to preterm birth have shown either no effect or small effects. Female fetuses are smaller than male fetuses but are at no greater risk for preterm delivery. Nulliparous women are at increased risk for intrauterine growth retardation but not for preterm birth. Cigarette smoking is a very potent determinant of intrauterine growth retardation, but a weak one for preterm birth. Severe pregnancy-induced hypertension is one of the few factors that have a strong etiologic relation to both of these outcomes. Maternal diabetes increases the risk of preterm birth but is actually protec-

Table 1 Well-established determinants of intrauterine growth retardation and preterm birth[a]

Variable	Intrauterine growth retardation	Preterm birth
Nulliparity	+	0
Female fetus	+	0
Alcohol consumption	+	0
Short stature	+	±
Low pregnancy weight	+	±
Low gestational weight gain	+	±
Cigarette smoking	++	+
Cocaine use	+	+
Severe pregnancy-induced hypertension	++	++
Genital tract infection	0	+
Age ≥35 years	0	+
Low maternal education	0	+
Unmarried mother	0	+
Physically demanding work	0	+
Maternal diabetes	−	+

[a]Sources: Abrams and Newman, 1991; Barros et al., 1992; Chomitz et al., 1992; Kramer, 1987; Kramer et al., 1992; Wen et al., 1990.

tive against intrauterine growth retardation, because of the effects of maternal hyperglycemia on fetal growth. On the other hand, genital tract infection increases the risk for preterm birth but has no effect on intrauterine growth retardation. Similarly, advanced maternal age, low maternal education, being unmarried, and physically demanding work appear to be important determinants of preterm birth but do not affect the risk of intrauterine growth retardation once maternal nutrition, cigarette smoking, and other risk factors have been taken into account.

Among those less well-established potential determinants currently under study, chronic stress and other psychosocial factors appear to be more related to preterm birth than to intrauterine growth retardation. The reverse is true for caffeine and passive smoking (exposure to environmental tobacco smoke). Data are insufficient to infer favorable benefits of prenatal care for either adverse outcome.

EPIDEMIOLOGIC STUDY DESIGNS

Epidemiologic studies can be either descriptive or analytic, although some studies attempt to accomplish both goals. In descriptive studies, the purpose is to summarize information about one or more variables in a group of subjects. An inference is then made about the value or distribution of the variable(s) in the source population from which the study sample is derived. In analytic studies (Table 2), the purpose is to infer an association (usually causation) between two variables. The inference in analytic studies is about the association between these two variables in the source population, based on the degree of association observed in the study sample.

The two variables whose association is studied in an analytic study are usually referred to as *exposure* and *outcome.* The exposure is the putative causal agent; it can occur either naturally, as a result of self-selection, or by prescription. The outcome is the putative health effect the investigator believes may be caused by the exposure. The research question or hypothesis then becomes: Does the exposure cause the outcome? Analytic studies can be further subdivided into *observational studies* (also called surveys), which are characterized by the fact that the exposure is not assigned by the investigator, and *experimental studies* (also called *clinical trials*), in which the exposure is assigned by the study investigator.

Clinical trials always proceed in a forward direction, from (assigned) exposure (usually referred to as "treatment" in a clinical trial) to outcome. This type of longitudinal follow-up is also involved in *cohort studies*, which are the observational counterpart of the clinical trial; the only difference is the fact that the exposure is not assigned by the study investigator. In *case-control studies*, on the other hand, the investigator begins with the presence or absence of the outcome (the cases and controls, respectively) and enquires about prior exposure. Cross-sectional studies represent the weakest design for causal inferences, because the ascertained exposure and outcome refer to the same point in time, and thus it is often impossible to be sure that the exposure preceded the outcome, rather than the other way around.

ESTIMATES OF EFFECT

In cohort studies and randomized trials, the measurement of effect depends on whether the outcome is measured on a *continuous* or *dichotomous* scale. For continuous outcomes, the effect of exposure can be expressed as the difference in mean outcomes between the exposed and unexposed groups of subjects (or the groups exposed to two different types or levels of exposure). When the outcome is dichotomous, the effect can be expressed as either the *incidence (risk) difference* or the *incidence (risk) ratio* (called the *relative risk*) between the two groups.

In case-control studies, the exposure can be measured on either a continuous or dichotomous scale. Although comparing the difference in mean exposures between the cases and controls is a valid means of assessing the exposure-outcome association, such a comparison is not very useful for predicting outcome from exposure. Thus, even when exposure is naturally measured on a continuous scale, it is often dichotomized for the purpose

Table 2 Analytic studies

Study type	Strengths	Weaknesses	Uses
Experimental			
Randomized clinical trial	Methodologically strongest evidence of causality. Randomization minimizes bias. Can directly estimate relative risk.	Complex, expensive, and time-consuming. Differential losses to follow-up may introduce bias.	Performed to demonstrate efficacy of an intervention when observational studies have shown an association between an exposure and an outcome. *Example*: ACTG 076
Observational			
Cohort study	Observational equivalent of randomized clinical trial. Prospective selection minimizes selection and information bias. Outcome follows exposure. Can directly estimate relative risk.	Large cohorts usually necessary, particularly for uncommon diseases. Relatively high cost because of time involved. Differential losses to follow-up may introduce bias.	Most suitable for frequent diseases. Used to follow up findings from case-control or cross-sectional studies. *Example*: Framingham Heart Study
Case-control study	Can be done more quickly and at lower cost than cohort studies because outcome has already occurred. Cost-effective for study of rare diseases.	More subject to information and selection biases than cohort study. Cannot directly estimate relative risk.	Often used as an initial step in examining association of an exposure and outcome. *Example*: Association of tampons and toxic shock syndrome
Cross-sectional study	Inexpensive, rapidly performed "snapshot."	Difficult to sort out chronological relationship between exposure and outcome, as they are measured simultaneously.	Most useful for describing disease patterns. *Example*: HIV seroprevalence studies

of effect estimation. The principal effect measure in case-control studies is the *odds ratio*, which is the ratio of the odds of exposure in the cases to the odds of exposure in controls. Provided that the outcome is reasonably uncommon, the odds ratio is a very good estimate of the relative risk that would have been obtained had the study been performed as a cohort study. Relative risk cannot be estimated directly from a case-control study, because the study does not begin with two representative groups of exposure, and thus the absolute risks, risk difference, and risk ratio cannot be directly ascertained; instead, the number of cases of the outcome is determined by the investigator.

ERROR IN EFFECT ESTIMATION

Sample Size

Required sample sizes for a given study depend upon the question being asked. Specifically, the frequency with which both the exposure and the outcome occur in a population determines the number of people that must be studied. In general, if either exposure or outcome is rare, then a large sample size is needed.

A *type I error* is the result of rejecting the null hypothesis when it is true (identifying a relationship between exposure and outcome when none exists). A *type II error* is the result of accepting the null hypothesis when it is false (no relationship is identified between exposure and outcome when a relationship actually exists).

All of the above-mentioned estimates of effect are subject to error. The two broad types of error can be characterized as *random error* and *systematic error.*

Random Error

Random error is due to *sampling variation* and is a reflection of the fact that samples randomly selected from a source population will differ in their degree of exposure-outcome association by chance from the true degree of association in the source population. The potential for random error is greatest when the size of the sample is small. An adequate sample size is important not only so that the effect estimate will be "statistically significant," but also so that we can be reasonably certain of its magnitude.

The required sample size depends on the incidence of the outcome under study. For example, intrauterine growth retardation, which is customarily defined as a birthweight less than the 10th percentile for gestational age, has an expected incidence of 10%. Preterm birth is also reasonably common, occurring in about 6 or 7% of all pregnancies. Fetal and neonatal mortality rates, however, are usually in the range of several per thousand, and for serious congenital malformations, the incidence may be another order of magnitude lower.

Tests of statistical significance examine the role of random error in producing the observed effect by chance under the assumption that the null hypothesis (there is no relationship between the exposure and the outcome in the source population) is true. But one must distinguish between statistical significance and clinical importance. As illustrated in Fig. 1A, with a small sample size, even clinically important effects may fail to achieve statistical significance. The risk of *type II error* here is large, as shown by the wide confidence interval compatible with either a clinically important reduction or increase in risk of preterm birth associated with the STD under study. At the other extreme, with very large sample sizes, random error is minimized and even trivial effects may achieve statistical significance (Fig. 1B). Thus, even though statistical tools are used to quantitate the probability of random error, the importance of a given degree of association is a clinical decision, not a statistical one.

Because etiologic studies are expensive and time-consuming, they are often used to answer several questions, including the effect of exposure on several outcomes, or the effect of multiple exposures on a given outcome. At a threshold probability (*P*) value of 0.05, 1 of 20 independent tests of the null hypothesis will be "significant" by chance alone; this is known as a *type I error*. If 100 independent associations are examined and 10 yield *P* values below 0.05, it is impossible to know which are chance findings and which are "truly" significant. This problem of multiple comparisons is particularly dangerous if the research hypotheses are examined post hoc,

A. Cohort study

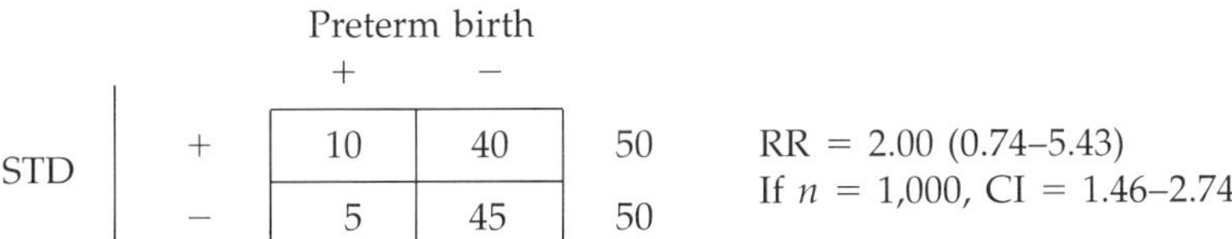

		Preterm birth +	Preterm birth −		
STD	+	10	40	50	RR = 2.00 (0.74–5.43)
	−	5	45	50	If n = 1,000, CI = 1.46–2.74

B. Randomized trial

	Preterm birth +	Preterm birth −		
Drug	10	40	50	RR = 0.91 (0.42–1.95)
Placebo	11	39	50	If n = 1,000, CI = 0.71–1.16 If n = 10,000, CI = 0.84–0.98

Figure 1 Random error: the effect of sample size. RR, relative risk; n, sample size; CI, confidence interval.

i.e., by analyzing associations that "look interesting." Research hypotheses should therefore be stated a priori and should be limited in number to reduce the potential for false-positive results.

Systematic Error (Bias)

There are four primary sources of systematic error: information bias, selection bias, confounding bias, and reverse causality bias. *Information bias* occurs when the true degree of association between exposure and outcome is systematically under- or overestimated because of errors in the measurement of exposure and/or outcome. When the errors are nondifferential (i.e., the direction and magnitude of the error in measurement of outcome do not differ according to exposure, and the error in measurement of exposure does not differ by outcome), the bias in effect estimate is generally towards the null. For example, perinatal epidemiologic studies of such outcomes as gestational age depend upon how accurately gestational age is measured. Menstrual date-based estimates, for example, are fraught with error. Thus, effects of exposures on gestational age and preterm birth might go undetected because of errors in recollection of the last menstrual period, as well as variation in time of ovulation, inapparent spontaneous abortions, or nonmenstrual bleeding early in pregnancy. On the other hand, if a particular exposure is associated with intrauterine growth retardation and the gestational age estimate is not based solely on dates, but is influenced by fetal size (e.g., fundal height), a false association with preterm birth would be made.

Two illustrative examples of information bias are shown in Fig. 2. Figure 2A shows a 2-by-2 table summarizing results of a cohort study comparing the incidence of congenital malformations in two large hypothetical cohorts of 10,000 pregnant women each, one with and one without a given STD of interest. Assuming no misclassification of exposure or outcome, the true relative risk is 2.00. In Fig. 2B, a comparable 2-by-2 table is shown in which there is nondifferential misclassification of the outcome, based on a clinical diagnosis of the congenital malformation that is 90% sensitive and 98% specific. The misclassification is nondifferential because the 10% underascertainment of outcome occurs equally among women with and without the STD, and the 2% false-positive diagnoses also occur nondifferentially according to exposure. As can be seen, this nondifferential misclassification of outcome results in a relative risk of 1.49, i.e., an underestimate of the true relative risk. Finally, in Fig. 2C, we have an example of differential misclassification of outcome. In this example, increased detection of the congenital malformation is seen in those women with the STD because of closer examination of their babies. This leads to a complete ascertainment of the cases occurring among the exposed women, but only a 75% ascer-

A. "Truth"

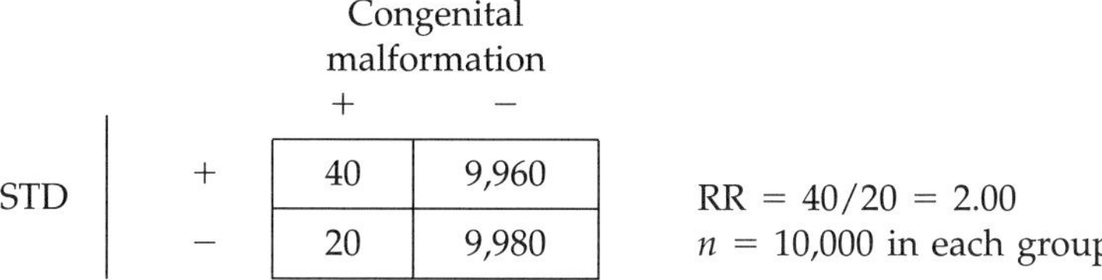

		Congenital malformation +	Congenital malformation −
STD	+	40	9,960
	−	20	9,980

RR = 40/20 = 2.00
n = 10,000 in each group

B. Nondifferential misclassification of outcome: measurement is 90% sensitive and 10% specific

		Congenital malformation +	Congenital malformation −
STD	+	55	9,945
	−	37	9,963

RR = 55/37 = 1.49
n = 10,000

C. Differential misclassification of outcome: ↑ detection among exposed

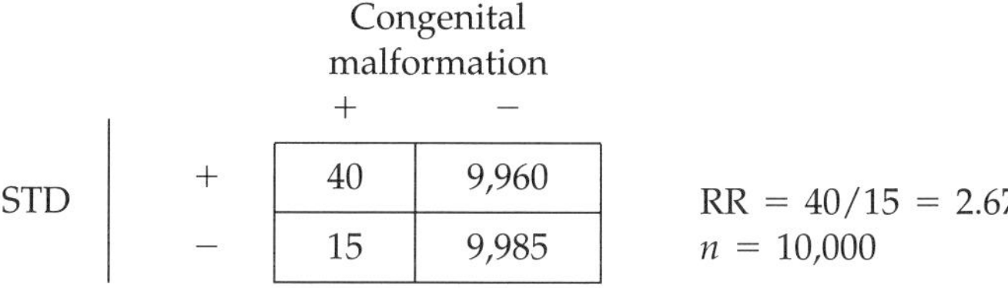

		Congenital malformation +	Congenital malformation −
STD	+	40	9,960
	−	15	9,985

RR = 40/15 = 2.67
n = 10,000

Figure 2 Information bias: illustrative examples. RR, relative risk; n, sample size.

tainment among the unexposed, yielding an overestimate of the true relative risk of 2.67.

In *selection bias,* those subjects selected for study and who remain in follow-up to be included in the analysis differ in their joint distribution of exposure and outcome from those not selected or those lost to follow-up. For example, Fig. 3A shows the "true" relationship between an STD and miscarriage in a source population of 22,000 pregnant women. A total of 9% of both the exposed and unexposed women in the population develop a (recognized) miscarriage, and the true relative risk is therefore 1.00. Figure 3B shows a case-control study of 200 cases and 200 controls randomly selected from the 2,000 and 20,000 in the source population who do and do not, respectively, develop a miscarriage. Because the study sample has been randomly selected from the source population, the rates of exposure and nonexposure to the STD remain identical (at least within sampling varia-

A. "Truth" source population

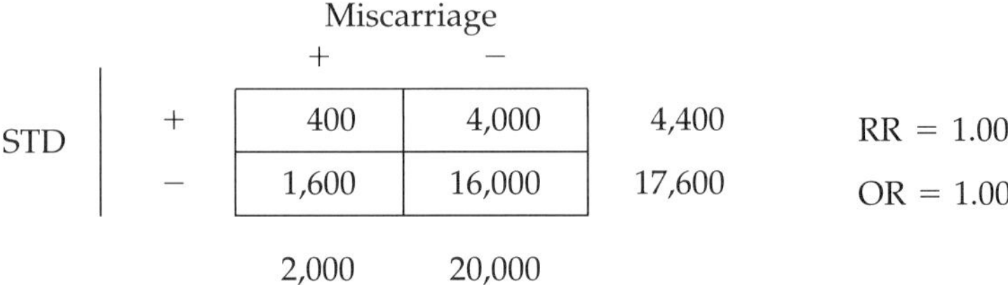

		Miscarriage +	Miscarriage −	
STD	+	400	4,000	4,400
	−	1,600	16,000	17,600
		2,000	20,000	

RR = 1.00
OR = 1.00

B. Random sample: case-control study

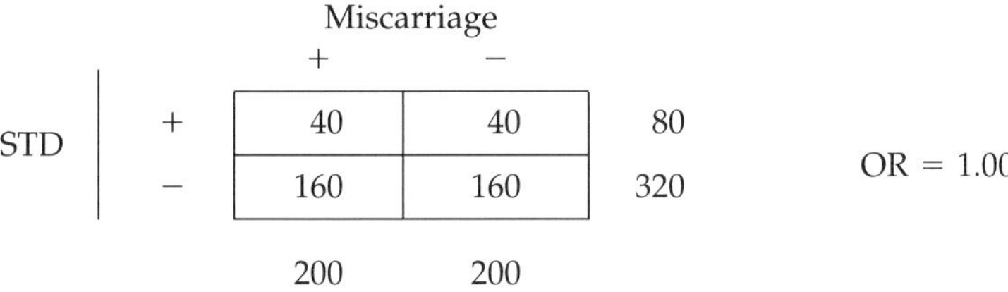

		Miscarriage +	Miscarriage −	
STD	+	40	40	80
	−	160	160	320
		200	200	

OR = 1.00

C. Biased sample: gynecologist cases

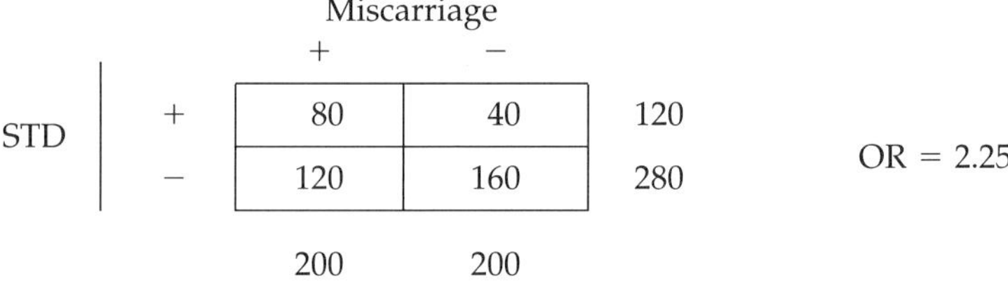

		Miscarriage +	Miscarriage −	
STD	+	80	40	120
	−	120	160	280
		200	200	

OR = 2.25

Figure 3 Selection bias: illustrative example. RR, relative risk; OR, odds ratio.

tion) to the 20% exposure rate in both cases and controls. In Fig. 3C, the sampling procedure is biased, because the cases are obtained from STD clinics, whereas the controls are obtained from antenatal clinics. The rate of exposure among the controls remains the expected 20%, whereas the proportion of exposed cases is 40%, since many of the women probably consulted their gynecologists because of symptoms of the STD. The resulting odds ratio of 2.25 is entirely artifactual because of the different selection procedures for cases and controls.

Selection bias can be a particularly important problem in case-control studies, especially if they are hospital-based and if exposed cases are either more or less likely to be hospitalized than exposed controls. One particular type of selection bias is called *Berkson's bias,* in which the association between two conditions is inflated as a result of the fact that patients with both conditions have a greater chance of being referred (and therefore studied) than those with one or the other condition but not both. Such a bias could create an association between an STD and, say, preterm labor, if the occurrence of the STD or of preterm labor can each result in referral to the study hospital.

In *confounding bias*, the true association between the exposure and outcome is either under- or overestimated because of a third factor. This third factor, which is also called a *confounding factor* (or merely a *confounder*), must satisfy the following three criteria: (i) it must be a determinant (cause) of the outcome; (ii) it must be associated with the exposure; (iii) it must not lie on the causal pathway between exposure and outcome. If women with a certain STD, for example, are more likely to use cocaine, an overall association (Fig. 4A) between STD and abruptio placentae might well be confounded by cocaine use. In other words, it may be the cocaine use that leads to the placental abruption. The fact that cocaine users are more likely to develop the STD under suspicion would create a spurious association between the STD and preterm birth. Control for confounding can occur

A. Overall results

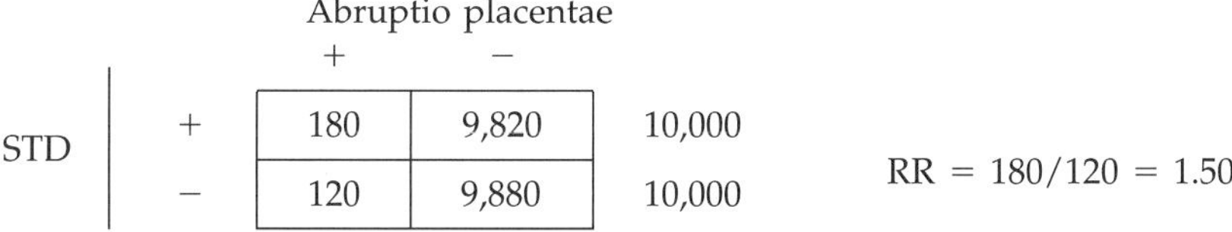

		Abruptio placentae +	Abruptio placentae −		
STD	+	180	9,820	10,000	RR = 180/120 = 1.50
	−	120	9,880	10,000	

B. Cocaine users

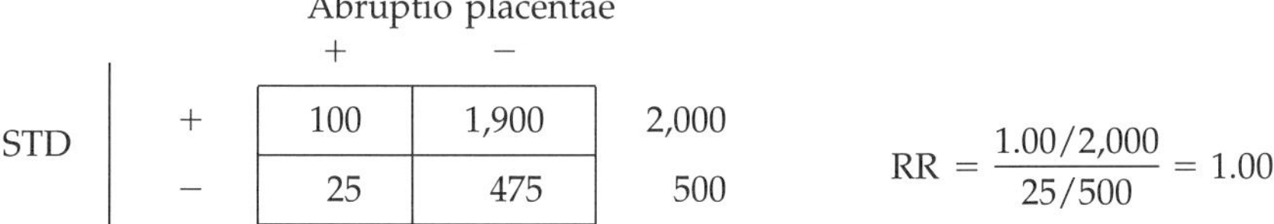

		Abruptio placentae +	Abruptio placentae −		
STD	+	100	1,900	2,000	$RR = \frac{1.00/2{,}000}{25/500} = 1.00$
	−	25	475	500	

C. Cocaine nonusers

		Abruptio placentae +	Abruptio placentae −		
STD	+	80	7,920	8,000	$RR = \frac{80/8{,}000}{95/9{,}500} = 100$
	−	95	9,405	9,500	

Figure 4 Confounding: illustrative example. RR, relative risk.

either at the design phase of the study (by matching or restriction), to ensure that study women with the STD are no more likely to be cocaine users than those without the STD, or in the analysis phase, by means of stratification or multivariate statistical adjustment. In Fig. 4B and 4C, the apparent association between the STD and abruptio placentae is eliminated when the analysis is stratified by cocaine use. Unfortunately, confounders may not be identified at the start or the end of the study.

Finally, in *reverse causality bias*, the "cart" and "horse" are reversed; the effect is taken as the cause. Reverse causality bias is particularly likely to occur in cross-sectional studies. Consider the example of preterm labor or preterm ruptured membranes and the presence of amniotic fluid infection. If amniotic fluid samples are analyzed only after a woman develops preterm labor or preterm ruptured membranes, one cannot be sure whether prior amniotic fluid infection led to the adverse outcome or whether preterm labor or ruptured membranes led to colonization and subsequent infection of the amniotic fluid by organisms previously confined to the lower genital tract.

RANDOMIZED TRIALS

Many of the above-noted sources of systematic error can be reduced or eliminated by use of a *randomized clinical trial* design. Random assignment of exposure (treatment) ensures that potential confounding variables are randomly distributed between the two exposure groups. The potential for selection bias is also reduced, provided that differential losses to follow-up do not occur between the treatment arms. Reverse causality is eliminated by ensuring that exposure occurs prior to the development of the outcome. Finally, differential information bias can be minimized by ensuring adequate blinding of subjects, investigators, and care givers.

The mere use of a randomized clinical trial design, however, does not guarantee that a study is free of analytic bias (Chalmers, 1989). Treatment assignment should be truly random, i.e., not merely haphazard, alternate, alphabetical, according to chart number, or based on other mechanisms susceptible to influence by subjects, investigators, or care givers. Losses to follow-up should be minimized to prevent possible selection bias, and analysis of trials should be based on the intention-to-treat principle. In other words, all subjects randomized to a given treatment should be analyzed according to the assigned treatment. Analyses based on good compliers only, or on those whose STD is prevented or cured, vitiate the scientific benefits of randomization and essentially turn an experimental study into an observational study. Such analyses are fraught with danger for biased inferences.

Blinding of subjects to treatment received, when feasible and ethical, is important to avoid the placebo effect. Blinding of investigators (i.e., those who assess the outcome) is essential to minimize differential information bias, especially for subjective outcomes or outcomes capable of influence by observers, e.g., neonatal gestational age assessment. Finally, it is also often useful to blind care givers to avoid the occurrence of co-interventions, i.e., additional interventions in one of the treatment arms capable of influencing the outcome and thereby confounding the effect of the study treatment.

With adequate attention to these methodologic features, the randomized trial is clearly the design of choice in minimizing systematic error. Nowhere is this truer than for studies of STDs and adverse outcomes of pregnancy. The potential sources of bias are rampant in such studies, and the "proof of the pudding" must be the demonstration in intervention trials where reduction in incidence of the outcome is measured with prevention or cure of the STD under study. Trials should be sufficiently large to minimize random error as well. Thus, large, rigorously designed, randomized clinical trials represent the most promising strategy for advancing knowledge about the effects of STDs and thereby reducing the risk of adverse pregnancy outcomes.

Acknowledgments
M.S.K. is a Distinguished Scientist of the Medical Research Council of Canada.

REFERENCES

Abrams, B., and V. Newman. 1991. Small-for-gestational-age birth: maternal predictors and comparison with risk factors of spontaneous preterm delivery in the same cohort. *Am. J. Obstet. Gynecol.* **161:**785–790.

Barros, F. C., S. R. A. Huttly, C. G. Victora, B. R. Kirkwood, and J. P. Vaughan. 1992. Comparison of the causes and consequences of prematurity and intrauterine growth retardation: a longitudinal study in Southern Brazil. *Pediatrics* **90:**238–244.

Chalmers, I. 1989. Evaluating the effects of care during pregnancy and childbirth, p. 3–38. *In* I. Chalmers, M. Enkin, and M. J. N. C. Keirse (ed.), *Effective Care in Pregnancy and Childbirth.* Oxford University Press, Oxford, United Kingdom.

Chomitz, V. R., E. Lieberman, and L. Cheung. 1992. Healthy mothers—healthy beginnings. Center for Health Communications, Harvard School of Public Health, Cambridge, Mass.

Hogue, C. J. R., J. W. Buehler, L. T. Strauss, and J. C. Smith. 1987. Overview of the National Infant Mortality Surveillance (NIMS) project—design, methods, results. *Public Health Rep.* **102:**126–138.

Keirse, M. J. N. C. 1984. Epidemiology and aetiology of the growth retarded baby. *Clin. Obstet. Gynaecol.* **11:**415–437.

Kessel, S. S., J. Villar, H. W. Berendes, and R. P. Nugent. 1984. The changing pattern of low birth weight in the United States: 1970 to 1980. *JAMA* **25:**1978–1982.

Kramer, M. S. 1987. Determinants of low birth weight: methodological assessment and meta-analysis. *Bull. W.H.O.* **65:**663–737.

Kramer, M. S. 1990. Birth weight and infant mortality: perceptions and pitfalls. *Paediatr. Perinat. Epidemiol.* **4:**381–390.

Kramer, M. S., M. Olivier, F. H. McLean, D. M. Willis, and R. H. Usher. 1990. The impact of intrauterine growth retardation and body proportionality on fetal and neonatal outcome. *Pediatrics* **85:**707–713.

Kramer, M. S., F. H. McLean, E. Eason, and R. H. Usher. 1992. Maternal nutrition and spontaneous preterm birth. *Am. J. Epidemiol.* **136:**574–583.

Stein, Z. A., and M. Susser. 1984. Intrauterine growth retardation: epidemiological issues and public health significance. *Sem. Perinatol.* **8:**5–14.

Wen, S. W., R. L. Goldenberg, G. R. Cutter, J. H. Hoffman, and S. P. Cliver. 1990. Intrauterine growth retardation and preterm delivery: prenatal risk factors in an indigent population. *Am. J. Obstet. Gynecol.* **162:**213–218.

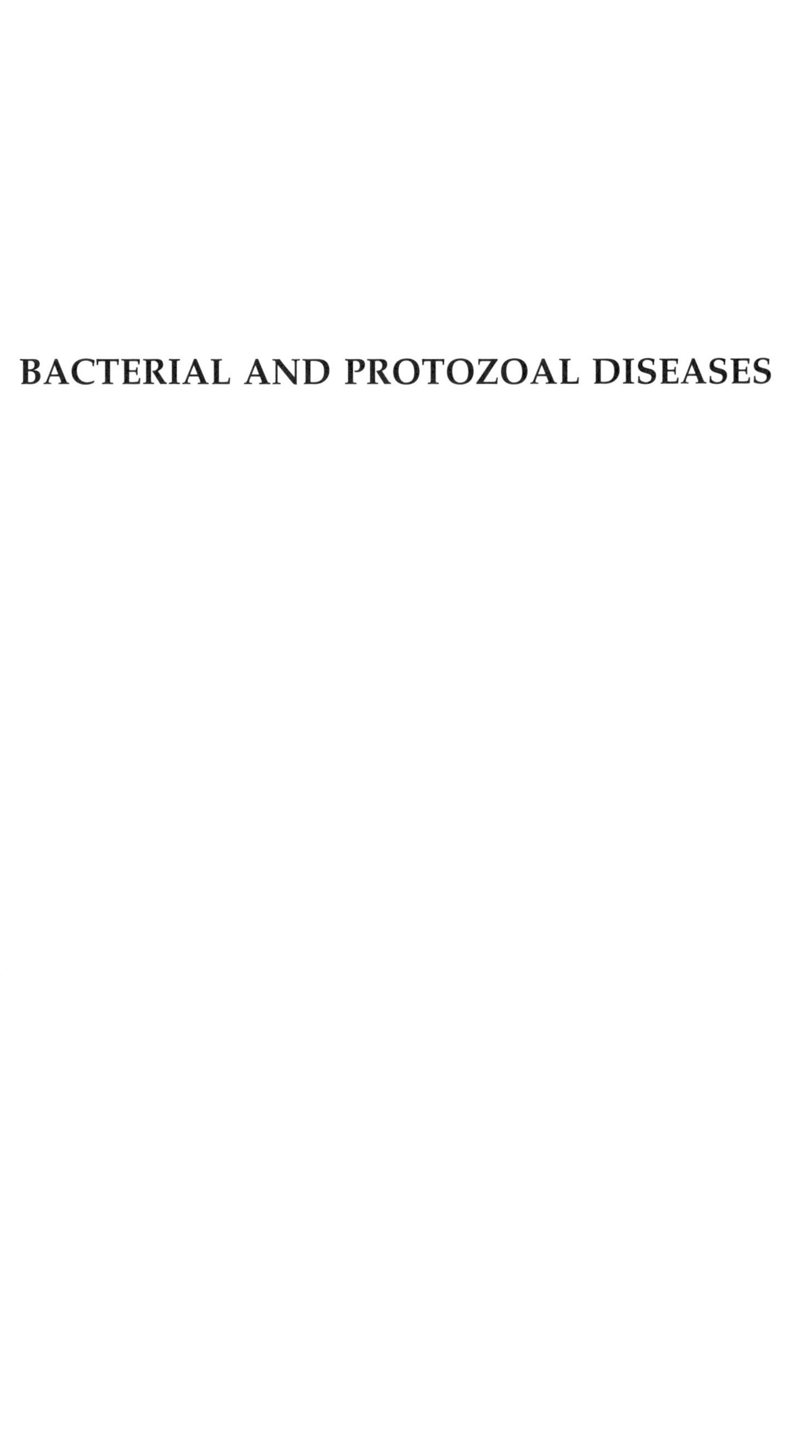

BACTERIAL AND PROTOZOAL DISEASES

7
Bacterial Vaginosis

David A. Eschenbach

Bacterial vaginosis (BV) is the name of a syndrome formerly called nonspecific vaginitis, *Haemophilus vaginalis* vaginitis, and *Gardnerella vaginalis* vaginitis, among others. It represents a disruption of a normal ecosystem and a shift in bacterial population with changes in normal flora, a vaginal pH shift, and susceptibility to sexually transmitted infectious diseases. In the healthy vagina, the normal vaginal flora consists predominantly of *Lactobacillus* species, which make up about 95% or more of the total bacterial count (Hillier et al., 1993a). *Lactobacillus* is usually found at 10^5 to 10^8 bacteria per ml of vaginal secretion (Hillier et al., 1993a; Hill et al., 1984). The majority of women with a *Lactobacillus*-dominant flora have lactobacilli that produce hydrogen peroxide (Eschenbach et al., 1989; Hillier et al., 1992a). Hydrogen peroxide inhibits bacteria which lack an enzyme (catalase), and hydrogen peroxide, together with a host enzyme peroxidase (present in the cervix and endometrium) and a halide ion, takes part in a potent mechanism by which neutrophils kill bacteria (Klebanoff, 1979). *Lactobacillus* also produces lactic acid from glycogen, which in turn produces a low vaginal pH (range, 3.8 to 4.2), although the pH does vary during the menstrual cycle and immediately after intercourse (Wagner and Ottesen, 1992). The acidic vaginal environment further inhibits the growth of pathogenic bacteria and maintains the predominance of lactobacilli. Further, *Lactobacillus* spp. produce other molecules that kill bacterial pathogens (Barefood and Klaenhammer, 1983) and interfere with bacterial adherence to uroepithelial cells (Chan et al., 1985). The net result of a *Lactobacillus*-dominant flora is

David A. Eschenbach, Department of Obstetrics and Gynecology, University of Washington, Seattle, WA 98195.

Sexually Transmitted Diseases and Adverse Outcomes of Pregnancy
Edited by P. J. Hitchcock, H. T. MacKay, J. N. Wasserheit, and R. Binder
©1999 American Society for Microbiology, Washington, D.C.

both the suppression of the vaginal flora (*G. vaginalis, Bacteroides* species, *Peptostreptococcus,* and *Mycoplasma hominis*) that are associated with BV and a reduced risk of gonorrhea and yeast infection (Hillier et al., 1992a, 1992b).

The detectable vaginal flora in women with normal concentrations of *Lactobacillus* consists of about 5 to 15 bacterial species per patient (Hill et al., 1984), usually at or below 10^4 bacteria per ml of vaginal fluid (Hillier et al., 1993a). However, these other bacteria account for only 5% or less of the number of bacteria in vaginas with a *Lactobacillus*-dominant flora. Women in whom *Lactobacillus* spp. are the dominant members of the flora have other bacteria such as diphtheroid species (30 to 70%), *Staphylococcus epidermidis* (40 to 90%), alpha- and beta-hemolytic streptococci (20 to 60%), and bacteria with slightly more pathogenic potential such as *G. vaginalis* (50%) and *Enterococcus* (25 to 35%) (Hillier et al., 1993a; Hill et al., 1984; Holst et al., 1987). Recognized pathogens such as group B streptococci, *Escherichia coli,* and *Bacteroides* probably account for less than 1% of the total number of bacteria in these women.

In contrast to women with a *Lactobacillus*-dominant flora, patients with BV have a reversal in the ratio of *Lactobacillus* to other flora. One-third to one-half of women with BV have no lactobacilli (Eschenbach et al., 1989; Hillier et al., 1992a); the remainder have a reduced concentration of *Lactobacillus* (Hillier et al., 1993a), and only about 5% have hydrogen peroxidase-producing lactobacilli (Eschenbach et al., 1989; Hillier et al., 1992a). Women with BV have an increased prevalence of anaerobic bacteria, *G. vaginalis, Mobiluncus* spp., and *M. hominis* (Hillier et al., 1993a; Holst et al., 1987; Spiegel et al., 1980, 1983b), and the prevalence of these bacteria is statistically related to BV (Martius et al., 1988). The most important aspect of BV in causing vaginitis is the tremendous increase in the concentration of the bacteria in the vagina. The increased concentration of bacteria explains, in part, the relationship between BV and preterm delivery/low birth weight and infection of the amniotic fluid and chorioamnion. Women with BV have a 20- to 100-fold increase in the concentration of *G. vaginalis,* a 20- to 1,000-fold increase in the concentration of anaerobic bacteria, and a 20- to 1,000-fold increase in the concentration of *M. hominis* compared to women with a *Lactobacillus*-dominant flora (Hillier et al., 1993a; Holst et al., 1987; Spiegel et al., 1980). A well-established principle of infectious disease is that increased rates of disease occur when the concentration of virulent bacteria is greatly increased over that of normal flora. This principle is well established for the skin and mucous membranes elsewhere in the body, and it appears to apply to the lower genital tract of women. In pregnant women, this can result in adverse outcomes.

The factors that contribute to the ascent of bacteria from the lower genital tract (cervix and vagina) to the upper genital tract (amniotic fluid, chorioamnion, and decidua) during pregnancy are unknown. Because of its mechanical and antibacterial properties, cervical mucus is a relative barrier to the ascent of bacteria through the cervical canal. The chorioamnion is a membranous barrier located immediately inside the cervix. It adheres tightly to the uterine lining and impedes the movement of bacteria high into the uterus. However, microorganisms can potentially overcome these relative barriers by producing exotoxins such as mucinase, collagenase, protease, and other products that are capable of degrading cervical mucus and membranes. In fact, these products are made by microorganisms associated with BV and are present in measurable quantities in the vaginas of women with BV (McGregor et al., 1990; Briselden et al., 1992).

The time when BV-related bacteria move from the lower to the upper genital tract is not known. This phenomenon could occur at a constant rate throughout pregnancy, but indirect information suggests otherwise. High rates of spontaneous abortion occur in the first trimester, but these may be more closely related to genetic abnormalities than to infection (Simpson, 1996). Low rates of premature delivery occur in the early second trimester until 22 to 26 weeks gestation, after which time the rate of premature delivery increases until term or 37 weeks (Simpson, 1996). If the rate of invasion into the upper genital tract was constant throughout pregnancy, the rate of infection-induced premature delivery over the entire 40 weeks of pregnancy would also be relatively constant. In fact, because the cervix becomes shorter and wider as pregnancy progresses (Iams et al., 1996), one would expect more invasion of the upper genital tract in late pregnancy than in early pregnancy. However, an inverse relationship exists between upper genital tract infection and gestational age from 22 to 34 weeks.

The lower-genital-tract flora changes very little during pregnancy, and there is no evidence of increased virulence over time during pregnancy (Hillier et al., 1993a; Goplerud et al., 1976). Pregnant patients also appear to have a somewhat stable flora with respect to BV. During cytological evaluation of vaginal ecosystems, BV is characterized by the presence of epithelial cells covered with pathogenic bacteria (clue cells). None of 100 patients without clue cells in the first trimester had clue cells in the third trimester; therefore, by inference, patients with a normal flora in the first trimester will usually have a normal flora in the third trimester (Platz-Christensen et al., 1993b). Conversely, about half of the patients with evidence of BV in the first trimester, based upon increased vaginal alkalinity (pH $>$ 4.5) and the presence of clue cells, had these characteristics in the third trimester (Hillier et al., 1993a; Platz-Christensen et al., 1993b).

The frequency of upper genital tract infection decreases with increasing gestational age at delivery. The proportion of preterm deliveries with evidence of infection is high when the preterm delivery occurs from 23 to 30 weeks, intermediate in deliveries from 30 to 34 weeks, and low beyond 34 weeks gestation. The inverse relationship between infection and gestational age at delivery has been reported for amniotic fluid infection (Watts et al., 1992), chorioamnion infection (Hillier et al., 1988), and histologic chorioamnionitis (Hillier et al., 1988; Russell, 1979). Since the morbidity and survival of the neonate are directly affected by gestational age at birth and since a higher rate of infection occurs in the more premature deliveries, infection of the upper genital tract accounts for a greater impact on the morbidity and mortality of the neonate than one would predict if one considered only a constant rate of infection.

The entire issue of the causes of "idiopathic" preterm birth is complicated and is the subject of intensive investigation. In addition, while upper genital tract infection undoubtedly contributes to preterm birth, as one can appreciate from the above discussion, the infectious process itself is complicated. The role of immunity is complicated. The fetus can be considered an allograft of the mother that is maintained by as yet unidentified factors. By contrast, an immunologic response to amniotic fluid infection (Romero et al., 1989a; Hillier et al., 1993b) and to histologic chorioamnionic infection (Hillier et al., 1993b) does occur as judged by the presence of a cytokine response in the amniotic fluid. These cytokines are produced by macrophages that recognize bacteria in the amniotic fluid of infected patients. The cytokine concentration in the amniotic fluid of infected patients is equal to or higher than the concentration of cytokines in the cerebrospinal fluid of children with meningitis (Mustafa et al., 1989) or in the abdominal fluid of adults with peritonitis (Table 1) (Zeni et al., 1993; Hillier et al., 1993b; Romero et al., 1987a, 1989b, 1992, 1993; Greig, 1993; Mustafa et al., 1990). Prostaglandin E_2, presumably produced in response to bacterial infection, has been associated not only with amniotic fluid infection, but also with meningitis. It is not clear whether the cytokine-producing macrophages are derived from decidual, chorioamnion, or other tissue or are of fetal or maternal origin.

The impact of infection and the immune response upon preterm birth may be even more complicated. A consistent phenomenon of preterm delivery is the exceptionally large number of women who have repetitive preterm deliveries. Women with a prior preterm delivery have a five- to sixfold increased rate of preterm delivery and account for about 30% of previously pregnant women who deliver preterm (McGregor et al., 1990). The history of a preterm delivery is one of the most consistent risk factors for this adverse pregnancy outcome (National Center for Health Statistics, 1976; Hay et al., 1994). The explanation for repetitive preterm delivery is unknown. Host immunogenetics is a possible reason; it is known to play a role in pathogenesis in several diseases. For example, in human lymphocyte antigen (HLA)-identical siblings, graft-versus-host disease, which normally occurs in HLA-mismatched patients, occurs in the recipient sibling when the HLA-identical donor sibling has a high frequency of host-specific

Table 1 Cytokine and prostaglandin concentrations in various infections[a]

Cytokine or prostaglandin	Concn. (pg/ml) in:		
	Amniotic fluid (median)	Cerebrospinal fluid[b] (mean ± SD)	Peritoneum[c] (mean ± SD)
Tumor necrosis factor	400–1,016[d,e,f]	787 ± 3,358	400 ± 129
Interleukin-1β	250[d]	944 ± 1,293	
Interleukin-1α	175[d]		71 ± 22
Interleukin-6	2,590–41,000[d,g,h]	170 × 10^6	
Prostaglandin E_2	>86–3140[d,i]	424–500[j]	

[a]There are "normal" values established for amniotic fluid, but the concentration is different for each cytokine. Normal values in cerebrospinal fluid and the peritoneum are probably near zero and have not been established. Since this table compares the absolute concentration of cytokine at the three sites, values should differ for each cytokine and normal levels are not established.
[b]Mustafa et al., 1989.
[c]Zeni et al., 1993.
[d]Hillier et al., 1993b.
[e]Romero et al., 1989b.
[f]Romero et al., 1992.
[g]Romero et al., 1993.
[h]Greig et al., 1993.
[i]Romero et al., 1987a.
[j]Mustafa et al., 1990.

interleukin-2-secreting T-cell precursors (Theobald et al., 1992). This suggests that a population of individuals with high-reacting T cells exists and that transplantation of their cells can cause graft-versus-host disease. Another example of a genetically determined response has been found in relatives of patients with meningococcal infection. Relatives of patients who died of meningococcal sepsis had a significantly increased production of tumor necrosis factor alpha when blood was stimulated with lipopolysaccharide compared to relatives of survivors (Westendorp et al., 1997).

A current working hypothesis for acute or chronic chlamydia infection is that a component(s) of the immune response to chlamydia heat shock protein cross-reacts with the analogous human heat shock protein and somehow results in infertility or first-trimester spontaneous abortion (Witkin and Ledger, 1992) and even preterm delivery. Although the theory is attractive, to date no one has been able to demonstrate a mechanism of pathogenesis.

Of all the emerging diseases associated with sexual behavior, perhaps the strongest links characterized to date are the relationships of BV and trichomoniasis with adverse outcomes of pregnancy. Trichomoniasis is discussed in detail in chapter 12. The remainder of this chapter specifically discusses the relationship between BV and preterm and low-birth-weight delivery. Both clinical and Gram stain criteria can be used to diagnose BV (Amsel et al., 1983; Eschenbach et al., 1988; Spiegel et al., 1983a; Nugent et al., 1991). The correlation between Gram stain and clinical criteria for diagnosis of BV is high (Eschenbach et al., 1988; Nugent et al., 1991). The Gram stain is particularly suited to screen large populations of pregnant women in settings where interpretive error is minimized by well-trained individuals, ensuring quality control. In fact, in the most recent studies of BV in pregnancy, BV has been diagnosed by Gram stain (Hay et al., 1994; Hillier et al., 1995; Kurki et al., 1992; Riduan et al., 1993; Holst et al., 1994).

BV was found in 12 to 22% of about 16,000 pregnant patients (summarized in Table 2) (Martius et al., 1988; Hay et al., 1994; Hillier et al., 1995; Kurki et al., 1992; Riduan et al., 1993; Gravett et al., 1986b). These patients were derived from cohorts of pregnant patients from various countries and from various socioeconomic groups. BV is roughly twice as common as gonorrhea, chlamydia infection, and urinary tract infection combined. The population attributable risk of BV for preterm delivery is 6% because of the high prevalence of BV (Hillier et al., 1995). This number was calculated in the Vaginal Infection in Prematurity Study and is based upon the preterm and low-birth-weight delivery rate of the population without BV, the preterm and low-birth-weight delivery rate among the untreated group with BV, and the proportion of patients with BV. Given the increased susceptibility of very-low-birth-weight babies to many diseases, the impact of BV in terms of infant morbidity and mortality is probably very high.

Table 2 Estimated frequency of BV in pregnancy

Study	Location	Method used to define BV[a]	No. of patients	No. (%) of patients with BV
Gravett et al., 1986b	United States	GLC	534	102 (19)
McGregor et al., 1990	United States	GS	139	26 (16)
Hillier et al., 1995	United States	GS	13,331	2,154 (16)
Kurki et al., 1992	Finland	GS	779	173 (22)
Riduan et al., 1993	Indonesia	GS	490	84 (17)
Hay et al., 1994	England	GS	718	87 (12)

[a] GLC, gas-liquid chromatography; GS, Gram stain.

BV was consistently related to preterm and low-birth-weight delivery in all eight studies listed in Table 3 in which BV was diagnosed prior to delivery (Martius et al., 1988; Hay et al., 1994; Hillier et al., 1995; Kurki et al., 1992; Riduan et al., 1993; Holst et al., 1994; Gravett et al., 1986b). BV has generally been present in 25 to 35% of those who deliver preterm and in 10 to 20% of those who deliver at term. Four of the studies monitored women with and without BV to delivery (Hay et al., 1994; Hillier et al., 1995; Kurki et al., 1992; Riduan et al., 1993), and in three of these studies, logistic regression analyses were used to adjust for potentially confounding demographic or microbial variables (Hay et al., 1994; Hillier et al., 1995; Gravett et al., 1986b). In the reports summarized in Table 3, the relative risk of preterm and low-birth-weight delivery in women with BV is 1.5 to 2.3. This association between BV and preterm and low-birth-weight delivery is very consistent. The only reported study where BV was not related to preterm and low-birth-weight delivery originated from Kenya, where patients who delivered neonates of <2,500 g had vaginal swabs taken for Gram stain after delivery. These findings are difficult to interpret because the accuracy of detecting BV in patients with heavy postpartum bleeding is com-

Table 3 Association between BV and preterm delivery

Study	Definition of preterm delivery	No. of patients with BV/ total no. (%) undergoing:		Relative risk (95% confidence interval)
		Preterm delivery	Term delivery	
Gravett et al., 1986b	<37 wk	24/77 (31)	78/457 (17)	2.2 (1.3–3.8)
Martius et al., 1988	<37 wk	21/61 (34)	21/115 (18)	2.3 (1.1–5.0)
McGregor et al., 1990	<37 wk	1/4 (25)	23/131 (18)	1.5 (0.3–14)
Hillier et al., 1995	<2,500 g	151/661 (23)	1,221/6,777 (18)	1.6 (1.3–2.0)
Kurki et al., 1992	<37 wk	11/17 (65)	151/716 (21)	6.9 (2.5–19)
Riduan et al., 1993	<37 wk	17/65 (26)	67/425 (16)	2.0 (1.0–3.9)
Holst et al., 1994	<37 wk	9/22 (41)	4/38 (11)	2.8 (1.5–5.3)
Hay et al., 1994	Preterm delivery	8/26 (31)	75/673 (11)	3.5 (1.5–8.9)
Elliott et al., 1990	<2,500 g	30/145 (21)	27/131 (21)	1.0 (0.5–1.8)

promised (Elliot et al., 1990). The largest of these studies is noteworthy in that potential confounding variables in the association between BV and premature and low-birth-weight delivery such as demographic factors, smoking, prior preterm delivery, and the recovery of other microbes were adjusted by logistic regression analysis (Hillier et al., 1995). The fact that adjustment for these potential confounding variables had little effect upon the relationship between BV and preterm and low-birth-weight delivery indicates the strength of the association. In the same study, women with BV who were given metronidazole, ampicillin, and amoxicillin had a reduced rate of preterm and low-birth-weight deliveries, suggesting that treatment of BV may reduce preterm delivery (Hillier et al., 1995).

In addition, the presence of the normal flora appears to have a protective effect. *Lactobacillus* in at $\geq 10^7$ CFU/ml in vaginal fluid was associated with a reduced rate of preterm delivery (Table 4). In contrast, anaerobic bacteria associated with BV, particularly *Bacteroides (Prevotella)* species, have been associated with an increased rate of preterm delivery (Table 4).

The data on whether BV is related to rupture of membranes in either the preterm or term patient are mixed. Rupture of membranes occurs in about one-third of preterm deliveries. In two reports, preterm rupture of the membranes was related to BV (Kurki et al., 1992; Gravett et al., 1986b), but in one stratified study, rupture of membranes did not change the odds ratio between BV and preterm delivery (Martius et al., 1988). In the largest study, BV was not related to rupture of membranes in either the preterm or term patient (Hillier et al., 1995).

If BV causes preterm delivery, one would expect an association between BV and upper genital tract infection. In fact, upper genital tract infection has now been highly associated with preterm delivery. BV is associated with a 2.7-fold-increased risk of bacterial amnionitis (infection of amniotic fluid) (Gravett et al., 1986a), with a 3.2-fold-increased risk of chorioamnion infection (Hillier et al., 1988), and with a 2.6-fold-increased risk of histologic chorioamnionitis (Hillier et al., 1988) among patients in preterm labor (Table 4) (Watts et al., 1992; Hillier et al., 1988, 1991; Krohn et al., 1991; Minkoff et al., 1984).

Further, vaginal bacteria associated with BV are the most common bacteria isolated from the upper genital tract of women in preterm labor. The most common isolates are *Fusobacterium*, *Bacteroides*, and *G. vaginalis* (Table 5) (Watts et al., 1992; Gravett et al., 1986a; Wahbeh et al., 1984; Romero et al., 1989c). About half the bacteria isolated from amniotic fluid during preterm labor were associated with BV (Martius et al., 1988) (Table 5). The anaerobes associated with BV, *G. vaginalis* and *M. hominis*, are commonly isolated from the chorioamnion (Hillier et al., 1991). In addition, *Bacteroides (Prevotella)* species, *Porphyromonas*, and *Fusobacterium* in the chorioamnion were associated with preterm delivery (Table 4).

Table 4 Data linking anaerobic infection with prematurity[a]

Study and infection	Organisms linked to prematurity	Probability or odds ratio (95% confidence interval) for prematurity
Vaginal flora		
Krohn et al., 1991	Facultative lactobacilli, $>10^7$/ml	0.6 (0.4–0.9)
Krohn et al., 1991	*Prevotella bivia*, $>10^4$/ml	2.0 (1.4–2.9)
Krohn et al., 1991	Any *Prevotella* species, $>10^{4.4}$/ml	1.6 (1.1–2.2)
Minkoff et al., 1984	*Prevotella* species	1.8 (1.0–3.2)
Amniotic fluid infection		
Watts et al., 1992	Anaerobes (in 55% of patients)	$P < 0.001$ (χ^2 for trend)
Chorioamnion infection		
Hillier et al., 1988	Organisms associated with BV[b]	9.5 (2.6–38.2)
Hillier et al., 1991	*Prevotella* species	$P = 0.05$ (Fisher's exact test)
Hillier et al., 1991	*Porphyromonas* species	4.6 (1.3–17.3)
Hillier et al., 1991	*Fusobacterium* species	$P = 0.03$ (Fisher's exact test)
Histologic chorioamnionitis		
Hillier et al., 1988	Organisms associated with BV[b]	2.6 (1.0–6.0)

[a] Modified from Eschenbach (1993).
[b] *G. vaginalis*, *M. hominis*, and *Mobiluncus*, *Prevotella*, and *Porphyromonas* species.

Table 5 Bacteria isolated from amniotic fluid of women in preterm labor with intact membranes

Microorganism	No. of patients with the microorganism isolated[a] in the study by:			
	Wahbeh et al., 1984 (n = 7)[b]	Gravett et al., 1986a (n = 13)	Romero et al., 1989c (n = 24)	Watts et al., 1992 (n = 20)
BV associated				
Fusobacterium, Bacteroides (± others)	4	3	8	10
G. vaginalis (± *M. hominis*)	0	2	3	0
M. hominis (alone)	ND[c]	1	2	1
Total	4	6	13	11
Non-BV associated				
Group B *Streptococcus, E. coli*	0	0	1	0
Other aerobes, *Candida*	3	1	3	3
Other anaerobes	0	0	6	2
Ureaplasma urealyticum (alone)	ND	6	1	4
Total	3	7	11	9

[a] The numbers listed represent the number of patients with the organism isolated from amniotic fluid. In many patients, more than one microorganism was isolated.
[b] Total number of patients with microorganisms isolated from the amniotic fluid.
[c] ND, not determined.

Infection of the amniotic fluid and chorioamnion has been consistently related to preterm delivery. Bacteria in the amniotic fluid of women in preterm labor with intact membranes is highly associated with preterm birth. Women with amniotic fluid infection tend to deliver within 24 h of the amniocentesis, while women with sterile amniotic fluid tend to deliver about 4 weeks later (Watts et al., 1992; Gravett et al., 1986a; Romero et al., 1989c). Bacteria are also more commonly isolated from the chorioamnion after preterm than term delivery (Hillier et al., 1988, 1991). As mentioned above, the presence of bacterial species associated with BV in the chorioamnion is also related to preterm delivery (Table 4). Presumably, the cytokines and prostaglandins that are produced as a result of bacterial infection act to trigger preterm labor (Romero et al., 1987a).

BV is not associated with an increased number of neutrophils in the vagina (Gardner and Dukes, 1955). Because of the lack of a purulent discharge, this condition was erroneously not considered to represent an infection. However, recent data indicate that an immune response to BV occurs in the lower genital tract. Pregnant women with BV have increased concentrations of endotoxin and interleukin-1α in the cervical mucus and vaginal fluid (Platz-Christensen et al., 1993a). There was correlation between the number of vaginal mononuclear cells and interleukin-1α levels in the vagina (Platz-Christensen et al., 1993a). In addition, BV is positively correlated with prostaglandins E_2 and $F_{2\alpha}$ in the cervixes of pregnant women (Platz-Christensen et al., 1992).

In afebrile women in preterm labor with intact membranes, the presence of bacteria in the amniotic fluid has been highly correlated with cytokines in amniotic fluid. Tumor necrosis factor, interleukin-1α, interleukin-6, interleukin-8, and prostaglandin E_2 levels in amniotic fluid have all correlated with the presence of bacteria in the amniotic fluid (Table 6) (Romero et al., 1987a, 1989a, 1989b, 1990, 1991, 1992, 1993; Hillier et al., 1993b; Cherouny et al., 1993; Pankuch et al., 1989). Elevated concentrations of tumor necrosis factor and interleukin-1α are present in over 85% of those with amniotic fluid infection and in about 20% or fewer of those with sterile amniotic fluid. Interleukin-6, interleukin-8, and prostaglandin E_2 are present in virtually all women with amniotic fluid infection (Table 6). This group with sterile amniotic fluid may have sites of upper genital infection other than the amniotic fluid or another reason for the cytokine response.

Women in preterm labor with bacteria and cytokines in the amniotic fluid deliver rapidly, usually within 24 h and virtually always within 7 days of the amniocentesis (Watts et al., 1992; Hillier et al., 1993b; Romero et al., 1993; Gravett et al., 1986a). In contrast, women in preterm labor with no bacteria or cytokines in the amniotic fluid usually deliver a week or more later (Hillier et al., 1993b) at a mean time of about 1 month after the amniocentesis (Watts et al., 1992; Gravett et al., 1986a). Presumably the bacteria, endotoxin from the bacteria (Romero et al., 1987b), or other bacterial products stimulate macrophages to produce cytokines and prostaglandins. These data suggest an immune response to the presence of bacteria in the amniotic fluid.

Two interesting models probably explain the limited response of infected individuals to treatment. The first is an elegant experimental monkey model of infection in pregnancy (Gravett et al., 1994), where experimental inoculation of the amniotic fluid with group B streptococci produced infection. This was manifested by increasing concentrations of group B streptococci, followed by a cytokine response (a tumor necrosis factor response rapidly followed by an interleukin-1 and interleukin-6 response). Maternal contractions began about a day after the cytokine response. If this scenario occurs in women, presentation of preterm labor occurs after the upper genital tract infection is well established and the cytokine burst has occurred. Cessation of labor would probably not occur, even if antibiotics eliminated the infection.

In another infection, the same cytokine response, including elevated levels of tumor necrosis factor, interleukin-1β, and prostaglandin E_2, has

Table 6 Association between amniotic fluid infection and cytokines in the amniotic fluid

Cytokine and study	Cytokine concn in amniotic fluid	No. with amniotic fluid infection/total no. (%)	No. with sterile amniotic fluid/total no. (%)	*P*
Tumor necrosis factor				
Romero et al., 1989b	>200 pg/ml	8/9 (89)	0/39 (0)	<0.001
Romero et al., 1992	>12 pg/ml	12/13 (92)	3/16 (19)	<0.001
Hillier et al , 1993b	>20 pg/ml	8/9 (89)	9/41 (22)	<0.001
Interleukin-1α				
Romero et al., 1989a	>1 U/ml	13/15 (87)	0/38 (0)	<0.001
Hillier et al , 1993b	>50 pg/ml	7/8 (88)	9/40 (23)	0.002
Interleukin-6				
Romero et al., 1990	>5,000 pg/ml	14/15 (93)	9/38 (24)	<0.001
Hillier et al , 1993b	>1,500 pg/ml	9/9 (100)	21/40 (53)	0.008
Romero et al., 1993	>1,700 pg/ml	11/11 (100)	51/109 (47)	0.002
Greig et al., 1993	>500 pg/ml	10/10 (100)	5/35 (14)	<0.001
Interleukin-8				
Romero et al., 1991	>300 pg/ml	13/13 (100)	23/49 (47)	0.002
Cherouny et al., 1993	>1,000 pg/ml	20/20 (100)	15/36 (42)	<0.001
Pankuch et al., 1989	Leukotaxis assay	8/8 (100)	6/24 (25)	<0.001
Prostaglandin				
Romero et al., 1987a[a]		2,238 ± 434 pg/ml	444 ± 78 pg/ml	<0.001
Hillier et al., 1993b	>10 pg/ml	9/9 (100)	16/41 (39)	0.002

[a] Patients with membrane rupture.

been found in the cerebrospinal fluid of children with meningitis (Mustafa et al., 1989, 1990). Children with meningitis given high corticosteroid doses prior to antibiotics had significantly lower levels of interleukin-1β and lower levels of tumor necrosis factor in the cerebrospinal fluid 18 to 30 h after the administration of antibiotics than did children given placebo and antibiotics (Table 7) (Mustafa et al., 1990). Prostaglandin E_2 levels also tended to be lower in the corticosteroid / antibiotic group than in the placebo / antibiotic group (Table 7) (Mustafa et al., 1990). Long-term neurologic damage occurred more often in children who received antibiotics alone than in those who received the corticosteroid-antibiotic combination (Mustafa et al., 1990).

Thus, one might expect that antibiotics would have to be given very early in the infection process to prevent preterm labor. This poses a difficult problem, because these women are asymptomatic before labor onset. Most of the antibiotics given to women in preterm labor are bacteriocidal. Ironically, bacteriocidal antibiotics may result in rapid deterioration of the bacteria and production of even more cell wall fragments, giving rise to a heightened endotoxin-cytokine response. Arguably, inhibition of preterm labor (Morales et al., 1988) may be enhanced by the use of a bacteriostatic antibiotic (McGregor et al., 1991). Additional measures may be needed to down-regulate the cytokine response if the infection-induced labor process is to be successfully inhibited. Studies have not included high doses of corticosteroids to stop labor but, rather, have concentrated on the doses given to reduce respiratory disease in the preterm infant. The effect of steroids on infection and preterm labor has not been well studied.

BV causes two other diseases in pregnant women. Clinical amnionitis at term occurs 1.5 times more commonly in patients with than without BV (Silver et al., 1989). The relative risk of developing postpartum uterine infection (endometritis) following cesarean section among patients with BV is 5.8 times as common as in those with a *Lactobacillus*-dominant flora (Watts et al., 1990). In this latter report, age and the duration of membrane rupture (adjusted for the duration of labor) were also related to postpartum endometritis (Watts et al., 1990). These data suggest that BV is an important risk factor for postpartum endometritis and that it is independent of other risk factors such as the duration of labor and membrane rupture. A high postpartum endometritis infection rate of 55% following cesarean section was noted in women with BV despite the routine use of antibiotic prophylaxis in the study (Watts et al., 1990). Apparently, the bacteria that contaminate the upper genital tract at the time of cesarean section and the bacteria that cause postpartum endometritis are similar and are not eliminated by antibiotic prophylaxis. The importance of BV in pregnancy is supported by the finding that 60% of the women with postpartum endometritis have the anaerobic bacteria associated with BV; *G. vaginalis* was recovered in com-

Table 7 Cytokine and prostaglandin concentrations in cerebrospinal fluid before and after treatment of meningitis with dexamethasone plus antibiotics or antibiotics alone[a]

Cytokine or prostaglandin	Initial concn in CSF of:		Concn in CSF 18–30 h after therapy		
	Dexamethasone (n = 40)	Placebo (n = 40)	Dexamethasone	Placebo	P
Interleukin-1β (IL-1β)					
Mean (pg/ml)	1,378 ± 422	1,151 ± 237	23 ± 13	192 ± 30	<0.001
% with IL-1β	98	98	35	98	<0.001
Tumor necrosis factor (TNF)					
Mean (pg/ml)	710 ± 282	885 ± 357	21 ± 10	82 ± 32	0.2
% with TNF	58	85	45	60	0.3
Prostaglandin E_2 (PGE_2)					
Mean (pg/ml)	424 ± 77	500 ± 107	5 ± 2	47 ± 16	0.06
% with PGE_2	90	90	13	40	0.01

[a] Data from Mustafa (1990).
[b] CSF, cerebrospinal fluid.

bination or separately from endometrial cultures and from blood cultures (Watts et al., 1989). BV is also associated with a 2.2-fold increased risk of postpartum endometritis among women who deliver vaginally (Newton et al., 1990). Thus, the impact of BV on pregnancy extends from the second and third trimesters to the postpartum period.

Several important issues have emerged based on two studies of women at high risk for preterm delivery. In these randomized double-blinded trials, treatment of BV demonstrated a reduced rate of preterm and low-birth-weight delivery (Morales et al., 1988; Hauth et al., 1995). These data support a causal relationship between BV and preterm and low-birth-weight delivery. Key issues in future treatment trials are (i) what antimicrobial agent to use; (ii) whether to administer therapy by the oral or vaginal route; (iii) when to treat the infection; (iv) whether to use anti-inflammatories; and (v) whether to treat women at low risk as well as women at high risk for preterm delivery. Within the trial, it would be important to know whether the antibiotic eliminated the infection. Other important issues include (i) the secondary impact on pregnancy in women coinfected with *Trichomonas vaginalis*, group B *Streptococcus*, *Chlamydia trachomatis*, and *Neisseria gonorrhoeae*; and (ii) the pregnancy outcome in patients with recurrent BV. The rate of amniotic fluid infection and postpartum endometritis should be studied by identifying and characterizing bacterial species to delineate virulent bacteria as well as drug-resistant bacteria.

More information is needed on the immune response of pregnant women, both with and without BV as well as other infections. For example, it is now becoming apparent that amniotic fluid infection is primarily a fetal infection (Eschenbach, 1997). An immunologic fetal response correlates with increased rates of respiratory distress (Grether and Nelson, 1997) and may be associated with cerebral palsy (Hitti et al., 1997). It is apparent that infection and the immune response may be key components in adverse outcomes of pregnancy.

Additional studies are needed to determine if the natural history of BV includes subclinical upper genital tract infection in nonpregnant women and, if so, whether this type of infection persists when these women become pregnant. If these bacteria ascend into the upper genital tract during pregnancy, we must know when in the pregnancy this occurs and whether it influences first-trimester abortion as well as second- and early-third-trimester preterm delivery.

There remain other major gaps in our knowledge about BV in particular. Does BV act as a cofactor for other infections, and, conversely, how effective is the normal flora, including *Lactobacillus* spp., in preventing infection? Does BV in conjunction with other bacterial species increase the relative risk of preterm delivery compared to BV alone? What is the role of new sexual partners, antibiotics, and douching in the acquisition and recurrence of BV in the nonpregnant patient? What property of the microorganisms or which of their metabolic products is important in upper genital tract infection, especially amniotic fluid and chorioamnion infection? We also need a complete understanding of interactions between the various microorganisms associated with BV, including *M. hominis*. What is the relationship between single and multiple infections to immunity, infertility, spontaneous abortions, and preterm delivery? How does one prevent BV in pregnancy? Are infected preterm-born infants at increased risk of respiratory distress, systemic infection, other complications of prematurity, and long-term chronic lung disease compared to uninfected preterm infants?

Recommendations for future research include the conduct of a randomized double-blinded treatment trial sufficiently large and detailed to answer the many clinical questions about BV and preterm and low-birth-weight delivery. Funding of basic research of the microbiology of BV and the immune response in both infected and uninfected pregnant patients is also critical. The natural history of BV in the nonpregnant patient must be elucidated. Natural history studies of women with and without BV who will attempt pregnancy are needed.

REFERENCES

Amsel, R., P. A. Totten, C. A. Spiegel, K. C. S. Chen, D. A. Eschenbach, and K. K. Holmes. 1983. Nonspecific vaginitis: diagnostic criteria and microbial and epidemiologic associates. *Am. J. Med.* **74:**14–22.

Barefood, S. F., and T. R. Klaenhammer. 1983. Detection and activity of lactacin B, a bacteriocin produced by *Lactobacillus acidophilus*. *Appl. Environ. Microbiol.* **45:** 1808–1815.

Briselden, A. M., B. J. Moncla, C. E. Stevens, and S. L. Hillier. 1992. Sialidases (neuraminidases) in bacterial vaginosis and bacterial vaginosis-associated microflora. *J. Clin. Microbiol.* **30:**663–666.

Chan, R. C. Y., G. Reid, R. T. Irvin, A. W. Bruce, and J. W. Costerton. 1985. Competitive elusion of uropathogens from human uroepithelial cells by *Lactobacillus* whole cells and cell wall fragments. *Infect. Immun.* 47:84–89.

Cherouny, P. H., G. A. Pankuch, R. Romero, J. J. Botti, D. C. Kuhn, L. M. Demers, and P. C. Appelbaum. 1993. Neutrophil attractant/activating peptide-1 interleukin-8: association with histologic chorioamnionitis, preterm delivery, and bioactive amniotic fluid leukoattractants. *Am. J. Obstet. Gynecol.* **169:**1299–1303.

Elliott, B., R. C. Brunham, M. Laga, P. Piot, J. O. Ndinya-Achola, G. Maitha, M. Cheang, and F. A. Plummer. 1990. Maternal gonococcal infection as a preventable risk factor for low birth weight. *J. Infect. Dis.* **161:**531–536.

Eschenbach, D. A. 1993. Bacterial vaginosis and anaerobes in obstetric-gynecologic infection. *Clin. Infect. Dis.* **16**(Suppl. 4):S282–S287.

Eschenbach, D. A. 1997. Amniotic fluid infection and cerebral palsy: focus on the fetus. *JAMA* **278:**247–248. (Editorial.)

Eschenbach, D. A., S. L. Hillier, C. W. Critchlow, C. E. Stevens, L. A. Koutsky, T. DeRouen, and K. K. Holmes. 1988. Diagnosis and clinical features associated with bacterial vaginosis. *Am. J. Obstet. Gynecol.* **158:**819–828.

Eschenbach, D. A., P. R. Davick, B. L. Williams, S. J. Klebanoff, K. Young-Smith, C. W. Critchlow, and K. K. Holmes. 1989. Prevalence of hydrogen peroxide producing *Lactobacillus* species in normal women and women with bacterial vaginosis. *J. Clin. Microbiol.* **27:**251–256.

Gardner, H. L., and C. D. Dukes. 1955. *Haemophilus vaginalis* vaginitis: a newly defined specific infection previously classified "nonspecific vaginitis." *Am. J. Obstet. Gynecol.* **69:**962.

Goplerud, C. P., M. J. Ohm, and R. P. Galask. 1976. Aerobic and anaerobic flora of the cervix during pregnancy and the puerperium. *Am. J. Obstet. Gynecol.* **126:**858–865.

Gravett, M. G., D. Hummel, D. A. Eschenbach, and K. K. Holmes. 1986a. Preterm labor associated with subclinical amniotic fluid infection and with bacterial vaginosis. *Obstet. Gynecol.* **67:**229–237.

Gravett, M. G., H. P. Nelson, T. DeRouen, C. W. Critchlow, D. A. Eschenbach, and K. K. Holmes. 1986b. Independent association of bacterial vaginosis and *Chlamydia trachomatis* infection with adverse pregnancy outcome. *JAMA* **256:**1899–1903.

Gravett, M. G., S. S. Witkin, G. J. Haluska, J. L. Edwards, M. J. Cook, and M. J. Novey. 1994. An experimental model for intraamniotic infection and preterm labor in rhesus monkeys. *Am. J. Obstet. Gynecol.* **171:**1660–1667.

Greig, P. C., J. M. Ernest, L. Teot, M. Erikson, and R. Talley. 1993. Amniotic fluid interleukin-6 levels correlate with histologic chorioamnionitis and amniotic fluid cultures in patients in premature labor with intact membranes. *Am. J. Obstet. Gynecol.* **169:**1035–1044.

Grether, J. K., and K. B. Nelson. 1997. Maternal infection and cerebral palsy in infants of normal birth weight. *JAMA* **278:**207–211.

Hauth, J. C., R. L., Goldenberg, W. W. Andrews, M. B. Dubard, and R. L. Copper. 1995. Reduced incidence of preterm delivery with metronidazole and erythromycin in women with bacterial vaginosis. *N. Engl. J. Med.* **333:**1732–1736.

Hay, P. E., R. F. Lamont, D. Taylor-Robinson, D. J. Morgan, C. Ison, and J. Peason. 1994. Abnormal bacterial colonisation of the genital tract and subsequent preterm delivery and late miscarriage. *Br. Med. J.* **308:**295–298.

Hill, G. B., D. A. Eschenbach, and K. K. Holmes. 1984. Bacteriology of the vagina. *Scand. J. Urol. Nephrol. Suppl.* **86:**23–39.

Hillier, S. L., J. Martius, M. A. Krohn, N. B. Kiviat, K. K. Holmes, and D. A. Eschenbach. 1988. A case-control study of chorioamniotic infection and chorioamnionitis in prematurity. *N. Engl. J. Med.* **319:**972–978.

Hillier, S. L., M. A. Krohn, N. B. Kiviat, D. H. Watts, and D. A. Eschenbach. 1991. Microbiologic causes and neonatal outcomes associated with chorioamnion infection. *Am. J. Obstet. Gynecol.* **165:**955–961.

Hillier, S. L., M. A. Krohn, S. J. Klebanoff, and D. A. Eschenbach. 1992a. The relationship of hydrogen peroxide producing lactobacilli to bacterial vaginosis and genital microflora in pregnant women. *Obstet. Gynecol.* **79:**369–373.

Hillier, S. L., M. A. Krohn, R. P. Nugent, and R. S. Gibbs. 1992b. Characteristics of three vaginal flora patterns assessed by gram stain among pregnant women. Vaginal Infections and Prematurity Study Group. *Am. J. Obstet. Gynecol.* **166:**938–944.

Hillier, S. L., M. A. Krohn, L. K. Rabe, S. J. Klebanoff, and D. A. Eschenbach. 1993a. Normal vaginal flora, H_2O_2-producing lactobacilli and bacterial vaginosis in pregnant women. *Clin. Infect. Dis.* **16**(Suppl. 4)**:**S273–S281.

Hillier, S. L., S. S. Witkin, M. A. Krohn, D. H. Watts, N. B. Kiviat, and D. A. Eschenbach. 1993b. The relationship of amniotic fluid cytokines and preterm delivery, amniotic fluid infection, histologic chorioamnionitis and chorioamnion infection. *Obstet. Gynecol.* **8:**941–948.

Hillier, S. L., R. P. Nugent, D. A. Eschenbach, M. A. Krohn, R. S. Gibbs, D. H. Martin, M. F. Cotch, R. Edelman, J. Pastorek, A. V. Rao, D. McNellis, J. A. Regan, J. C. Carey, and M. A. Klebanoff. 1995. The association of bacterial vaginosis, bacteroides and *Mycoplasma hominis* with preterm low birth weight delivery. *N. Engl. J. Med* **333:**1737–1742.

Hitti, J., M. J. Krohn, D. L. Patton, P. Tarczy-Hornoch, S. L. Hillier, E. M. Cassen, and D. A. Eschenbach. 1997. Amniotic fluid tumor necrosis factor-α and the risk of respiratory distress syndrome among preterm infants. *Am. J. Obstet. Gynecol.* **177:**50–56.

Holst, E., B. Wathne, B. Hovelius, and P.-A. Mårdh. 1987. Bacterial vaginosis: microbiological and clinical findings. *Eur. J. Clin. Microbiol.* **6:**536–541.

Holst, E., A. R. Goffeng, and B. Andersch. 1994. Bacterial vaginosis and vaginal microorganisms in idiopathic premature labor and association with pregnancy outcome. *J. Clin. Microbiol.* **32:**176–186.

Iams, J. D., R. L. Goldenberg, P. J. Meis, B. M. Mercer, A. Moawad, A. Das, E. Thom, D. McNellis, R. L. Copper, F. Johnson, and J. M. Roberts. 1996. The length of the cervix and the risk of spontaneous premature delivery. *N. Engl. J. Med.* **334:** 567–572.

Klebanoff, S. J., and D. C. Smith. 1970. Peroxidase-medicated antimicrobial activity of rat uterine fluid. *Gynecol. Invest.* **1:**21–30.

Krohn, M. A., S. L. Hillier, M. L. Lee, L. K. Rabe, and D. A. Eschenbach. 1991. Vaginal *Bacteroides* species are associated with an increased rate of preterm delivery among women in preterm labor. *J. Infect. Dis.* **164:**88–93.

Kurki, T., A. Sivonen, O. Renkonen, E. Savia, and O. Ylikorkala. 1992. Bacterial vaginosis in early pregnancy and pregnancy outcome. *Obstet. Gynecol.* **80:**173.

Martius, J., M. A. Krohn, S. L. Hillier, W. E. Stamm, K. K. Holmes, and D. A. Eschenbach. 1988. Relationship of vaginal *Lactobacillus* species, cervical *Chlamydia trachomatis*, and bacterial vaginosis to preterm birth. *Obstet. Gynecol.* **71:**89–95.

McGregor, J. A., J. I. French, R. Richter, A. Franco-Buff, A. Johnson, S. L. Hillier, F. N. Judson, and J. K. Todd. 1990. Antenatal microbiologic and maternal risk factors associated with prematurity. *Am. J. Obstet. Gynecol.* **163:**1465–1473.

McGregor, J. A., J. I. French, and K. Seo. 1991. Adjunctive clindamycin therapy for preterm labor. Results of a double-blind, placebo-controlled trial. *Am. J. Obstet. Gynecol.* **165:**867–875.

Minkoff, H., A. N. Grunebaum, R. H. Schwarz, J. Feldman, M. Cummings, W. Crombleholme, L. Clark, G. Pringle, and W. M. McCormack. 1984. Risk factors for prematurity and premature rupture of membranes: a prospective study of the vaginal flora in pregnancy. *Am. J. Obstet. Gynecol.* **150:**965.

Morales, W. J., J. L. Angel, W. F. O'Brien, R. A. Knuppel, and M. Finazzo. 1988. A randomized study of antibiotic therapy in idiopathic preterm labor. *Obstet. Gynecol.* **72:**829–833.

Mustafa, M. M., M. H. Lebel, O. Ramilo, K. D. Olsen, J. S. Reisch, B. Beutler, and G. H. McCracken, Jr. 1989. Correlation of interleukin-1b and cachectin concentrations in cerebrospinal fluid and outcome from bacterial meningitis. *J. Pediatr.* **115:** 208–213.

Mustafa, M. M., O. Ramilo, X. Sáez-Llorens, K. D. Olsen, R. R. Magness, and G. H. McCracken, Jr. 1990. Cerebrospinal fluid prostaglandins, interleukin 1b, and tumor necrosis factor in bacterial meningitis. *Am. J. Dis. Child.* **144:**883–887.

National Center for Health Statistics. 1976. Factors associated with low birthweight: United States. U.S. Dept. of Health, Education and Welfare Publication no. 80-1915. U.S. Government Printing Office, Washington, D.C.

Newton, E. R., T. J. Prihoda, and R. S. Gibbs. 1990. A clinical and microbiologic analysis and risk factors for puerperal endometritis. *Obstet. Gynecol.* **75:**402–406.

Nugent, R. P., M. A. Krohn, and S. L. Hillier. 1991. Reliability of diagnosing bacterial vaginosis is improved by a standardized method of Gram stain interpretation. *J. Clin. Microbiol.* **29:**297–301.

Pankuch, G. A., P. H. Cherouny, J. J. Botti, and P. C. Appelbaum. 1989. Amniotic fluid leukotaxis assay as an early indicator of chorioamnionitis. *Am. J. Obstet. Gynecol.* **161:**802–807.

Platz-Christensen, J., A. Brandberg, and N. Wiqvist. 1992. Increased prostaglandin concentrations in the cervical mucus of pregnant women with bacterial vaginosis. *Prostaglandins* **43:**133.

Platz-Christensen, J., I. Mattsby-Baltzer, P. Thomsen, and N. Wiqvist. 1993a. Endotoxin and interleukin-1a in the cervical mucus and vaginal fluid of pregnant women with bacterial vaginosis. *Am. J. Obstet. Gynecol.* **169:**1161–1166.

Platz-Christensen, J., P. Pernevi, B. Hagmar, E. Andersson, A. Brandberg, and N. Wiqvist. 1993b. A longitudinal follow-up of bacterial vaginosis during pregnancy. *Acta Obstet. Gynecol. Scand.* **72:**99–102.

Riduan, J. M., S. L. Hillier, B. Utomo, G. Wiknjosastro, M. Linnan, and N. Kandung. 1993. Bacterial vaginosis and prematurity in Indonesia: association in early and late pregnancy. *Am. J. Obstet. Gynecol.* **169:**175–178.

Romero, R., M. Emamian, M. Wan, R. Quintero, J. C. Hobbins, and M. D. Mitchell. 1987a. Prostaglandin concentrations in amniotic fluid of women with intra-amniotic infection and preterm labor. *Am. J. Obstet. Gynecol.* **157:**1461–1467.

Romero, R., N. Kadar, J. C. Hobbins, and G. W. Duff. 1987b. Infection and labor: the detection of endotoxin in amniotic fluid. *Am. J. Obstet. Gynecol.* **157:**815–819.

Romero, R., D. T. Brody, E. Oyarzun, M. Mazor, Y. K. Wu, J. C. Hobbins, and S. K. Durum. 1989a. Infection and labor. III. Interleukin-1: a signal for the onset of parturition. *Am. J. Obstet. Gynecol.* **160:**1117–1123.

Romero, R., K. R. Manogue, M. D. Mitchell, Y. K. Wu, E. Oyarzun, J. C. Hobbins, and A. Cerami. 1989b. Infection and labor. IV. Cachectin-tumor necrosis factor in the amniotic fluid of women with intra-amniotic infection and preterm labor. *Am. J. Obstet. Gynecol.* **161:**336–341.

Romero, R., M. Sirtori, E. Oyarzun, C. Avila, M. Mazor, R. Callahan, V. Sabo, A. P. Athanassiadis, and J. C. Hobbins. 1989c. Infection and labor. V. Prevalence, microbiology, and clinical significance of intra-amniotic infection in women with preterm labor and intact membranes. *Am. J. Obstet. Gynecol.* **161:**817–824.

Romero, R., C. Avila, U. Santhanam, and P. B. Sehgal. 1990. Amniotic fluid interleukin 6 in preterm labor. *J. Clin. Invest.* **85:**1392–1400.

Romero, R., M. Ceska, C. Avila, M. Mazor, E. Behnke, and I. Lindley. 1991. Neutrophil attractant/activating peptide-1/interleukin-8 in term and preterm parturition. *Am. J. Obstet. Gynecol.* **165:**813–820.

Romero, R., M. Mazor, W. Sepulveda, C. Avila, D. Copeland, and J. Williams. 1992. Tumor necrosis factor in preterm and term labor. *Am. J. Obstet. Gynecol.* **166:** 1576–1587.

Romero, R., B. H. Yoo, M. Mazor, R. Gomez, M. P. Diamond, J. S. Kenney, M. Ramirez, P. L. Fidel, Y. Sorokin, D. Cotton, and P. B. Sehgal. 1993. The diagnostic and prognostic value of amniotic fluid white blood cell count, glucose, interleukin-6, and Gram stain in patients with preterm labor and intact membranes. *Am. J. Obstet. Gynecol.* **169:**805–816.

Russell, P. 1979. Inflammatory lesions of the human placenta. I. Clinical significance of acute chorioamnionitis. *Am. J. Diagn. Gynecol. Obstet.* **1:**127–137.

Silver, H. M., R. S. Sperling, P. J. St. Clair, and R. S. Gibbs. 1989. Evidence relating bacterial vaginosis to intra-amniotic infection. *Am. J. Obstet. Gynecol.* **161:**808–812.

Simpson, J. L. 1996. Fetal wastage, p. 717–742. *In* S. Gabbe, J. R. Niebyl, and J. L. Simpson (ed.), *Obstetrics: Normal and Problem Pregnancies.* Livingstone, New York, N.Y.

Spiegel, C. A., R. Amsel, D. A. Eschenbach, F. Schoenknecht, and K. K. Holmes. 1980. Anaerobic bacteria in nonspecific vaginitis. *N. Engl. J. Med.* **303:**601–607.

Spiegel, C. A., R. Amsel, and K. K. Holmes. 1983a. Diagnosis of bacterial vaginosis by direct Gram stain of vaginal fluid. *J. Clin. Microbiol.* **18:**170–177.

Spiegel, C. A., D. A. Eschenbach, R. Amsel, and K. K. Holmes. 1983b. Curved anaerobic bacteria in nonspecific vaginosis and their response to antibiotic therapy. *J. Infect. Dis.* **148:**817–822.

Theobald, M., T. Nierle, D. Bunjes, R. Arnold, and H. Heimpel. 1992. Host-specific interleukin-2-secreting donor t-cell precursors as predictors of acute graft-versus-host disease in bone marrow transplantation between HLA-identical siblings. *N. Engl. J. Med.* **327:**1613–1617.

Wagner, G., and B. Ottesen. 1992. Vaginal physiology during menstruation. *Ann. Intern. Med.* **96:**921–923.

Wahbeh, C. J., G. B. Hill, R. D. Eden, and S. A. Gall. 1984. Intra-amniotic bacterial colonization in premature labor. *Am. J. Obstet. Gynecol.* **148:**739–743.

Watts, D. H., D. A. Eschenbach, and G. E. Kenny. 1989. Early postpartum endometritis: the role of bacteria, genital mycoplasmas and *Chlamydia trachomatis. Obstet Gynecol.* **73:**52–60.

Watts, D. H., M. A. Krohn, S. L. Hillier, and D. A. Eschenbach. 1990. Bacterial vaginosis as a risk factor for postcesarean endometritis. *Obstet. Gynecol.* **75:**52–58.

Watts, D. H., M. A. Krohn, S. L. Hillier, and D. A. Eschenbach. 1992. The association of occult amniotic fluid infection with gestational age and neonatal outcome among women in preterm labor. *Obst. Gynecol.* **79:**351–357.

Westendorp, R. G. J., J. A. M. Langermans, T. W. J. Huizinga, A. H. Elouali, C. L. Verweij, D. I. Boomsma, and J. P. Vandenbrouke. 1997. Genetic influence on cytokine production and fatal meningococcal disease. *Lancet* **349:**170–173.

Witkin, S. S., and W. J. Ledger. 1992. Antibodies to *Chlamydia trachomatis* in sera of women with recurrent spontaneous abortions. *Am. J. Obstet. Gynecol.* **167:**135–139.

Zeni, F., B. Tardy, M. Vindimian, C. Comtet, Y. Page, I. Cusey, and J. C. Bertrand. 1993. High levels of tumor necrosis factor-a and interleukin-6 in the ascitic fluid of cirrhotic patients with spontaneous bacterial peritonitis. *Clin. Infect. Dis.* **17:** 218–223.

8
Syphilis and Pregnancy

Pablo J. Sánchez

Syphilis is a systemic infection caused by the spirochete *Treponema pallidum*. Despite years of clinical experience with this disease, syphilis remains a global problem of major medical and public health consequences. The disease can profoundly affect pregnancy outcome (Ingraham, 1951; Fiumara et al., 1952) and act as a cofactor for the sexual transmission of the human immunodeficiency virus (HIV) (Wasserheit, 1992; Dickerson et al., 1996). Untreated syphilis during pregnancy is associated with spontaneous abortion, stillbirth, nonimmune hydrops, premature delivery, and perinatal death (Wendel, 1988). Moreover, congenital infection with *T. pallidum* can result in two syndromes in infants and children, early and late congenital syphilis, both of which can adversely affect neurodevelopment (Ingall et al., 1994).

EPIDEMIOLOGY

Syphilis in the United States is currently found among racial and ethnic minorities who live in poverty. People who live in the inner cities on the east coast and in the rural south bear a disproportionate burden. In fact, the majority of the total reported cases of primary and secondary syphilis occur in southeastern states, which contain only 19% of the total U.S. population (Fig. 1) (Nakashima et al., 1996; CDC, 1996b). Large numbers of cases occur in inner cities of New York City (CDC, 1989), Los Angeles (Cohen et al., 1990), Miami (Ricci et al., 1989), Houston (Risser and Hwang, 1996), Dallas (Sánchez et al., 1991a, 1992), Detroit (Berry and Dajani, 1992;

Pablo J. Sánchez, Divisions of Neonatal-Perinatal Medicine and Pediatric Infectious Diseases, University of Texas Southwestern Medical Center at Dallas, 5323 Harry Hines Blvd., Dallas, TX 75235-9063.

Sexually Transmitted Diseases and Adverse Outcomes of Pregnancy
Edited by P. J. Hitchcock, H. T. MacKay, J. N. Wasserheit, and R. Binder
©1999 American Society for Microbiology, Washington, D.C.

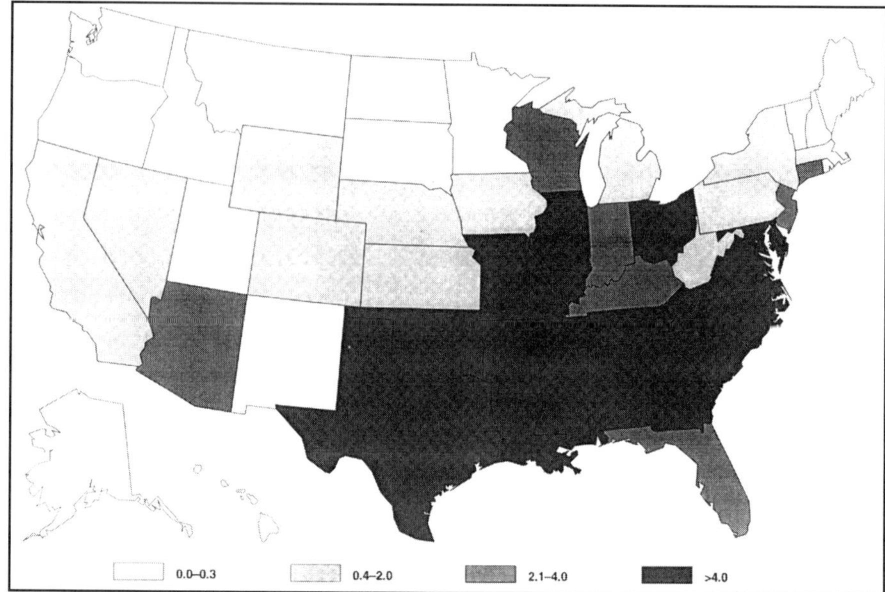

Figure 1 Reported cases of primary and secondary syphilis per 100,000 population in the United States, 1996 (CDC, 1996).

Reyes et al., 1993), and Baltimore (CDC, 1996a). In 1995, the rate of primary and secondary syphilis for non-Hispanic blacks (i.e., 30.2 cases per 100,000 population) was 50-fold greater than that for non-Hispanic whites (Fig. 2).

A major contributor to the increased incidence of syphilis in the late 1980s and early 1990s was the use of crack cocaine and the exchange of illegal drugs for sex (Rolfs et al., 1990; Sison et al., 1997; Ikeda and Jenson, 1990; CDC, 1991). Among these populations, medical care is poor and the identities of sexual partners are often unknown; this makes sexual partner notification, a traditional syphilis control strategy, virtually impossible (Andrus et al., 1990; Cates et al., 1996). This problem has been compounded by the reduction in resources for syphilis control programs that are coordinated in sexually transmitted disease clinics of local public health departments. Recent attention also has focused on the induced migration that results when public housing projects are dismantled and infected individuals move to less impoverished areas that surround the inner city; this results in infection of new sexual partners, who often lack a history of drug use. Finally, the use of spectinomycin for treatment of penicillinase-producing *Neisseria gonorrhoeae* has also been implicated in the resurgence, since spectinomycin is not effective against incubating syphilis (Petzoldt, 1975).

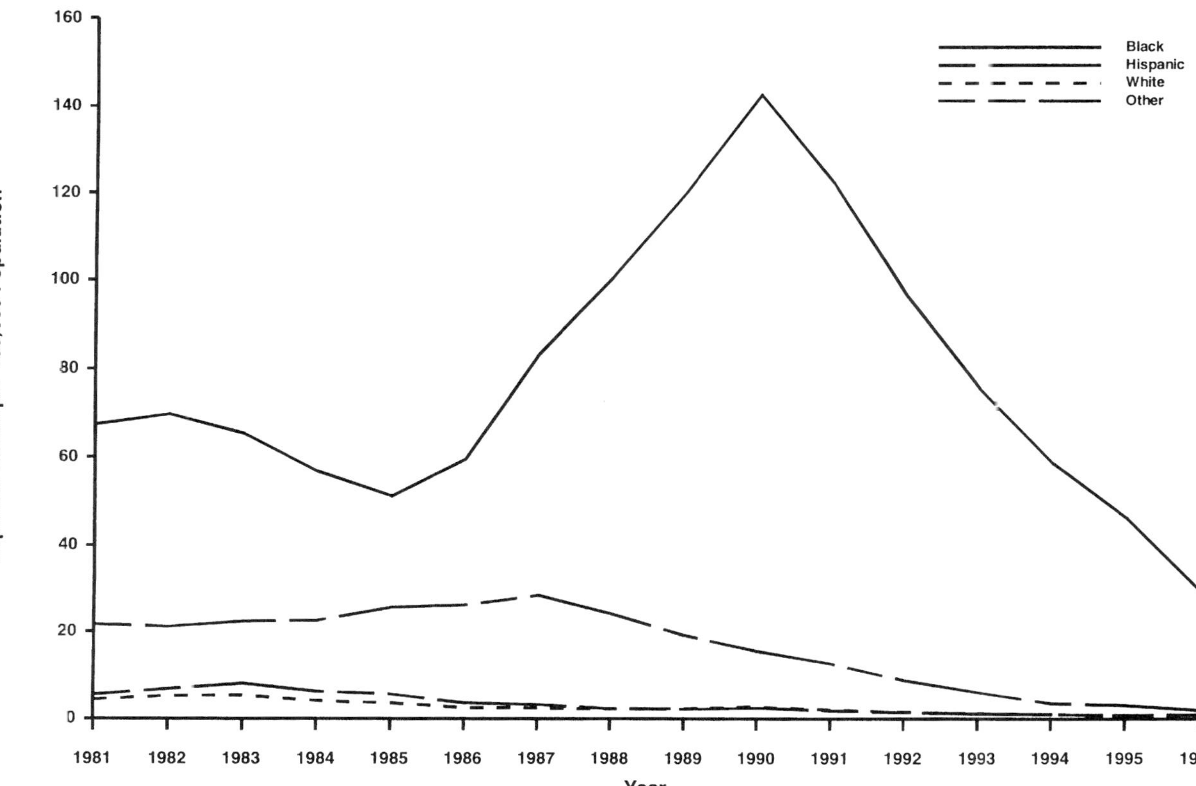

Figure 2 Reported cases of primary and secondary syphilis per 100,000 population by race and ethnicity in the United States, 1981 to 1996 (CDC, 1996).

In the past several years, the incidence of primary and secondary syphilis has decreased (Fig. 2). There are currently heightened expectations for the possibility of the eventual control and even elimination of syphilis in the United States. However, the rate of primary and secondary syphilis in 1996 was still 4.3 per 100,000 population, higher than the national *Healthy People 2000* objective of ≤4.0 per 100,000 population (CDC, 1996b). The reasons for this recent downward trend remain unclear (Nakashima et al., 1996). Certainly, the awareness of the syphilis epidemic has led to wider screening practices and identification of infected persons. More recently, it also has been attributed to a combination of innovative, community-based programs which identify particular locations with a high prevalence of syphilis and with core populations at high risk for infection (CDC, 1991, 1993). The recognition of these demographics has allowed presumptive treatment of syphilis based on epidemiologic indications. At the same time, it has facilitated identification, testing, and follow-up of infected individuals and their sexual partners by public health workers. Other reasons for the recent decline include a decrease in cocaine use, AIDS prevention programs which target prevention of other STDs, and immunity that developed among high-risk populations when syphilis was more prevalent.

Gestational syphilis primarily affects women who are young and unmarried and who receive inadequate or no prenatal care (CDC, 1989; Ricci et al., 1989; Rawstron et al., 1993; Mascola et al., 1985; Webber et al., 1993). The dramatic increase in the number of cases of congenital syphilis that occurred in the late 1980s and early 1990s is due to both an increase in actual cases and the adoption of revised reporting guidelines by the CDC in 1989. These guidelines broadened the surveillance case definition for congenital syphilis (Fig. 3; Table 1) (CDC, 1989; Cohen et al., 1990; Sánchez, 1992; Ikeda and Jenson, 1990; Zenker and Berman, 1991). Reported cases now include not only all infants with clinical evidence of congenital syphilis (Kaufman et al., 1977) but also asymptomatic infants and stillbirths born to women with untreated or inadequately treated syphilis (Table 1). Use of these guidelines increases the sensitivity for reporting cases of congenital syphilis by almost fourfold (Ricci et al., 1989; Sánchez, 1992), although clearly some uninfected cases will be reported.

VERTICAL TRANSMISSION AND PATHOGENESIS

A pregnant woman with syphilis can transmit the infection to her unborn infant in utero, presumably by a transplacental route or possibly during delivery by contact with a genital lesion. In utero infection has been documented by the isolation of the organism from umbilical cord blood (Wendel et al., 1991; Grimprel et al., 1991; Sánchez et al., 1993) and amniotic fluid (Wendel et al., 1991; Grimprel et al., 1991; Lucas et al., 1991, 1989; Nathan et al., 1993) as well as by the detection of specific immunoglobulin M (IgM)

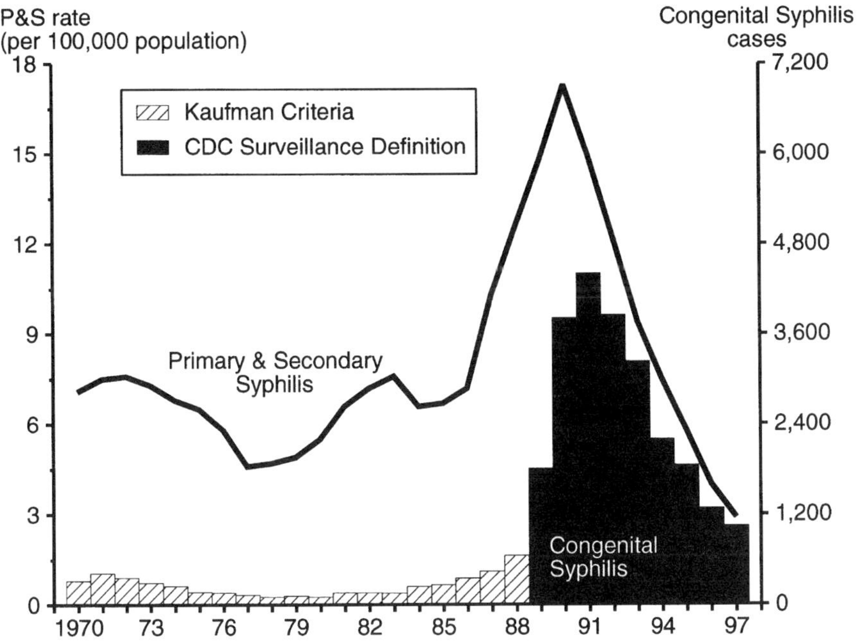

Figure 3 Congenital syphilis cases in infants younger than 1 year of age, 1970 to 1997 (CDC, 1998). P & S, primary and secondary syphilis among women. Note: the surveillance case definition for congenital syphilis changed in 1988.

antibody to *T. pallidum* in neonatal serum obtained at birth (Sánchez et al., 1989; Dobson et al., 1988). A transplacental route of infection is further supported by the detection of spirochetes in the placenta and umbilical cord in association with typical histopathologic changes (Benirschke, 1974; Russel and Altshuler, 1974; Fojaco et al., 1989; Qureshi et al., 1993; Jacques and Qureshi, 1992; Bromberg et al., 1993). An important intermediary step in fetal infection may be invasion of the amniotic fluid by *T. pallidum*, since spirochetes can be recovered from as many as 74% of amniotic fluid samples from women with early syphilis (Lucas et al., 1991). It is possible that nasopharyngeal and/or gastrointestinal colonization with *T. pallidum* from in utero exposure to infected amniotic fluid is another mechanism for neonatal infection. The latter mechanism may explain why some exposed infants are born without clinical manifestations of congenital syphilis yet develop characteristic signs later in life if they are not treated appropriately during the newborn period (Ikeda and Jenson, 1990; Ingall et al., 1995). Breastfeeding does not result in transmission of syphilis unless an infectious lesion is present on the breast.

Table 1 Surveillance case definition for congenital syphilis[a]

A **confirmed case** of congenital syphilis is an infant in whom *T. pallidum* is identified by dark-field microscopy, fluorescent antibody, or other specific stains in specimens from lesions, placenta, umbilical cord, or autopsy material.

A **presumptive case** of congenital syphilis is either of the following.

A. Any infant whose mother had untreated or inadequately treated[b] syphilis at delivery, regardless of findings in the infant; or

B. Any infant or child who has a reactive treponemal test for syphilis and any one of the following:

1. any evidence of congenital syphilis on physical examination; or
2. any evidence of congenital syphilis on long bone radiograph; or
3. reactive CSF in a nontreponemal test such as the VDRL test; or
4. elevated CSF cell count or protein (without other cause); or
5. quantitative nontreponemal serologic titers which are fourfold higher than the mother's (both drawn at birth).

A **syphilitic stillbirth** is defined as a death of a fetus weighing >500 g or having a gestational age of >20 weeks in which the mother had untreated or inadequately treated syphilis at delivery.

[a] Adapted from CDC (1989).

[b] Inadequate treatment consists of any nonpenicillin therapy or penicillin given <30 days prior to delivery.

T. pallidum is able to cross the placenta at any time during gestation, although the risk of fetal infection is believed to increase as the stage of pregnancy advances. Formerly, it was believed that fetal infection did not occur before the fourth month of pregnancy, inasmuch as pathologic changes in fetal tissues could not be demonstrated before this time. It was believed that the Langhans' cell layer of the cytotrophoblast formed a placental barrier against treponemal invasion of the fetus (Harter and Benirschke, 1976). This theory, however, has been disproved by electron microscopic demonstration of the persistence of the Langhans' cell layer throughout pregnancy (Benirschke, 1974) and by the detection of spirochetes by silver staining and immunofluorescence techniques in fetal tissue from spontaneous abortions at 9 and 10 weeks of gestation (Harter and Benirschke, 1976). Recently, Lee et al. (1994) detected spirochetes by silver staining by using the Steiner technique in endometrial tissue of a woman with syphilis who had an incomplete abortion at 11 weeks gestation, further suggesting that treponemal infection can cause fetal morbidity during early gestation. Moreover, Nathan et al. (1994) have demonstrated spirochetes in amniotic fluid as early as 14 weeks of pregnancy, further proving that *T. pallidum* can gain access to the fetal compartment early in gestation. Fetal immunoincompetence during early gestation may explain the lack of characteristic pathologic changes in fetal tissues prior to the fifth month of pregnancy (Silverstein, 1962).

The effect of concurrent maternal infection with *T. pallidum* and HIV on the risk of fetal infection with *T. pallidum* and HIV remains to be elucidated (Sánchez et al., 1990; Pollack et al., 1990). However, the recent finding that virulent *T. pallidum* can directly promote the induction of HIV gene expression in macrophages and possibly result in increased systemic HIV levels and more rapid progression of the HIV infection (Theus et al., 1998) raises concern about the possible increased vertical transmission of HIV from a coinfected mother to the fetus. Concern also exists that the cellular immune dysfunction associated with HIV infection may result in a greater degree of treponemal proliferation and lead to a higher rate of fetal infection. HIV-infected women who acquire syphilis during pregnancy may not adequately respond to currently recommended benzathine penicillin therapy (Lukehart et al., 1988), thereby increasing the risk of fetal infection with *T. pallidum*.

CLINICAL MANIFESTATIONS

Pregnancy

Pregnancy has no known effect on the clinical course of syphilis. The appearance of a painless chancre with local lymphadenopathy marks the primary stage. The secondary stage represents more widespread hematogenous and lymphatic dissemination of *T. pallidum* and is characterized by systemic symptoms such as low-grade fever, malaise, sore throat, headache, adenopathy, and cutaneous or mucosal rash. Alopecia, mild hepatitis, and even nephrotic syndrome may develop. Latent syphilis refers to infection in individuals who have reactive serologic tests for syphilis but no clinical manifestations. Latency is further subdivided into early (≤1 year from onset of infection) and late (>1 year) latent stages based on the time when mucocutaneous lesions may still recur and the infection may still be transmitted. After years of untreated disease, approximately one-third of adults may develop tertiary syphilis, consisting of benign gummatous syphilis, cardiovascular syphilis, and neurosyphilis.

One of the most common outcomes of syphilis during pregnancy that is recognized worldwide is spontaneous abortion during the second and early third trimesters (Schulz et al., 1987; McKown and Kapernick, 1988; Hira et al., 1990; Lindstrand et al., 1993). In 1917, Osler observed that syphilis accounted for 20% of all stillbirths in the United States (Radolf et al., 1999). In England in 1917, Harman reported that 9% of the pregnancies complicated by syphilis resulted in miscarriages, 8% in stillbirths, 23% in infant deaths, 21% in infected infants, and only 39% in healthy uninfected infants (Radolf et al., 1999). Subsequently, in 1944, Dippel (Dippel, 1976) detected spirochetes in 16 (24%) of 67 fetuses of mothers with syphilis who aborted or miscarried between 18 and 27 weeks gestation. In Zambia, 19 to 42% of all stillbirths have been attributed to syphilis, and in Ethiopia, an estimated 5% of all pregnancies result in abortion or stillbirth due to syphilis (Schulz et al., 1987; Watts et al., 1984). Moreover, in these two countries, approximately 1% of pregnancies that extend beyond 20 to 27 weeks gestation result in a perinatal or postneonatal death due to syphilis. More recently, in a rural aboriginal community in Australia, 28% of 71 pregnancies were complicated by maternal syphilis; the presence of maternal syphilis was associated significantly with stillbirth and preterm delivery (odds ratios of 4 and 22, respectively) (How and Bowditch, 1994). Similar associations continue to be found in the United States today. From 1986 to 1988 in Miami, 34% of 56 infants born with congenital syphilis were stillborn and preterm delivery was more commonly seen in pregnancies complicated by syphilis (Ricci et al., 1989). Between 1988 and 1989 in Brooklyn, 40 (53%) of 75 infants with congenital syphilis were stillborn and the overall case fatality rate among infants with congenital syphilis was 57% (Rawstron et al., 1993). In Detroit, 6 (8%) of 72 infants born to mothers with untreated syphilis were stillborn, and these infants also had a significantly lower mean gestational age than those born to mothers who had received treatment for syphilis before delivery (Reyes et al., 1993). The problem of congenital syphilis in South America is only now being unraveled. In a recent study in Buenos Aires, 10% of women with reactive serologic tests for syphilis had a history of stillbirth that was believed to be secondary to syphilis (Pereyra et al., 1997). In 1996 in Bolivia, 26% of women who delivered stillborn infants had syphilis, compared to only 4% of mothers of liveborn infants (Southwick et al., 1997). The tragedy behind these data is that the majority of these adverse pregnancy outcomes are completely preventable.

The risk of prematurity, perinatal death, and congenital infection is directly related to the stage of maternal syphilis during pregnancy (Ingraham, 1951; Fiumara et al., 1952). In 1951, Ingraham studied a cohort of 1,959 pregnant women with syphilis, 1,063 of whom had received penicillin either before or during their pregnancy, and compared them to a control group consisting of 10,323 pregnant women without syphilis. He reported that for 220 women who had untreated early syphilis (up to 4 years duration), 41% of their infants were liveborn and had congenital syphilis, 25% were stillborn, 14% died in the neonatal period, 21% were premature (defined as birth weight less than 5 lb) but had no evidence of congenital syphilis, and only 18% were normal, full-term living infants. These outcomes were all significantly different from those observed among nonsyphilitic women. Untreated early syphilis resulted in a dead or diseased infant in approximately 82% of cases and increased the possibility of neonatal death 6-fold and increased the possibility of stillbirth at term 32-fold over the normal control group. In contrast, only 2% of infants born to 82 mothers with untreated late syphilis (over 4 years duration) had congenital syphilis and the likelihood of a normal full-term living infant was 75%. The stillbirth rate at 12.2% continued to remain higher than that of the normal control group.

Subsequently, Fiumara et al. (1952) reported that premature delivery occurred twice as frequently among mothers with recent or old infection than among uninfected mothers. Table 2 highlights the importance of early syphilis in contributing to adverse pregnancy outcomes and increasing the rate of vertical transmission of *T. pallidum*. Sánchez et al. (1993) documented similar infection rates in a small cohort of 19 infants. In their series, two of two infants born to mothers with primary syphilis had laboratory evidence of infection (reactive serum IgM immunoblot, positive serum or cerebrospinal fluid [CSF] PCR result, or positive rabbit infectivity testing), as did six of six infants born to mothers with secondary syphilis. In contrast, only 6 (55%) of 11 infants born to mothers with early latent infection had evidence of infection.

Infants

An early clue to the diagnosis of congenital syphilis is provided by examination of the placenta. The infected placenta is often large, thick, and pale; the histologic findings consist of focal villitis, endovascular and perivascular proliferation in villous vessels, and relative immaturity of the villi (Benirschke, 1974; Russell and Altshuler, 1974; Qureshi et al., 1993). The umbilical cord also may be involved; a deeply seated inflammatory process within the matrix of the umbilical cord termed necrotizing funisitis

Table 2 Syphilis in pregnancy: outcome by stage of infection[a]

Outcome	% of pregnancies with outcome at stage:		
	Primary or secondary	Early latent	Late latent
Prematurity	50[b]	20	9[c]
Stillbirth		10	10
Neonatal death		4	1[c]
Congenital syphilis	50	40	10
Normal	0	20	70

[a] Adapted from Fiumara et al. (1952).
[b] Prematurity, stillbirth, and neonatal death together.
[c] Not increased beyond the expected rate among women without syphilis.

has been described and may be specific for syphilis (Fojaco et al., 1989; Jacques and Qureshi, 1992). Microscopically, there is an abscess-like focus of necrosis located within Wharton's jelly and centered around the umbilical vessels. Macroscopically, the umbilical cord resembles a "barber pole"; the edematous portions have a spiral striped zone of red and pale blue discoloration, interspersed with streaks of chalky white.

Congenital infection with *T. pallidum* results in two characteristic syndromes of clinical disease, arbitrarily designated as early and late congenital syphilis (Ingall et al., 1995; Radolf et al., 1999). Early congenital syphilis refers to clinical manifestations that appear within the first 2 years of life. Features that occur after 2 years, and usually are manifested near puberty, constitute late congenital syphilis. The clinical manifestations of early congenital syphilis and their relative frequencies of occurrence are given in Table 3. These signs and symptoms are a consequence of active infection with *T. pallidum* and the resultant inflammatory response induced in various body organs and tissues. The severity of these manifestations is extremely variable and can range from overwhelming involvement of multiple organs and body systems, as seen in fetal hydrops, to only laboratory or radiographic abnormalities in an otherwise normal-appearing newborn. Although as many as one-third of severely affected fetuses will die either in utero or shortly after birth, the majority of liveborn infants, if not hydropic, will survive the neonatal period. This is most probably due not only to early identification and treatment of infected infants but also to improved neonatal care.

The malformations or stigmata of late congenital syphilis represent scars induced by the initial lesions of early congenital syphilis or reactions to persistent inflammation. The clinical manifestations of late congenital syphilis are given in Table 4. Late congenital syphilis is not infectious.

DIAGNOSIS

The diagnosis of antepartum syphilis is most often made by serologic screening at the first prenatal visit. This practice has been shown to be cost-effective even in areas with a low prevalence of syphilis (Schmid, 1996). Whenever possible, an attempt to visualize the characteristic motile spirochetes by dark-field microscopy in clinical lesions such as a chancre should be undertaken. In early primary syphilis, a chancre may be present yet the serologic tests are nonreactive.

Serologic tests for syphilis are classified as either nontreponemal tests (the Venereal Disease Research Laboratory [VDRL] test and the rapid plasma reagin [RPR] test) or treponemal tests (the fluorescent treponemal antibody-absorption [FTA-ABS] test and *T. pallidum* hemagglutination tests [microhemagglutination assay for *T. pallidum* antibody {MHA-TP} and *T. pallidum* particle agglutination {TP-PA} tests]) (Larsen et al., 1995). Non-

Table 3 Clinical findings and their frequencies in infants with early congenital syphilis[a]

Finding	Frequency[b]
Nonimmune hydrops (fetalis)	+
Intrauterine growth retardation	+
Reticuloendothelial system	
Jaundice	+++
Hepatitis	++
Hepatosplenomegaly	[+++]
Anemia	+++
Thrombocytopenia	++
Adenopathy	++
Mucocutaneous lesions	
Rhinitis (snuffles)	±
Skin rash	[+++]
Mucus patch	±
Condylomata lata	±
Bone abnormalities	[+++]
Periostitis, osteochondritis, pseudoparalysis of Parrot	
Eyes	
Chorioretinitis	±
Cataract	±
Glaucoma/uveitis	±
Central nervous system	
Asymptomatic invasion	++
Acute leptomeningitis	±
Chronic meningovasculitis	±
Hydrocephalus	±
Cranial nerve palsies	±
Cerebral infarction	±
Seizures	±
Hypopituitarism	±
Nephrotic syndrome	±
Pancreatitis	++
Pneumonia alba	+
Myocarditis	±
Fever	±
Gastrointestinal malabsorption	±

[a] From Sánchez and Wendel (1997).
[b] ±, rare; +, 5 to 20%; ++, 20 to 50%; +++, more than 50%; boxes indicate prominent feature.

Table 4 Clinical findings in late congenital syphilis

System	Finding
Dentition	Hutchinson's teeth,[a] mulberry molars
Eyes and ears	Interstitial keratitis,[a] healed chorioretinitis, eighth nerve deafness[a]
Mucocutaneous system	Rhagades
Central nervous system	Mental retardation, hydrocephalus, seizures, optic nerve atrophy, juvenile general paresis, cranial nerve palsies
Musculoskeletal	Frontal bossing, saddle nose deformity, protuberant mandible, saber shin, sternoclavicular joint thickening (Higouménakis' sign), Clutton's joints

[a]These findings comprise Hutchinson's triad.

treponemal tests use an antigen composed of lipids, including lecithin, cholesterol, and purified cardiolipin (diphosphatidylglycerol—a component of both mammalian and treponemal cell membranes), to detect an antibody against cardiolipin that is present in the sera of patients with syphilis. The RPR test is more sensitive than the VDRL test and is preferred for routine serologic screening of pregnant women. A fourfold decrease in titer of the same nontreponemal test is a useful indicator that treatment was adequate. The VDRL test is recommended for use on CSF. False-positive nontreponemal test results can occur and have been associated with collagen vascular diseases (systemic lupus erythematosus), viral infections (Epstein-Barr, varicella-zoster, and hepatitis viruses), narcotic addiction, malignancy, advanced age, immunizations, and even pregnancy.

The nontreponemal test results become reactive approximately 4 to 8 weeks after the infection is acquired and several days to 1 week after the appearance of a chancre. Overall, nonreactive results occur in approximately one-fourth of patients with primary, latent, and late syphilis (Larsen et al., 1995). On the other hand, with secondary syphilis, the nontreponemal test results are almost always reactive. However, about 1 to 2% of serum samples from patients with secondary syphilis are nonreactive (Larsen et al., 1995; Berkowitz et al., 1990). This immunologic reaction is called prozone and is due to an excess amount of cardiolipin antibody in the patient's undiluted serum that prevents flocculation and results in a false-negative reaction. The prozone effect can be overcome by diluting the serum before testing, after which the serum will usually exhibit titers of 1:16 or greater.

Specific treponemal antibody tests include the FTA-ABS test and hemagglutination tests (MHA-TP and TP-PA tests) which utilize lyophilized *T. pallidum* or a lysate of pathogenic *T. pallidum*, respectively (Larsen et al.,

1995). These tests are both more sensitive and specific than the nontreponemal tests and are used to confirm reactive nontreponemal test results. Since the treponemal tests remain reactive indefinitely even after appropriate treatment in most adults infected with syphilis, they cannot be used to distinguish active infection from past infection or to assess the adequacy of treatment. Positive results obtained from the FTA-ABS and hemagglutination tests are not quantified. The FTA-ABS test may be nonreactive in up to 18% of adults with primary syphilis and in up to 5% of those with latent and late syphilis (Larsen et al., 1981). The sensitivity of the MHA-TP test is less than that of the FTA-ABS test in primary syphilis; nonreactivity of up to 36% has been reported. It appears to be as sensitive as the FTA-ABS test with the other stages of syphilis. False-positive treponemal test results are infrequent but can occur in mixed connective tissue and autoimmune diseases, viral infections, and even pregnancy (Larsen et al., 1995). In many clinical laboratories, the hemagglutination tests have replaced the FTA-ABS test since they are easier to perform, are less time-consuming, and require less specialized equipment and personnel. The MHA-TP test, however, is no longer commercially available. The TP-PA test uses the same treponemal antigen as the MHA-TP test, but utilizes gelatin particles rather than sheep red blood cells, which may eliminate nonspecific reactions with serum/plasma samples. The TP-PA test was developed in Japan; its performance has been comparable to that of the MHA-TP and FTA-ABS tests (Deguchi et al., 1994). Investigational tests which detect treponemal IgG antibodies include enzyme-linked immunosorbent assays (ELISA) and immunoblotting (Norgard, 1993).

Fetal syphilis can be diagnosed by ultrasonography, which identifies hydrops fetalis in the presence of maternal syphilis (Wendel et al., 1991; Nathan et al., 1993; Hallak et al., 1992). The sonographic findings of fetal hydrops include skin thickening, placental thickening, serous cavity effusions, hepatomegaly, and hydramnios. Hill and Maloney (1991) also reported noncontinuous gastrointestinal tract obstruction in association with hepatosplenomegaly and placentomegaly in a fetus with syphilis. Satin et al. (1992) described the ultrasonographic findings of dilated small bowel and hepatomegaly in a fetus who was subsequently delivered stillborn to a mother whose amniotic fluid had spirochetes visualized by dark-field microscopy. At autopsy, spirochetes were detected within the intestinal wall. Antenatal sonography may also detect fetal hepatomegaly in syphilitic pregnant women, and this may be a useful marker of amniotic fluid or fetal infection. Using rabbit infectivity testing to confirm the presence of *T. pallidum* in amniotic fluid, Nathan et al. (1993) associated the finding of spirochetes in amniotic fluid with the presence of hepatomegaly by antenatal sonography. Sampling of the umbilical cord has also been used to diagnose fetal syphilis (Wendel et al., 1991; Hallak et al., 1992). Wendel et al. (1991)

obtained fetal blood by cordocentesis at 24 weeks gestation; the fetal blood sample showed anemia, thrombocytopenia, and elevated levels of liver enzymes. The diagnosis of congenital syphilis was confirmed by rabbit infectivity testing with fetal blood as well as by immunoblot analysis revealing fetal IgM directed against the immunogenic lipoproteins of *T. pallidum*.

A diagnosis of congenital syphilis must be considered in infants born to mothers who have reactive nontreponemal and treponemal test results. The diagnosis can be established by the demonstration of spirochetes in infant's lesions, body fluids, or tissues by dark-field microscopy, direct fluorescent-antibody testing (Bromberg et al., 1993), or histologic examination. Use of these techniques has demonstrated the typical spiral organisms in mucocutaneous lesions, nasal discharge, vesicular fluid, placenta, umbilical cord, and tissue obtained at autopsy. The sensitivity of these tests in neonates, however, is generally low because the organism often is present in low concentrations. Consequently, the diagnosis must rest on the findings of the physical examination of the infant and on the results of other laboratory and radiographic tests.

Infants born to mothers with reactive serologic tests for syphilis should be evaluated by the same nontreponemal test that was performed on the mother (Ingall et al., 1995; Rawstron and Bromberg, 1991; Chhabra et al., 1993; Sánchez, 1998). The Centers for Disease Control and Prevention (CDC) has recommended that serum from the infant (rather than from umbilical cord blood obtained at birth) be used for serologic testing because the rates of false-positive and false-negative results are lower. However, due to its ease of collection, umbilical cord blood continues to be a readily available specimen. Appropriate care in collection of umbilical cord blood should be taken to avoid contamination with maternal blood. Since the currently available nontreponemal and treponemal tests detect mostly transplacentally acquired IgG antibody that is maternal in origin, treponemal tests do not have to be performed in the newborn, since they will only reflect the maternal status. On the other hand, comparison of the maternal nontreponemal serologic titer obtained at delivery to that of the newborn infant may provide a clue to the infant's infection status (Sánchez, 1998; CDC, 1998). A diagnosis of congenital syphilis is supported if an infant's nontreponemal antibody level is fourfold or greater than that of the mother's serum (Sánchez et al., 1993). More commonly, however, the maternal and infant serologic titers are similar. In that case, a probable diagnosis of congenital syphilis is made if the infant or stillbirth has a reactive nontreponemal test result and clinical, laboratory, or radiographic manifestations consistent with congenital syphilis. If the infant's physical examination, laboratory tests, and bone radiographs are normal, a diagnosis of congenital syphilis at birth is virtually impossible to determine by current serologic testing. In these cases, a retrospective diagnosis of congenital syphilis can be made when a reactive treponemal antibody test result persists beyond 15 months of age; however, this occurs in only 30% of infants who had documented evidence of syphilis as determined by the isolation of spirochetes from blood and/or CSF by rabbit infectivity testing (Taber and Baughn, 1991; Sánchez et al., 1994).

Diagnosis of congenital syphilis based on results of commercially available tests for specific IgM antibodies is not reliable due to the low sensitivity of the assays (Stoll et al., 1993). These tests are not recommended by the CDC for evaluation or management of infants born to mothers with syphilis (CDC, 1998). Several investigators have used immunoblotting techniques to detect and characterize the specific neonatal IgM (Sánchez et al., 1989, 1993; Dobson et al., 1988; Lewis et al., 1990; Schmitz et al., 1994) and IgA (Schmitz et al., 1994) antibody responses to *T. pallidum*. Specific IgM antibody directed against *T. pallidum* antigens with apparent molecular masses ranging from 93 to 15 kDa has been detected in sera from infants with clinical and laboratory evidence of congenital syphilis. Sanchez et al. (1993) noted that reactivity against the 47-kDa antigen has been uniformly present in all the reactive serum IgM immunoblots; this membrane lipoprotein is a major immunogen in both human and experimental syphilis. IgM reactivity to the 47-kDa antigen also has been detected in the CSF of infants with congenital syphilis (Sánchez et al., 1992). IgM immunoblotting, although currently limited to research laboratories, may represent the most important technological advance for the diagnosis of congenital syphilis.

PCR has been used by several investigators for the detection of *T. pallidum* DNA in clinical specimens, including genital ulcers, from adults and infants (Grimprel et al., 1991; Sánchez et al., 1993; Burstain et al., 1991; Hay et al., 1990; Noordhoek et al., 1991; Wicher et al., 1992; Genest et al., 1996; Zoechling et al., 1997; Centurion-Lara et al., 1997; Orle et al., 1996). For amniotic fluid obtained from 12 pregnant women with early syphilis, Grimprel et al. (1991) found a sensitivity of 91% and specificity of 100% for PCR compared to recovery of spirochetes by rabbit infectivity testing. With respect to infant blood and CSF, sensitivities of 74 and 71% and specificities of 96 and 99%, respectively, have been found (Sánchez et al., 1993).

TREATMENT

Penicillin remains the drug of choice for treatment of both acquired and congenital syphilis (Table 5; Fig. 4) (CDC, 1998). Penicillin resistance has not been reported. Pregnant women with reactive serologic tests for syphilis should be counseled about the risks of HIV infection, tested for HIV antibody, and treated with the penicillin regimen appropriate for the stage of syphilis (Table 2).

Approximately 5 to 10% of pregnant women with syphilis report a history of penicillin allergy. Wendel et al. (1985) have demonstrated the

Table 5 Treatment guidelines for acquired syphilis during pregnancy

Stage of infection	Regimen[a]
Primary, secondary, early latent (≤1 yr)	Benzathine penicillin G, 2.4 mU i.m. × 1
Late latent (>1 yr), unknown duration	Benzathine penicillin G, 2.4 mU i.m. q week × 3
Neurosyphilis	Aqueous penicillin G, 3–4 mU i.v. q 4 h × 10–14 days[b]
	or
	Procaine penicillin G, 2.4 mU i.m. q.i.d., and probenicid, 500 mg p.o. q.i.d. × 10–14 days[b]

[a] i.m., intramuscularly; i.v., intravenously; p.o., orally.
[b] Some experts recommend following this regimen with benzathine penicillin G, 2.4 mU intramuscularly.

safety of oral desensitization to penicillin in pregnant women. This method is currently recommended so that all pregnant women with syphilis can receive penicillin therapy (CDC, 1998), since no other antimicrobial agent has been shown to be as effective for treatment of syphilis during pregnancy. Tetracycline and doxycycline are contraindicated in pregnancy; both can result in staining of decidual teeth and impairment of long-bone growth. Moreover, tetracycline use during pregnancy has been associated with hepatic toxicity when there is concomitant renal dysfunction. Erythromycin should not be used because of reports of treatment failure (Fenton and Irwin, 1976; South et al., 1964; Hashiasaki et al., 1983). Patient noncompliance with erythromycin therapy, as a result of gastrointestinal side effects, has been a major problem. Moreover, there remains concern about unpredictable levels in maternal serum and erratic transplacental transfer of the drug (Philipson et al., 1973). Insufficient data exist to recommend azithromycin or ceftriaxone (CDC, 1998).

The Jarisch-Herxheimer reaction commonly occurs after treatment of acquired early syphilis in adults. It consists of fever, chills, myalgias, headache, hypotension, tachycardia, and transient accentuation of the cutaneous lesions. It typically begins within several hours of treatment and resolves by 24 to 36 h. The etiology is not fully known; however, since *T. pallidum* lacks lipopolysaccharides, the release of *T. pallidum* lipoproteins that may cause acute inflammation has been implicated as the cause of this clinical phenomenon. Klein et al. (1990) have shown that another manifestation of the Jarisch-Herxheimer reaction is uterine contractions in pregnant women, possibly mediated secondarily by prostaglandins. By fetal monitoring during the episode, they demonstrated evidence of fetal stress with tachycardia and decelerations along with a marked decrease in fetal activity. No pro-

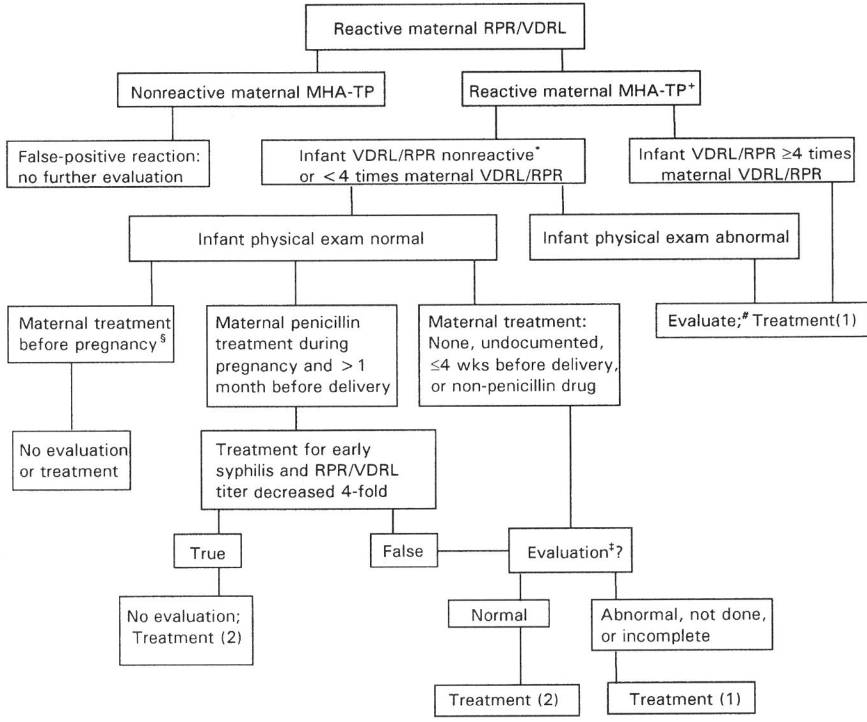

+ Test for HIV-antibody. Infants of HIV-Ab ⊕ mothers do not require different evaluation or treatment.

* Infant's VDRL may be nonreactive due to low maternal VDRL titer or recent maternal infection. If the mother has untreated or inadequately treated syphilis and infant's physical exam is normal, some experts would not perform diagnostic evaluation but would treat infant with a single IM injection of benzathine penicillin (50,000 U/kg).

Evaluation consists of CBC, platelet count; CSF examination for cell count, protein, and quantitative VDRL; Other tests as clinically indicated (eye exam, long-bone films; chest X-ray; liver function tests; cranial ultrasound; auditory brainstem response).

§ Women who maintain a VDRL titer ≤1:2 beyond 1 year following successful treatment are considered serofast.

‡ CBC, platelet count; CSF examination for cell count, protein, and quantitative VDRL; Long bone films.

TREATMENT:

(1) Aqueous penicillin G 50,000 U/kg IV q 12 hr (≤1 wk of age), q 8 hr (> 1 wk), or procaine penicillin G 50,000 U/kg IM single daily dose x 10 days.

(2) Benzathine penicillin G 50,000 U/kg IM x 1 dose.

Figure 4 Algorithm for management of infants born to mothers with reactive serologic tests for syphilis.

phylactic measure or treatment is currently available. For these reasons, some authorities recommend sonographic evaluation of the fetus before initiation of penicillin therapy if early syphilis is diagnosed in the third trimester. If the sonographic evaluation is normal, appropriate penicillin therapy is initiated and the mother is sent home with appropriate warnings of uterine contractions and fetal activity. If the sonographic evaluation is abnormal and consistent with fetal infection, the mother is hospitalized for fetal monitoring during the first 24 h following treatment. This allows early and timely intervention if fetal distress occurs. If fetal compromise is already present before treatment and the fetus is viable, delivery followed by treatment of the mother and infant may result in an improved outcome.

Despite administration of recommended penicillin therapy to pregnant women, as many as 14% will deliver dead fetuses or infants with clinical evidence of congenital syphilis (Ingall et al., 1995; Alexander et al., 1999; Mascola et al., 1984). Many of these women were treated for secondary syphilis late in pregnancy; this stage of syphilis is associated with a high degree of spirochetemia and widespread dissemination. For this reason, a second dose of benzathine penicillin G 1 week after the initial dose has been empirically recommended by some authorities (Sheffield et al., 1998). Whether such a regimen has superior efficacy in either preventing or treating fetal syphilis is not known. Concern also exists that in the final 4 weeks of pregnancy maternal treatment for syphilis by recommended regimens may be inadequate therapy for the fetus (Mascola et al., 1984). A possible explanation is that penicillin pharmacokinetics may be altered due to normal increases in renal clearance and plasma volume, leading to lower levels of penicillin in serum and CSF in both the mother and fetus (Nathan et al., 1993). Moreover, maternal treatment in the final weeks of pregnancy may not allow sufficient time for the fetus to be adequately treated, thus necessitating penicillin therapy for the newborn infant. Because currently available methods for diagnosis of congenital syphilis do not accurately identify infants with active infection, the majority of these so-called treatment failures could reflect resolving abnormalities from treated fetal infection. It is well known that the clinical and laboratory abnormalities seen in infants infected with *T. pallidum* may require months for complete resolution even after prolonged intravenous penicillin therapy. Recently, improper use of the new CDC surveillance case definition (CDC, 1989) as a diagnostic criterion for congenital syphilis has led to the erroneous labeling of certain infants as congenitally infected, further complicating the issue. Nonetheless, it is clear that some treatment failures do occur, as evidenced by autopsy findings in stillborn infants.

The decision to treat an infant for congenital syphilis is based on the clinical presentation, previous serologic test results and treatment of the mother, as well as results of serologic testing of the mother and infant at the time of delivery (Fig. 4) (CDC, 1998; American Academy of Pediatrics, 1997; Finelli et al., 1998). Maternal infection with syphilis late in pregnancy may result in the infant having a nonreactive nontreponemal serologic test for syphilis; these infants should be treated to prevent development of disease (Sánchez et al., 1991b; Dorfman and Glaser, 1990). Moreover, infants born to mothers who develop secondary or early latent syphilis within 1 year after delivery should be tested and treated if their serologic test results are reactive. Infants born to mothers coinfected with syphilis and HIV do not require more aggressive or prolonged penicillin therapy. The necessity for serologic follow-up of these high-risk infants cannot be overemphasized.

Fewer than 1% of infants who are treated for presumed congenital syphilis develop, within several hours of initiation of penicillin therapy, a Jarisch-Herxheimer reaction, consisting of fever, tachypnea, tachycardia, hypotension, accentuation of the cutaneous lesions, and/or death due to cardiovascular collapse. Other than supportive care, there is no specific treatment or prophylaxis.

PREVENTION

Prevention of syphilis among pregnant women has remained an elusive public health goal. Adverse outcomes of pregnancy including congenital syphilis can be effectively prevented by routine prenatal serologic screening and penicillin treatment of infected women and their sexual partners. All pregnant women should be given a nontreponemal serologic test for syphilis during the first trimester (CDC, 1998). In areas with a high prevalence of syphilis, serologic screening also should be performed at the beginning of the third trimester (28 weeks) and at delivery. Serologic screening tests should be performed on maternal serum and not on the infant's serum or umbilical cord blood (Ingall et al., 1995; Rawstron and Bromberg, 1991). An infant's serologic titer is often 1 to 2 dilutions less than that of the mother's serum; therefore, an infant may have a nonreactive umbilical cord VDRL test even though the mother has a reactive serologic test for syphilis at delivery. It is prudent not to discharge an infant before the results of maternal serologic screening at delivery are known. With the practice of early discharge at 24 h or less becoming more common, it becomes the responsibility of the infant's health care worker to have adequate follow-up arrangements for infants who are discharged before the results of the maternal serologic test are known. If such close follow-up is not possible, early discharge cannot be recommended.

Limitations of current screening practices exist. A false-negative result in a nontreponemal test can occur from a prozone reaction (Berkowitz et al., 1990). Also, a negative nontreponemal maternal test at delivery may not exclude incubating syphilis or even primary syphilis, when nontreponemal and treponemal antibodies have not yet reached detectable levels (Larsen et al., 1995). By current methods, detection of treponemal infection in the asymptomatic infant is impossible. Infants born to such seronegative women are at risk of developing syphilis in the ensuing 3 to 14 weeks. For these reasons, in high-risk populations, repeated screening of the mother at the first postpartum visit at 4 weeks should be considered.

Reporting of cases to the local public health department will allow contact investigation and appropriate follow-up. Rapid investigation of named sexual partners is essential for effective treatment of partners. Individuals who have had sexual contact with an untreated person or with someone treated within the last 24 h should be tested serologically, treated prophylactically, and retested 3 months later (CDC, 1998). Issues of accessibility and use of health care facilities as well as behavioral practices by at-risk populations have prompted more community-based strategies for identification and treatment of infected individuals and high-risk populations. As partner notification has become more challenging due to anonymous sex and the inability to locate sexual partners, attention has focused on identifying core environments and populations in which syphilis transmission is occurring. Such knowledge has resulted in provision of prophylactic syphilis treatment to groups of people in high-risk populations.

Elimination of syphilis from the Western Hemisphere has recently been advocated by the CDC and the Pan American Health Organization. Seroprevalence studies which will help to identify the magnitude of the problem among pregnant women are under way in Latin America. The success of such efforts will then depend on the willingness of governments to fund different strategies that will successfully identify and provide treatment to infected individuals in a timely fashion. Such efforts can only assist the American prevention programs, since more and more cases in the United States are among immigrants who acquired the infection abroad.

Ultimately, the hidden epidemic of syphilis will be eliminated and conquered only when a national system of prevention of sexually transmitted diseases becomes a reality. Such a program would enlist community leaders and health care providers and would provide culturally sensitive preventive strategies that address the concerns of disadvantaged and minority populations, who are more likely to be infected with syphilis and other sexually transmitted diseases.

Acknowledgments

Supported by Public Health Service grant 1R29 AI 34932-01 from the National Institute of Allergy and Infectious Diseases and by Centers for Disease Control and Prevention contract C1000 689.

REFERENCES

Alexander, J. M., J. S. Sheffield, P. J. Sánchez, J. Mayfield, and G. D. Wendel. 1999. Efficacy of treatment of syphilis in pregnancy. *Obstet. Gynecol.* **93**:5–8.

American Academy of Pediatrics. 1997. *Report of the Committee on Infectious Diseases* (*Red Book*), 24th ed., p. 504–514. American Academy of Pediatrics, Elk Grove Village, Ill.

Andrus, J. K., D. W. Fleming, D. R. Harger, M. Y. Chin, D. V. Bennett, J. M. Horan, G. Oxman, B. Olson, and L. R. Foster. 1990. Partner notification: can it control epidemic syphilis? *Ann. Intern. Med.* **112:**539–543.

Benirschke, K. 1974. Syphilis: the placenta and fetus. *Am. J. Dis. Child.* **128:**142–143.

Berkowitz, K., L. Baxi, and H. E. Fox. 1990. False-negative screening: the prozone phenomenon, nonimmune hydrops, and diagnosis of syphilis during pregnancy. *Am. J. Obstet. Gynecol.* **163:**975–977.

Berry, M. C., and A. S. Dajani. 1992. Resurgence of congenital syphilis. *Infect. Dis. Clin. North Am.* **1:**19–29.

Bromberg, K., S. Rawstron, and G. Tannis. 1993. Diagnosis of congenital syphilis by combining *Treponema pallidum*-specific IgM detection with immunofluorescent antigen detection for *T. pallidum. J. Infect. Dis.* **168:**238–242.

Burstain, J. M., E. Grimprel, S. A. Lukehart, M. V. Norgard, and J. D. Radolf. 1991. Sensitive detection of *Treponema pallidum* by using the polymerase chain reaction. *J. Clin. Microbiol.* **29:**62–69.

Cates, W., R. B. Rothenberg, and J. H. Blount. 1996. Syphilis control: the historic context and epidemiolic basis for interrupting sexual transmission of *Treponema pallidum. Sex. Transm. Dis.* **23:**68.

Centers for Disease Control. 1989. Congenital syphilis, New York City, 1986–1988. *Morbid. Mortal. Weekly Rep.* **38:**825–829.

Centers for Disease Control. 1991. Alternative case-finding methods in a crack-related syphilis epidemic—Philadelphia. *Morbid. Mortal. Weekly Rep.* **40:**77–80.

Centers for Disease Control. 1993. Selective screening to augment syphilis case-finding—Dallas, 1991. *Morbid. Mortal. Weekly Rep.* **42:**424–427.

Centers for Disease Control and Prevention. 1996a. Outbreak of primary and secondary syphilis—Baltimore City, Maryland, 1995. *Morbid. Mortal. Weekly Rep.* **45**(8)**:**166–169.

Centers for Disease Control and Prevention. 1996b. Summary of notifiable diseases, United States. *Morbid. Mortal. Weekly Rep.* **45**(53)**:**58–61.

Centers of Disease Control and Prevention. 1998. Guidelines for treatment of sexually transmitted diseases. *Morbid. Mortal. Weekly Rep.* **47**(RR-1)**:**28–49.

Centurion-Lara, A., C. Castro, J. M. Shaffer, W. C. VanVoorhis, C. M. Marra, and S. A. Lukehart. 1997. Detection of *Treponema pallidum* by sensitive reverse transcriptase PCR. *J. Clin. Microbiol.* **35:**1348–1352.

Chhabra, R. S., L. P. Brion, M. Castro, L. Freundlich, and J. H. Glaser. 1993. Comparison of maternal sera, cord blood, and neonatal sera for detecting presumptive congenital syphilis: relationship with maternal treatment. *Pediatrics* **91:**88–91.

Cohen, D. A., D. Boyd, I. Prabhudas, and L. Mascola. 1990. The effects of case definition in maternal screening and reporting criteria on rates of congenital syphilis. *Am. J. Public Health* **80:**316–317.

Deguchi, M., H. Hosotsubo, N. Yamashita, T. Ohmine, and S. Asari. 1994. Evaluation of gelatin particle agglutination method for detection of *Treponema pallidum* antibody. *J. Jpn. Assoc. Infect. Dis.* **68:**1271–1277.

Dickerson, M. C., J. Johnston, T. E. Delea, A. White, and E. Andrews. 1996. The causal role for genital ulcer disease as a risk factor for transmission of human immunodeficiency virus. *Sex. Transm. Dis.* **23:**429–440.

Dippel, A. L. 1976. The relationship of congenital syphilis to abortion and miscarriage, and the mechanism of intrauterine protection. *Am. J. Obstet. Gynecol.* **47:**369.

Dobson, S. R. M., L. H. Taber, and R. E. Baughn. 1988. Recognition of *Treponema pallidum* antigens by IgM and IgG antibodies in congenitally infected newborns and their mothers. *J. Infect. Dis.* **157:**903–910.

Dorfman, D. H., and J. H. Glaser. 1990. Congenital syphilis presenting in infants after the newborn period. *N. Engl. J. Med.* **323:**1299–1302.

Fenton, L. J., and J. L. Irwin. 1976. Congenital syphilis after maternal treatment with erythromycin. *Obstet. Gynecol.* **47:**492–494.

Finelli, L., E. M. Crayne, and K. C. Spitalny. 1998. Treatment of infants with reactive syphilis serology, New Jersey: 1992 to 1996. *Pediatrics* **102:**e27.

Fiumara, N. J., W. L. Fleming, J. G. Downing, and F. L. Good. 1952. The incidence of prenatal syphilis at the Boston City Hospital. *N. Engl. J. Med.* **247:**48–52.

Fojaco, R. M., G. T. Hensley, and L. Moskowitz. 1989. Congenital syphilis and necrotizing funisitis. *JAMA* **12:**1788–1780.

Genest, D. R., S. R. Choi-Hong, J. E. Tate, F. Qureshi, S. M. Jacques, and C. Crum. 1996. Diagnosis of congenital syphilis from placental examination: comparison of histopathology, steiner stain, and polymerase chain reaction for *Treponema pallidum* DNA. *Hum. Pathol.* **27:**366–372.

Grimprel, E., P. J. Sánchez, G. D. Wendel, J. M. Burstain, G. H. McCracken, Jr., J. D. Radolf, and M. V. Norgard. 1991. Use of polymerase chain reaction and rabbit infectivity testing to detect *Treponema pallidum* in amniotic fluids, fetal and neonatal sera, and cerebrospinal fluid. *J. Clin. Microbiol.* **29:**1711–1718.

Hallak, M., J. F. Peipert, A. Ludomirsky, and J. Byers. 1992. Nonimmune hydrops fetalis and fetal congenital syphilis: a case report. *J. Reprod. Med.* **37:**173–176.

Harter, C. A., and K. Benirschke. 1976. Fetal syphilis in the first trimester. *Am. J. Obstet. Gynecol.* **124:**705–711.

Hashiasaki, P., G. G. Wertzberger, G. L. Conrad, and C. R. Nichols. 1983. Erythromycin failure in the treatment of syphilis in a pregnant woman. *Sex. Transm. Dis.* **10:**36–38.

Hay, P. E., J. R. Clarke, R. A. Strugnell, D. Taylor-Robinson, and D. Goldmeier. 1990. Use of the polymerase chain reaction to detect DNA sequences specific to pathogenic treponemes in cerebrospinal fluid. *FEMS Microbiol. Lett.* **68:**233–238.

Hill, L. M., and J. B. Maloney. 1991. An unusual constellation of sonographic findings associated with congenital syphilis. *Obstet. Gynecol.* **78:**895–897.

Hira, S. K., G. J. Bhat, D. Chikamata, B. Nkowane, G. Tembo, P. L. Perine, and A. Meheus. 1990. Syphilis intervention in pregnancy: Zambian demonstration project. *Genitourin. Med.* **66:**159–164.

How, J. H. Y., and J. D. P. Bowditch. 1994. Syphilis in pregnancy: experience from a rural aboriginal community. *Aust. N. Z. J. Obstet. Gynaecol.* **34:**383–389.

Ikeda, M. K., and H. B. Jenson. 1990. Evaluation and treatment of congenital syphilis. *J. Pediatr.* **117:**843–852.

Ingall, D., P. J. Sánchez, and D. Musher. 1995. Syphilis, p. 529–564. *In* J. S. Remington and J. D. Klein (ed.), *Infectious Disease of the Fetus and Newborn,* 4th ed. The W. B. Saunders Co., Philadelphia, Pa.

Ingraham, N. R. 1951. The value of penicillin alone in the prevention and treatment of congenital syphilis. *Acta Dermato-Venereol.* **31**(Suppl. 24)**:**60–88.

Jacques, S. M., and F. Qureshi. 1992. Necrotizing funisitis: a study of 45 cases. *Hum. Pathol.* **23:**1278–1283.

Kaufman, R. E., O. G. Jones, J. H. Blount, and P. J. Wiesner. 1977. Questionnaire survey of reported early congenital syphilis: problems in diagnosis, prevention and treatment. *Sex. Transm. Dis.* **4:**135–139.

Klein, V. R., S. M. Cox, M. D. Mitchell, and G. D. Wendel, Jr. 1990. The Jarisch-Herxheimer reaction complicating syphilotherapy in pregnancy. *Obstet. Gynecol.* **75:**375–380.

Larsen, S. A., E. A. Hambie, D. E. Pettit, M. W. Perryman, and S. J. Kraus. 1981. Specificity, sensitivity, and reproducibility among the fluorescent treponemal antibody-absorption test, the microhemagglutination assay for *Treponema pallidum* antibodies, and the hemagglutination treponemal test for syphilis. *J. Clin. Microbiol.* **14:**441–445.

Larsen, S. A., B. M. Steiner, and A. H. Rudolph. 1995. Laboratory diagnosis and interpretation of tests for syphilis. *Clin. Microbiol. Rev.* **8:**1–21.

Lee, W. K., D. A. Schwartz, J. R. Rice, and S. A. Larsen. 1994. Syphilitic endometritis causing first trimester abortion: a potential infectious cause of fetal morbidity in early gestation. *South. Med. J.* **87:**1259–1261.

Lewis, L. L., L. H. Taber, and R. E. Baughn. 1990. Evaluation of immunoglobulin M Western blot analysis in the diagnosis of congenital syphilis. *J. Clin. Microbiol.* **28:**296–302.

Lindstrand, A., S. Bergström, A. Bugalho, G. Zanconato, A. M. Helgesson, and B. Hedersted. 1993. Prevalence of syphilis infection in Mozambican women with second trimester miscarriage and women attending antenatal care in second trimester. *Genitourin. Med.* **69:**431–433.

Lucas, M. J., S. K. Theriot, and G. D. Wendel. 1991. Doppler systolic-diastolic ratios in pregnancies complicated by syphilis. *Obstet. Gynecol.* **77:**217–222.

Lukehart, S. A., E. W. Hook III, S. A. Baker-Zander, A. C. Collier, C. W. Critchlow, and H. H. Handsfield. 1988. Invasion of the central nervous system by *Treponema pallidum*: implications for diagnoses and therapy. *Ann. Intern. Med.* **109:**855–862.

Mascola, L., R. Pelosi, and C. E. Alexander. 1984. Inadequate treatment of syphilis in pregnancy. *Am. J. Obstet. Gynecol.* **150:**945–947.

Mascola, L., R. Pelosi, J. H. Blount, C. E. Alexander, and W. Cates, Jr. 1985. Congenital syphilis revisited. *Am. J. Dis. Child.* **139:**575–580.

McKown, R. R., and P. S. Kapernick. 1988. Syphilis in pregnancy. *South. Med. J.* **81:** 447–451.

Nakashima, A. K., R. T. Rolfs, M. L. Flock, P. Kilmarx, and J. R. Greenspan. 1996. Epidemiology of syphilis in the United States, 1941–1993. *Sex. Transm. Dis.* **23:**16–23.

Nathan, L., R. E. Bawdon, E. Sidawi, R. W. Stettler, D. M. McIntire, and G. D. Wendel, Jr. 1993. Penicillin levels following the administration of benzathine penicillin G in pregnancy. *Obstet. Gynecol.* **82:**338–342.

Nathan, L., D. M. Twickler, M. T. Peters, P. J. Sánchez, and G. D. Wendel. 1993. Fetal syphilis: correlation of sonographic findings and rabbit infectivity testing of amniotic fluid. *J. Ultrasound Med.* **2:**97–101.

Nathan, L., V. R. Bohman, P. J. Sánchez, N. K. Leos, D. M. Twickler, and G. D. Wendel. 1997. In utero infection with *Treponema pallidum* in early pregnancy. *Prenat. Diag.* **17**(2)**:**119–123.

Noordhoek, G. T., E. C. Wolters, M. E. J. DeJonge, and J. D. A. Van Embden. 1991. Detection by polymerase chain reaction of *Treponema pallidum* DNA in cerebrospinal fluid from neurosyphilis patients before and after antibiotic treatment. *J. Clin. Microbiol.* **29:**1976–1984.

Norgard, M. V. 1993. Clinical and diagnostic issues of acquired and congenital syphilis encompassed in the current syphilis epidemic. *Curr. Opin. Infect. Dis.* **6:**9–16.

Orle, K. A., C. A. Gates, D. H. Martin, B. A. Body, and J. B. Weiss. 1996. Simultaneous PCR detection of *Haemophilus ducreyi, Treponema pallidum,* and herpes simplex virus types 1 and 2 from genital ulcers. *J. Clin. Microbiol.* **34:**49–54.

Pereyra, N., A. Parisi, and G. Baptista. 1997. Situación de la sífilis congénita en un municipio del gran Buenos Aires tres años de evaluación 1994–97, San Isidro, p. 187. *In Program and Abstracts of the XI Latin American Congress on Sexually Transmitted Diseases/V Pan-American Congress on AIDS.*

Petzoldt, D. 1975. Effect of spectinomycin on *T. pallidum* in incubating syphilis. *Br. J. Vener. Dis.* **51:**305–306.

Philipson, A., L. D. Sabath, and D. Charles. 1973. Transplacental passage of erythromycin and clindamycin. *N. Engl. J. Med.* **288:**1219–1221.

Pollack, H., W. Borkowsky, and K. Kransinski. 1990. Maternal syphilis is associated with enhanced perinatal HIV transmission, abstr. 1274. *In Program and Abstracts of the 30th Interscience Conference on Antimicrobial Agents and Chemotherapy.* American Society for Microbiology, Washington, D.C.

Qureshi, F., S. M. Jacques, and M. P. Reyes. 1993. Placental histopathology in syphilis. *Hum. Pathol.* **23:**779–784.

Radolf, J. D., P. J. Sánchez, K. F. Schulz, and F. K. Murphy. 1999. Congenital syphilis, p. 1165–1189. *In* K. K. Holmes, P. F. Sparling, P.-A. Mårdh, S. M. Lemon, W. E. Stamm, P. Piot, and J. N. Wasserheit (ed.), *Sexually Transmitted Diseases,* 3rd ed. McGraw-Hill, New York, N.Y.

Rawstron, S. A., and K. Bromberg. 1991. Comparison of maternal and newborn serologic tests for syphilis. *Am. J. Dis. Child.* **145:**1383–1388.

Rawstron, S. A., S. Jenkins, S. Blanchard, P.-W. Li, and K. Bromberg. 1993. Maternal and congenital syphilis in Brooklyn, NY: epidemiology, transmission, and diagnosis. *Am. J. Dis. Child.* **147:**727–731.

Reyes, M. P., N. Hunt, E. M. Ostrea, Jr., and D. George. 1993. Maternal/congenital syphilis in a large tertiary-care urban hospital. *Clin. Infect. Dis.* **17:**1041–1046.

Ricci, J. M., R. M. Fojaco, and J. O'Sullivan. 1989. Congenital syphilis: the University of Miami/Jackson Memorial Medical Center experience, 1986–1988. *Obstet. Gynecol.* **74:**687–693.

Risser, W. L., and L.-Y. Hwang. 1996. Problems in the current case definitions of congenital syphilis. *J. Pediatr.* **129:**499–505.

Rolfs, R. T., M. Goldberg, and R. G. Sharrar. 1990. Risk factors for syphilis: cocaine use and prostitution. *Am. J. Public Health* **80:**853–857.

Russell, P., and G. Altshuler. 1974. Placental abnormalities of congenital syphilis: a neglected aid to diagnosis. *Am. J. Dis. Child.* **128:**160–163.

Sánchez, P. J. 1992. Congenital syphilis. *Adv. Pediatr. Infect. Dis.* **7:**161–180.

Sánchez, P. J. 1998. Laboratory tests for congenital syphilis. *Pediatr. Infect. Dis. J.* **17:** 70–71.

Sánchez, P. J., and G. D. Wendel. 1997. Syphilis in pregnancy. *Clin. Perinatol.* **24:**71–90.

Sánchez, P. J., G. H. McCracken, G. D. Wendel, K. Olsen, N. Threlkeld, and M. V. Norgard. 1989. Molecular analysis of the fetal IgM response to *Treponema pallidum* antigens: implications for improved serodiagnosis of congenital syphilis. *J. Infect. Dis.* **159:**508–517.

Sánchez, P. J., G. D. Wendel, G. H. McCracken, and M. V. Norgard. 1990. Congenital syphilis and HIV infection. *Pediatr. Res.* **27:**276A. (Abstract.)

Sánchez, P. J., G. D. Wendel, M. Hal, J. Mayfield, and M. Eason. 1991a. Congenital syphilis: the Dallas experience. *Pediatr. Res.* **29:**286A. (Abstract.)

Sánchez, P. J., G. D. Wendel, and M. V. Norgard. 1991b. Congenital syphilis associated with negative results of maternal serologic tests at delivery. *Am J. Dis. Child.* **145:**967–969.

Sánchez, P. J., G. D. Wendel, and M. V. Norgard. 1992. IgM antibody to *Treponema pallidum* in cerebrospinal fluid of infants with congenital syphilis. *Am. J. Dis. Child.* **146:**1171–1175.

Sánchez, P. J., G. D. Wendel, E. Grimprel, M. Goldberg, M. Hall, O. Arencibia-Mireles, J. D. Radolf, and M. V. Norgard. 1993. Evaluation of molecular methodologies and rabbit infectivity testing for the diagnosis of congenital syphilis and neonatal central nervous system invasion by *Treponema pallidum. J. Infect. Dis.* **167:**148–157.

Sánchez, P. J., G. D. Wendel, F. Zeray, N. K. Leos, and J. Mayfield. 1994. Serologic follow-up in congenital syphilis: what's the point? abstr. L22, p. 182. *In Abstracts of the 34th Interscience Conference on Antimicrobial Agents and Chemotherapy.* American Society for Microbiology, Washington, D.C.

Satin, A. J., D. M. Twickler, and G. D. Wendel, Jr. 1992. Congenital syphilis associated with dilation of fetal small bowel: a case report. *J. Ultrasound Med.* **11:**49–52.

Schmid, G. P. 1996. Serologic screening for syphilis. Rationale, cost, and realpolitik. *Sex. Transm. Dis.* **23:**45–50.

Schmitz, J. L., K. S. Gertis, C. Mauney, L. V. Stamm, and J. D. Folds. 1994. Laboratory diagnosis of congenital syphilis by immunoglobulin M (IgM) and IgA immunoblotting. *Clin. Diagn. Lab. Immunol.* **1:**32–37.

Schulz, K. F., W. Cates, Jr., and P. R. O'Mara. 1987. Pregnancy loss, infant death, and suffering: legacy of syphilis and gonorrhoea in Africa. *Genitourin. Med.* **63:**320–325.

Sheffield, J. S., J. Alexander, D. D. McIntire, P. Sanchez, and G. Wendel, Jr. 1998. Serologic response after antepartum secondary syphilis treatment with one vs. two doses of benzathine penicillin G. *Am. J. Obstet. Gynecol.* **178:**5210, abstr. 757.

Silverstein, A. M. 1962. Congenital syphilis and the timing of immunogenesis in the human fetus. *Nature* **194:**196–197.

Sison, C. G., E. M. Ostrea, Jr., M. P. Reyes, and V. Salari. 1997. The resurgence of congenital syphilis: a cocaine-related problem. *J. Pediatr.* **130:**289–292.

South, M. A., D. H. Short, and J. M. Knox. 1964. Failures of erythromycin estolate therapy in utero syphilis. *JAMA* **190:**70–71.

Southwick, K., S. Blanco, A. Santander, G. Seonae, M. Estenssoro, F. Torrico, W. Brady, V. Pope, J. Lewis, M. Fears, and W. Levine. 1997. Rapid assessment of maternal and congenital syphilis in Bolivia, 1996, p. 96. *In Program and Abstracts of the International Congress of Sexually Transmitted Diseases.*

Stoll, B. J., F. K. Lee, S. Larsen, E. Hale, D. Schwartz, R. J. Rice, R. Ashby, R. Holmes, and A. J. Nahmias. 1993. Clinical and serologic evaluation of neonates for congenital syphilis: a continuing diagnostic dilemma. *J. Infect. Dis.* **167:**1093–1099.

Taber, L., and B. Baughn. 1991. Long-term follow-up of infants born of mothers with past or active infection with *Treponema pallidum*, p. 155, abstr. 337. *In Program and Abstracts of the 31st Interscience Conference on Antimicrobial Agents and Chemotherapy.* American Society for Microbiology, Washington, D.C.

Theus, S. A., D. A. Harrich, R. Gaynor, J. D. Radolf, and M. V. Norgard. 1998. *Treponema pallidum*, lipoproteins, and synthetic lipoprotein analogues induce human immunodeficiency virus type 1 gene expression in monocytes via NF-kB activation. *J. Infect. Dis.* **177:**941–950.

Wasserheit, J. N. 1992. Epidemiological synergy. Interrelationships between human immunodeficiency virus infection and other sexually transmitted diseases. *Sex. Transm. Dis.* **19:**61–71.

Watts, T. E., S. A. Larsen, and S. T. Brown. 1984. A case-control study of stillbirths at a teaching hospital in Zambia, 1979–80: serological investigations for selected infectious agents. *Bull. W. H. O.* **62:**803–808.

Webber, M. P., G. Lambert, D. A. Bateman, and W. A. Hauser. 1993. Maternal risk factors for congenital syphilis: a case-control study. *Am. J. Epidemiol.* **137:**415–422.

Wendel, G. D. 1988. Gestational and congenital syphilis. *Clin. Perinatol.* **15:**287–303.

Wendel, G. D., Jr., B. J. Stark, R. B. Jamison, R. D. Molina, and T. J. Sullivan. 1985. Penicillin allergy and desensitization in serious infections during pregnancy. *N. Engl. J. Med.* **312:**1229–1232.

Wendel, G. D., M. C. Maberry, J. T. Christmas, M. S. Goldberg, and M. V. Norgard. 1989. Examination of amniotic fluid in diagnosing congenital syphilis with fetal death. *Obstet. Gynecol.* **74:**967–970.

Wendel, G. D., P. J. Sánchez, M. T. Peters, T. W. Harstad, L. L. Potter, and M. V. Norgard. 1991. Identification of *Treponema pallidum* in amniotic fluid and fetal blood from pregnancies complicated by congenital syphilis. *Obstet. Gynecol.* **78:**890–895.

Wicher, K., G. T. Noordhoek, F. Abbruscato, and V. Wicher. 1992. Detection of *Treponema pallidum* in early syphilis by DNA amplification. *J. Clin. Microbiol.* **40:**497–500.

Zenker, P. N., and S. M. Berman. 1991. Congenital syphilis: trends and recommendations for evaluation and management. *J. Pediatr. Infect. Dis.* **10:**516–522.

Zoechling, N., E. M. Schluepen, H. P. Soyer, H. Kerl, and M. Volkenandt. 1997. Molecular detection of *Treponema pallidum* in secondary and tertiary syphilis. *Br. J. Dermatol.* **136:**683–686.

9
Gonorrhea

Stephen A. Morse and Consuelo M. Beck-Sagué

Until 1994, gonorrhea was the most common reportable infectious disease in the United States (CDC, 1996). Nationwide, the incidence of gonorrhea has declined since 1975 (CDC, 1997). However, in some subpopulations, such as African American adolescents, it rose in the 1990s, consistent with reported increases in the proportion of adolescent women who report having had sexual intercourse and other social and behavioral factors (CDC, 1991, 1996; Webster et al., 1993). The highest rates per 100,000 population continue to occur among women of childbearing age (CDC, 1996).

The purpose of this chapter is (i) to review the pathophysiology of gonorrhea during pregnancy, (ii) to summarize epidemiologic data regarding gonorrhea among pregnant women, and (iii) to discuss the manifestations of maternal and infant infections, with special emphasis on principles of prevention and management.

PATHOPHYSIOLOGY

Neisseria gonorrhoeae is a sexually transmitted bacterium which infects columnar and transitional epithelium of the genitourinary tract, including the urethra, endocervix, and anal canal, and the conjunctivae and pharynx. Humans are the only natural hosts. Contiguous spread along mucosal surfaces in females may result in endometritis, salpingitis, peritonitis, and bartholinitis. Gonococci can also spread systemically (causing gonococcemia) and can cause complications which may include arthritis, tenosynovitis, dermatitis, endocarditis, and meningitis.

Stephen A. Morse and Consuelo M. Beck-Sagué, Division of AIDS, Sexually Transmitted Diseases and Tuberculosis Laboratory Research, and Office of Minority Health, National Center for Infectious Diseases, Centers for Disease Control and Prevention, Atlanta, GA 30333.

Sexually Transmitted Diseases and Adverse Outcomes of Pregnancy
Edited by P. J. Hitchcock, H. T. MacKay, J. N. Wasserheit, and R. Binder
©1999 American Society for Microbiology, Washington, D.C.

Mucosal Attachment

The most critical interactions of gonococci with their host occur at the mucosal surface. To survive in this environment, the gonococcus must first attach to epithelial cells and then multiply. The organism must also resist any natural host defense mechanisms, as well as acquired immune mechanisms that may be the result of a prior gonococcal infection or colonization with an antigenically related microorganism. Surface components of the gonococcus play an important role in the attachment of this microorganism to host cells and evasion of the host immune system.

Pili are involved in the initial phase of attachment (Swanson, 1973) and may help to overcome repulsive forces between two similarly charged cells (Heckels et al., 1976). Gonococcal pili undergo both phase and antigenic variation at a high frequency (So et al., 1985; Hagblom et al., 1985). There are several nonpilus surface ligands which are also involved in attachment, including opacity-associated (Opa) proteins (Bessen and Gotschlich, 1986) and a 37-kDa protein that binds to certain host cell glycolipids (Paruchuri et al., 1990). Opa proteins are members of a set of closely related outer membrane proteins. A single strain may have the ability to produce as many as 11 different Opa proteins; however, only a few, or none, of the Opa proteins are expressed at any one time. Specific Opa proteins appear to facilitate the attachment of gonococci to different host tissues, such as cervical, endometrial, and conjunctival (Kupsch et al., 1993; Simon and Rest, 1992; Dekker et al., 1990). Variation in the expression of these Opa proteins occurs at a rate of about 10^3 per cell per generation (Murphy et al., 1989). The molecular events responsible for the variation in Opa proteins and pili have been extensively studied and are not discussed further in this chapter. However, in the context of gonococcal pathogenesis, this high-frequency antigenic variation of Opa proteins and pili enables the organism to escape the host immune response as well as providing specific ligands for different cell receptors.

Gonococci attach to and subsequently invade epithelial cells in vitro (Makino et al., 1991; Weel et al., 1991) via a mechanism believed to involve parasite-directed endocytosis (McGee et al., 1988). Similarly, gonococci have been shown to adhere selectively to the nonciliated cells of human fallopian tube organ cultures (McGee et al., 1976). Approximately 20 h after infection of these organ cultures, gonococci are transported into the nonciliated epithelial cells. After ingestion, the gonococcus is transported across the epithelial cytoplasm to the basal side of the cell. Membrane fusion occurs, and viable gonococci are released into the subepithelial space (McGee et al., 1981; Gregg et al., 1981). Gonococcal infection results in loss of cilia activity followed by sloughing of the ciliated cells from the mucosa (Gregg et al., 1981).

Mucosal Damage

Rather than damaging the mucosa directly, gonococci elaborate one or more products that may be responsible for initiating this damage. Both lipooligosaccharide (LOS) (Gregg et al., 1981) and peptidoglycan fragments (Melly et al., 1984) have cytotoxic activity. Outer membrane proteins, such as protein I (Por), and some but not all Opa proteins may facilitate the invasion of epithelial cells by *N. gonorrhoeae.* All of the above-mentioned studies were carried out in vitro; however, there is evidence from in vivo studies which suggest that invasion of mucosal cells can occur during a natural infection. Harkness reported that histological examination of mucosal surfaces infected with gonococci revealed mucosal erosion and the presence of gonococci in submucosal tissues (Harkness, 1948). Examination of cervical biopsy specimens from women with culture-proven infection by light microscopy revealed a loss of surface columnar epithelial cells (Kiviat et al., 1990). Electron microscopic examination of endocervical sites from infected women has revealed intraepithelial gonococci (Ward et al., 1975).

Recent evidence suggests that gonococcal LOS is important in the pathogenesis of gonorrhea. McGee et al. (1992) have shown that LOS stimulated the production of tumor necrosis factor (TNF) by cells of the human fallopian tube mucosa. Epithelial damage appeared to be related to the production of TNF by fallopian tube lymphocytes. The addition of recombinant TNF-α damaged fallopian tube mucosa in a dose-dependent manner and produced epithelial damage with the same ultrastructural features as those observed during gonococcal infection. TNF may act in concert with other cytokines such as interleukin-1 (IL-1) and IL-6 to cause the tissue damage (McGee et al., 1992).

Pregnancy Complications

A similar mechanism may be responsible for the pregnancy complications caused by *N. gonorrhoeae.* The decidua, the epithelial lining of the endometrium lining the uterus, is macrophagelike in many of its properties. The decidual cell responds to bacterial endotoxin (and LOS) by producing large amounts of prostaglandins (Casey and MacDonald, 1988). Decidual tissue, in vitro, produces IL-1 and TNF-α (Casey and MacDonald, 1988), as do macrophages (Beutler and Cerami, 1986; Gery et al., 1972). It has been hypothesized that the activation of decidua is the penultimate event in the initiation of parturition (Casey and MacDonald, 1988). Therefore, gonococcal infection, which is known to stimulate the production of TNF-α and possibly other cytokines, may activate the decidua resulting in preterm labor.

An alternative mechanism was proposed by Elliott et al. (1990), who hypothesized that the ascending spread of gonococci to the chorioamnion might induce premature labor by directly activating the prostaglandin parturition pathway. This mechanism would require the activity of a gonococcal phospholipase A on host phospholipids with the subsequent release of arachidonic acid, a precursor of prostaglandin biosynthesis. Gonococci possess several outer membrane phospholipases which are capable of releasing arachidonic acid from phospholipids (Cacciapuoti et al., 1979). However, *N. gonorrhoeae* also incorporates exogenous arachidonic acid into its cellular phospholipids (Chen, 1988) and thus would reduce the concentration available for prostaglandin biosynthesis. Further studies are necessary to define the exact mechanism by which gonococcal infection induces premature labor.

EPIDEMIOLOGY OF GONORRHEA IN PREGNANT WOMEN

The prevalence of gonorrhea among pregnant women varies among populations in developing and developed countries (Table 1) (Charles et al., 1970; Brunham and Embree, 1992; Corman et al., 1974; Stutz et al., 1976; Jones et al., 1976; Amstey and Steadman, 1976; van der Lugt et al., 1980; Goh et al., 1981; Frau and Alexander, 1985; Welgemoed et al., 1986; Plummer et al., 1987; Vuyllsteke et al., 1993; Campos-Outcalt and Ryan, 1995; Behets et al., 1995; Mayoud et al., 1995). The prevalence of gonorrhea among screened U.S. pregnant women has ranged from <1 to 7.5%; in 1983, the last year for which national data were available, the prevalence of positive cervical cultures for *N. gonorrhoeae* from prenatal and obstetric clinics and hospital inpatient obstetrics services ranged from 2.2 to 2.9% (Frau and Alexander, 1985). In one recent study of minority women in a U.S. population, 1.2% had gonorrhea (Frau and Alexander, 1985). In antenatal populations in some developing countries, prevalence rates have varied considerably, ranging from 0.5% in the prenatal clinic at the University Hospital, Kuala Lumpur, Malaysia, to 15% in antenatal patients in Cameroon (Brunham and Embree, 1992; Goh et al., 1981). Some of these rates may be underestimates, since laboratory procedures varied by site.

The majority of pregnant women with gonorrhea are asymptomatic; the proportion of symptomatic patients among pregnant women with gonorrhea has been reported to be as low as 1.2% (Charles et al., 1970; Jones et al., 1976). Thus, syndromic approaches recommended for low-resource areas reportedly may have low sensitivity (Vuyllsteke et al., 1993; Behets et al., 1995; Mayoud et al., 1995); scoring systems that incorporate behavioral and demographic risk markers may represent an affordable alternative (Vuyllsteke et al., 1993; Mayoud et al., 1995). These indicators and predictors include behavioral risk factors for infection, such as young age and more than one partner over the last year, polygamous marriage, previous child born more than 5 years earlier (suggesting subfertility in a developing-country setting related to sexually transmitted diseases), any previous child (the absence of whom suggests recent initiation of sexual activity), and any

Table 1 Prevalence of *N. gonorrhoeae* infection in selected populations of pregnant women in developing and developed countries, 1970 to 1989[a]

Country	Year[a]	Prenatal population	Prevalence (no. infected/ total no. tested) (%)	Reference
United States	1970	Hospital clinic	158/2,160 (7.3)	Charles et al., 1970
Nigeria	1972	Prenatal clinic	7/208 (3.4)	Brunham and Embree, 1992[b]
United States	1974	University hospital/ clinic	29/723 (4.0)	Corman et al., 1974
Thailand	1976	U.S. Army hospital/ clinic	45/424 (10.6)	Stutz et al., 1976
United States	1976	Public clinic	92/1,229 (7.5)	Jones et al., 1976
United States	1976	Hospital/clinic	222/5,065 (4.4)	Amstey and Steadman, 1976
Netherlands	1980	Abortion clinic	13/1,688 (0.8)	van der Lugt et al., 1980
Cameroon	1980	Prenatal clinic	106/720 (14.7)	Brunham and Embree, 1992[b]
Malaysia	1981	University hospital	4/744 (0.5)	Goh et al., 1981
United States	1985	Health department/clinic	5,163/235,492 (2.2)	Frau and Alexander, 1985
United States	1985	Hospital inpatients	136/5,077 (2.7)	Frau and Alexander, 1985
United States	1985	Community health center	1,477/51,239 (2.9)	Frau and Alexander, 1985
South Africa	1986	Hospital/clinic	137/1,200 (11.4)	Welgemoed et al., 1986
Fiji	1987	Prenatal clinic	10/430 (2.3)	Brunham and Embree, 1992[b]
Kenya	1987	Maternity hospital	49/728 (6.7)	Plummer et al., 1987
South Africa	1989	Prenatal	11/193 (5.7)	Brunham and Embree, 1992[b]
Zaire	1993	Prenatal	19/1,160 (1.6)	Vuyllsteke et al., 1993
United States	1995	Prenatal	4/347 (1.2)	Campos-Outcalt and Ryan, 1995
Haiti	1995	Prenatal	36/898 (4.0)	Behets et al., 1995
Tanzania	1995	Prenatal	20/964 (2.1)	Mayaud et al., 1995

[a] Year of publication of study.
[b] Reference includes a summary of original studies in developing countries (1972 to 1989).

symptom related to genital infection (Mayoud et al., 1995). Douching may be associated with a higher risk of gonorrhea among pregnant women in some settings (Josef et al., 1996).

Cervical gonorrhea appears to be a significant risk factor for endocervical *Chlamydia trachomatis* coinfection in pregnant women (Christmas et al., 1989). Both of these infections are associated with vertical transmission and adverse pregnancy outcomes, as well as infant conjunctivitis and other evidence of perinatal infection (Alexander and Harrison, 1983; Schachter et al., 1986). The effects of coinfection on the course of either infection are unknown, but coinfection may increase the likelihood of vertical transmission in some populations (see below).

Pharyngeal infection appears to be somewhat higher in antenatal populations than in similar nonpregnant female populations; in two studies, the throat was the only infected site in 15 and 36% of pregnant women screened (Campos-Outcalt and Ryan, 1995; Behets et al., 1995). This finding has been associated with changes in sexual behavior during pregnancy, such as a relative increase in fellatio (Solberg et al., 1973). Since pharyngeal gonococcal infection has been diagnosed among even pregnant women who deny fellatio, some researchers have suggested that the pharynx, in addition to the endocervix, be cultured. Infections may be acquired after the first prenatal visit, so that cultures obtained late in pregnancy and during delivery may be needed to maximize the yield of prenatal screening (Solberg et al., 1973).

Surveillance of *N. gonorrhoeae* isolates has demonstrated the ability of this organism to readily develop resistance to antimicrobial agents (Lind, 1997; Gorwitz et al., 1993). Of isolates referred to the U.S. National Gonococcal Isolate Surveillance Project in 1996, 29% were resistant to penicillin, tetracycline, or both (CDC, 1997). Moreover, while no documented clinical treatment failures have been observed with the currently recommended ceftriaxone treatment regimen, the recently reported decreased susceptibility of gonococcal isolates to ciprofloxacin in the United States is worrisome; clinical treatment failures associated with resistant strains have been reported (Lind, 1997; Van Dyck et al., 1997; Gorwitz et al., 1993; CDC, 1995, 1997, 1998a).

ADVERSE MATERNAL OUTCOMES

Disseminated Gonococcal Infection

Although gonorrhea is frequently asymptomatic during pregnancy, disseminated gonococcal infection occasionally occurs, generally in the late third trimester or after delivery (Ross, 1996) (Table 2). Pregnancy has long been recognized as a precipitating factor to dissemination in 28 to 40% of women with gonococcal arthritis, and either pregnancy or menstruation precipitates dissemination in over 70% of women (Ross, 1996; Taylor et al., 1966). Al-

Table 2 Adverse outcomes of pregnancy associated with *N. gonorrhoeae* infection

Frequency	Outcome in:	
	Mother	Infant
High	Premature and/or prolonged rupture of membranes Preterm labor	Prematurity Fetal distress Low birth weight
Medium	Amnionitis	Ophthalmia
Low	Endometritis PID Disseminated gonococcal infection, arthritis	Disseminated gonococcal infection, arthritis
Rare	Meningitis, endocarditis	Sepsis Endocarditis, meningitis

though gonococcal arthritis has been diagnosed primarily in the third trimester, half of the pregnant women in one series were in the second trimester at the time of dissemination (Ross, 1996; Holmes et al., 1971).

Before the introduction of antimicrobial treatment for gonorrhea, disseminated gonococcal infection was considerably more common in men than in women (Graber et al., 1968). The predominance of women in most series since the availability of sulfonamides and penicillin appears to be related to the fact that women with gonorrhea are much more likely than men to be asymptomatic. They may therefore be less likely to receive early treatment when the infection is still confined to the pharynx or anogenital sites (Ross, 1996).

Arthritis is the most common manifestation of disseminated gonococcal infection; there are two clinical forms (Holmes et al., 1971; Keiser et al., 1968). One form presents with fever, chills, bacteremia, and polyarticular arthritis or tenosynovitis. This polyarthritis generally presents with scant effusion and affects the knees, wrists, ankles, elbow, and small joints of the hands. Typical skin lesions are usually seen with this type of gonococcal arthritis. The skin lesions begin as small red papules or petechiae that either resolve or evolve through vesicular, then pustular stages to form a necrotic center on a hemorrhagic base. The second, monarticular form typically presents with joint effusion, absence of bacteremia and skin lesions, and positive cultures for *N. gonorrhoeae* from the synovial fluid. These two clinical forms may represent successive stages of the same process, with the bacteremic stage preceding the septic joint stage.

Subacute gonococcal endocarditis, most frequently involving the aortic valve, has been found in pregnant women with disseminated gonococcal infection and is generally preceded by polyarthritis (Holmes et al., 1971; Niles and Lowe, 1966). Myocarditis and pericarditis are frequent findings in gonococcemic patients. Gonococcal meningitis has also been found during pregnancy.

Pelvic Inflammatory Disease

Pelvic inflammatory disease (PID), or acute salpingitis, is probably the most common severe complication of gonorrhea, and both gonorrhea and PID appear to be declining in developed countries (Kamwendo et al., 1996). Among the sequelae of PID are infertility due to tubal occlusion, chronic abdominal pain, and occasionally death, generally due to rupture of tubo-ovarian abscesses, resulting in generalized peritonitis. Ectopic pregnancy also appears to be strongly associated with past PID (odds ratios range, 2.0 to 7.5) and with gonorrhea (odds ratios range, 2.5 to 5.5) (Chow et al., 1987).

The number of hospitalizations for PID in the United States decreased during the 1980s, whereas the number of patients seen in physicians' offices did not vary significantly (Rolfs et al., 1992). This decrease may indicate a decrease in the incidence of the disease and/or of its more severe manifestations. The decreasing incidence of gonorrhea also may be related to a lower incidence of acute PID (CDC, 1996, 1997).

Although gonorrhea in pregnancy is generally asymptomatic, abnormal adnexal findings are not unusual in recently infected women, with some patients presenting with symptoms and findings suggestive of PID, including cervical motion tenderness. Although PID in pregnancy is uncommon, it must be considered in the differential diagnosis of the acute abdomen during pregnancy (Yip et al., 1993).

Most authorities consider that gonococcal PID rarely occurs during pregnancy because it is impossible for the gonococci to traverse the barrier of the intact cervix and uterus during pregnancy. Nevertheless, some possible mechanisms of infection in the pregnant patient have been proposed. They include infection at the time of fertilization or soon after, before the uterine cavity has become closed (about 12 weeks), vascular or lymphatic spread, flare-up of preexisting infection, instrumentation or ascending infection associated with threatened abortion, and intrauterine bleeding (Rolfs et al., 1992; Yip et al., 1993). While a pelvic abscess can be discovered at any time during gestation, acute PID in pregnant women, consistent with the mechanisms proposed, typically occurs in the first trimester (Blanchard et al., 1987). Since, in general, pelvic abscesses and acute PID can be managed medically, awareness of these entities may spare pregnant women unnecessary surgical procedures. Even with prompt medical treatment, fetal loss is common in pregnancies complicated by PID, approximating 50% (Yip et al., 1993).

Amnionitis and Perinatal Complications

Maternal gonorrhea without ascending infections is also associated with adverse effects on the course of pregnancy. This effect of maternal gonococcal infection was first established by the observation that recovery of gonococci from neonatal orogastric aspirates was associated with significantly increased risks of prematurity, premature rupture of the fetal membranes, maternal peripartum fever, and a clinical presentation consistent with sepsis in the infant (Handsfield et al., 1973). Perinatal mortality has been reported to be over twice as high among infants of mothers who were culture positive for *N. gonorrhoeae* than among infants of culture-negative mothers attending the same clinic (Handsfield et al., 1973). Studies have since confirmed the association of maternal gonorrhea with gonococcal chorioamnionitis, upper genital tract infections, intrauterine growth retardation, premature rupture of membranes, prematurity, low birth weight, fetal death or a complicated neonatal course, and endometritis following elective abortion (Plummer et al., 1987; Wendel and Wendel, 1993; Donders et al., 1993; Burkman et al., 1976; Yvert et al., 1985; Alger et al., 1988; Schulz et al., 1987; Elliott et al., 1990).

Maternal gonorrhea may not be the sole risk factor for these outcomes. Gonococcal infection may be a marker for other genital organisms that may adversely affect the course of pregnancy. However, the likelihood that gonorrhea and amnionitis due to *N. gonorrhoeae* truly have an independent adverse effect on the course of a pregnancy is suggested by the fact that timely specific treatment for asymptomatic gestational gonorrhea or gonococcal amnionitis appears to result in reduction of maternal infectious complications, reduction of some neonatal complications after delivery, or reduction of endometritis after abortion (Plummer et al., 1987; Elliott et al., 1990; Owen et al., 1993; Blackwell et al., 1993).

It is estimated that the odds ratios for prematurity and postpartum PID associated with maternal gonorrhea are 2.9 and 4.4, respectively (Brunham and Embree, 1992). Therefore, in a population with 1.2 million births and a prenatal gonorrhea prevalence of 6%, it was estimated that 10,000 cases of premature birth were due to gonococcal infections, of which 1,500 resulted in infant deaths, and that 40,000 mothers developed postpartum pelvic infection, of whom up to 8,000 became infertile as a result (Brunham and Embree, 1992).

ADVERSE INFANT OUTCOMES

Vertical Transmission

Gonococcal infection is probably only rarely transmitted through intact placental membranes, and contact with an infected birth canal is the most frequent mode of transmission of the infection from mother to child. The risk of transmission from an infected mother to her child in the absence of prophylaxis is estimated at 30 to 50% (Charles et al., 1970; Laga et al., 1989). Instillation of 2% silver nitrate drops in the newborn infant's eyes can reduce the risk to <2% if given shortly after birth. In one study, the transmission rate was significantly higher among mothers with concomitant chlamydial infection (68 and 31% in those with and without, respectively) or with endometritis (Laga et al., 1986). Penicillinase production by the infecting strain did not appear to affect the risk of transmission.

The most common manifestation of infant infection is gonococcal ophthalmia neonatorum. Recognized arthritis, sepsis, and meningitis are much less common.

Gonococcal Ophthalmia

Epidemiology

Before the introduction of silver nitrate prophylaxis in 1880, the incidence of gonococcal ophthalmia neonatorum varied from 1 to 4%, and 20 to 79% of children in institutions for the blind had a history of gonococcal ophthalmia (Armstrong et al., 1976).

The introduction of ocular prophylaxis in the decade of the 1880s resulted in a dramatic decline in the incidence of gonococcal ophthalmia in most of the developed world. Nevertheless, the risk of gonococcal ophthalmia remains high in many developing countries and in areas of developed countries with a high prevalence of gonorrhea among women of childbearing age (Armstrong et al., 1976; Frost et al., 1987; Doraiswamy et al., 1983; CDC, 1983). Prevalence rates of 2 to 4% are common in much of Africa (Schulz et al., 1992). A seasonal incidence has been observed in the incidence of gonococcal ophthalmia, with peaks in the third quarter of the year (Armstrong et al., 1976). In one study, 16% of neonates with gonococcal ophthalmia had corneal involvement, but in most series and case reports in both developing and developed countries, no evidence of corneal involvement has been noted (Armstrong et al., 1976; Frost et al., 1987; Doraiswamy et al., 1983; CDC, 1983; Schulz et al., 1992; Desenclos et al., 1992).

Gonococcal ophthalmia neonatorum caused by *N. gonorrhoeae* strains resistant to antimicrobial agents has been reported despite ocular prophylaxis with antimicrobial agents (Mabey et al., 1987). However, the occurrence of ophthalmia neonatorum due to susceptible strains after ocular prophylaxis suggests that factors other than antimicrobial resistance may play a role in the failure of prophylaxis, particularly prophylaxis with erythromycin, to prevent clinically apparent ophthalmia (CDC, 1983; Schulz et al., 1992); these factors include prolonged rupture of membranes, well-established infection at the time of birth, and, possibly, delay in application of the antimicrobial agent (Frost et al., 1987). In one series, 44 of 46 cases of gonococcal ophthalmia occurred in spite of silver nitrate prophylaxis, with chemical conjunctivitis providing confirmatory evidence of proper installation and onset of antiseptic activity (Frost et al., 1987).

Clinical Manifestations

The severity of gonococcal ophthalmia ranges from a mild conjunctivitis, similar to chemical conjunctivitis, to a devastating process resulting in corneal ulceration and perforation and eventually blindness if left untreated (Armstrong et al., 1976). Although occasionally seen in adults and in sexually abused children, gonococcal ophthalmia is most often seen in infants, generally within 4 to 6.5 days after birth (range, 1 to 28 days) (Armstrong et al., 1976; Frost et al., 1987; Desenclos et al., 1992).

Typically, gonococcal ophthalmia is bilateral and the discharge is generally purulent. Gonococcal ophthalmia tends to be more severe in terms of palpebral edema, conjunctival injection, and purulent discharge than is ophthalmia caused by *C. trachomatis* and ophthalmia not attributable to either pathogen (Armstrong et al., 1976; Mabey et al., 1987). Concomitant gonococcal and chlamydial ophthalmia does not appear to differ significantly in severity from that due to *N. gonorrhoeae* alone.

Severe inflammation of the conjunctivae is associated with a serosanguinous exudate and may produce inflammatory membranes which bleed if an attempt is made to remove them; these membranes are replaced by scar tissue in the conjunctivae as the disease resolves (Wilfert and Gutman, 1987). Corneal involvement presents initially as diffuse epithelial edema, giving the cornea a hazy, smoky-grey appearance. Infiltrations appear as coarse opacities in the sclera, which enlarge and then ulcerate within 2 to 3 weeks. Ulceration is followed by perforation. Corneal scarring generally follows ulceration and perforation and often results in blindness due to involvement of the central cornea.

Disseminated Gonococcal Infection

In most cases, gonococcal infection in newborns is localized, although cough, irritability, or poor feeding may accompany gonococcal conjunctivitis. Nonspecific symptoms commencing within 1 to 2 weeks of birth, giving way to fever, irritability, and poor feeding often herald the onset of dissemination. The incidence of dissemination is unknown, but is probably low. When dissemination does occur, it typically presents as polyarthritis, although a single joint may be most prominently involved (Glaser et al., 1966). Specific signs of joint involvement have been seen as early as 3 days of age but are more commonly seen 1 to 3 weeks after birth. The ankle and knee joints are the most commonly affected, but the hips, arms, hands, and feet may be involved. Generally, the infant presents with little or no spontaneous movement of the involved joint, and physical findings may include swelling, erythema, and tenderness. Skin lesions such as those seen in adults with disseminated gonococcal infections are rarely seen in neonates.

Many infants with disseminated infections have a recognized source of infection, usually ophthalmia. Severe panophthalmitis, caused by extensive local involvement, can serve as a portal of entry for bloodstream infection and can result in arthritis, meningitis, and even endocarditis, proctitis, or stomatitis (Frau and Alexander, 1985; Glaser et al., 1966; Bradford and Kelley, 1933). Meningitis has only rarely been recognized as a complication of dissemination (Frau and Alexander, 1985; D'Auria et al., 1975). Meningitis presents with nonspecific symptoms of sepsis, including irritability, fever or hypothermia, and poor feeding within the first weeks of life. Dissemination has also followed gonococcal infections of scalp wounds occurring during fetal monitoring (D'Auria et al., 1975). These wounds may produce extensive local inflammation and necrosis. Mucous membranes of the infant, including the oropharynx, vagina, rectum, and urethra, may serve as portals of entry for infection.

PREVENTION

Prenatal Screening

Ocular prophylaxis is not entirely effective in preventing neonatal complications and does not address the multiple prenatal and perinatal complications of gonorrhea among pregnant women. Therefore, the most important strategy in the prevention of these complications is screening and prompt treatment of pregnant women (Frau and Alexander, 1985).

Primary prevention through the use of barrier contraceptives has generally not been widely promoted during pregnancy, because of the difficulty in introducing such methods outside the context of contraception. However, the widespread promotion of condoms in relation to prevention of human immunodeficiency virus transmission may provide the impetus to introduce the use of condoms during pregnancy in some populations.

Screening with culture at the first prenatal visit is recommended as the ideal method of prevention, particularly in high-risk populations. However, poor results have been observed when cervical swabs for culture are transported to laboratories before inoculation of culture media (Jones et al., 1976). Therefore, prenatal screening with culture requires the ability to directly inoculate Thayer-Martin medium (or another appropriate selective medium) in the examining room and the ability to confirm the identity of *N. gonorrhoeae.* Selective screening in groups at highest risk may increase the cost-effectiveness of prenatal culture screening. Gram stain and rapid enzyme immunoassays have been disappointing due to low sensitivity and poor predictive value of negative results in female populations outside of sexually transmitted disease clinics, and they cannot substitute for culture screening (Donders et al., 1996). Probe-based assays are as sensitive as culture (Limberger et al., 1992). Nucleic acid amplification tests (such as PCR or ligase chain reaction) are commercially available and offer increased sensitivity for detecting the presence of *N. gonorrhoeae* in anogenital specimens (Quinn, 1997); however, the high cost of these tests may prohibit widespread usage. The use of noninvasive specimen collection, such as first-catch urine, together with a nucleic acid amplification test for *N. gonorrhoeae* and *C. trachomatis*, may be advantageous for screening pregnant women.

Since 18 to 30% of patients diagnosed during pregnancy reacquired gonococcal infections during pregnancy despite efforts to treat their sexual partners, all patients with evidence of gonococcal infection early in pregnancy should undergo repeat testing during the last weeks of gestation (Charles et al., 1970; Jones et al., 1976).

Prenatal care tends to be underutilized due to unavailability and/or multiple other factors in precisely those populations where a higher incidence of gonorrhea and other sexually transmitted diseases may be seen (CDC, 1994). For this reason, female partners of men diagnosed with gonorrhea should be aggressively sought and treated. Moreover, all women diagnosed with gonorrhea or any other pathogen that can be transmitted vertically should be questioned about the date of last menstrual period, and urine pregnancy testing should be offered, if appropriate.

Mass Treatment

In some populations where the prevalence of gonococcal infections in pregnant women exceeds 10% and adequate screening is possible, mass third-trimester treatment of pregnant women may be cost-effective (Laga et al., 1986). Such a decision should be contemplated only when the risk of bacterial antibiotic resistance, side effects, and failure to identify and treat infected sexual partners, resulting in unrecognized reinfections, can be taken into account.

Ocular Prophylaxis at Birth

The introduction of neonatal silver nitrate ocular prophylaxis has been heralded as one of the great public health triumphs and has resulted in well-recognized reduction of neonatal disease (Frau and Alexander, 1985; Laga et al., 1986; Coulaud, 1991; Rothenberg, 1979). Moreover, discontinuation of prophylaxis in populations with a big prevalence of gonorrhea generally results in prompt resurgence of gonococcal ophthalmia (Armstrong et al., 1976). Silver nitrate prophylaxis should be performed as soon after birth as possible in the delivery room, ideally before the infant opens her or his eyes. The infant's eyelids should be cleaned before instillation of the drops in the conjunctival sacs. No cleaning or rinsing of the infant's eyes should be performed after instillation of the drops.

The solution recommended is a 1% aqueous silver nitrate solution (Coulaud, 1991; Rothenberg, 1979; Laga et al., 1988; CDC, 1998b). In Crede's original study, a 2% solution was used, and most efficacy studies report the use of 2% solution (Rothenberg, 1979). Inadvertent use of higher concentrations of silver nitrate due to evaporation has reportedly caused damage to newborns' eyes.

In most settings, *C. trachomatis* is a more frequent cause of neonatal conjunctivitis than is *N. gonorrhoeae* (Armstrong et al., 1976; Frost et al., 1987). Silver nitrate prophylaxis does not appear to be as effective in preventing chlamydial conjunctivitis (reduction of incidence by 68%) as it is in preventing gonococcal conjunctivitis (reduction of incidence by 83 to 95%) among newborns exposed to maternal infection (Rothenberg, 1979; Laga et al., 1988). This finding has prompted studies to determine whether prophylaxis with antimicrobial agents effective against both organisms may be preferable.

Despite concern that tetracycline may not be effective in areas with a high prevalence of tetracycline-resistant organisms, tetracycline ointment has been shown to be very effective, resulting in a reduction in the incidence of gonococcal ophthalmia by 93% and reduction in the incidence of chlamydial ophthalmia by 77% (Laga et al., 1988). These data are limited by the lack of studies assessing the effect of tetracycline resistance on prophylaxis failure. There is even less data to support prophylaxis with erythromycin. Despite concerns about sensitization and drug susceptibility, both tetracycline ophthalmic ointment (1%) and erythromycin ophthalmic ointment (0.5%) in a single application are recommended as alternatives to silver nitrate for neonatal ocular prophylaxis (Quinn, 1997).

MANAGEMENT

Treatment of Pregnant Women with Gonorrhea

Pregnant women who are diagnosed with uncomplicated gonococcal infections or who are the sexual partners of men with gonorrhea should be treated with ceftriaxone (125 mg intramuscularly) in a single dose or with cefixime (400 mg orally) in a single dose (Table 3) (CDC, 1998b). Because of the higher risk of pharyngeal gonorrhea in pregnant women, it may be preferable to treat them with ceftriaxone, since the efficacy of cefixime for treating pharyngeal gonorrhea has not been established. Ceftriaxone may also abort incubating syphilis. Quinolones and tetracyclines should not be used in pregnant women.

Since gonorrhea frequently coexists with chlamydial infections, it is generally recommended that effective treatment for chlamydia be given to all candidates for gonorrhea treatment (CDC, 1993). Since doxycycline, ofloxacin, and erythromycin estolate are all contraindicated during preg-

Table 3 Recommended regimens for perinatal *N. gonorrhoeae* infection

Infection	Regimen for:	
	Mother[a]	Infant
Uncomplicated gonorrhea	Ceftriaxone 125 mg i.m. × 1 or Cefixime 400 mg p.o. × 1	
PID	Cefoxitin 2 g i.v. every 6 h[b] or Cefotetan 2 g every 12 h	
Maternal untreated gonorrhea		Ceftriaxone 25–50 mg/kg i.v. or i.m., × 1, not to exceed 125 mg
Gonococcal ophthalmia	Ceftriaxone 1 g i.m. × 1	Ceftriaxone 25–50 mg/kg i.v. or i.m., × 1, not to exceed 125 mg[c]
Disseminated gonococcal infection, infant scalp abscess	Ceftriaxone 1 g i.m. or i.v. daily continued for 24–48 h after improvement begins	Ceftriaxone 25–50 mg/kg/day i.v. or i.m. daily, × 7 days
Meningitis or endocarditis	Ceftriaxone 1–2 g i.v. every 12 h × 10–14 days (meningitis) or 4 wk (endocarditis)	Ceftriaxone 25–50 mg/kg/day for 10–14 days (meningitis)

[a] Treatment for *N. gonorrhoeae* infections should be accompanied by effective treatment for *C. trachomatis* (CDC, 1998b). i.m., intramuscularly; i.v., intravenously.

[b] Treatment for PID should include a minimum of two antimicrobial agents to ensure coverage for *N. gonorrhoeae*, *C. trachomatis*, and gram-negative facultative bacteria, anaerobes, and streptococci (CDC, 1998b).

[c] Many pediatricians continue treatment until cultures are negative at 48 to 72 h; ceftriaxone should be administered with caution among infants with elevated bilirubin levels, particularly premature infants. Ceftriaxone regimens for disseminated gonococcal infection and scalp abscess are also available (CDC, 1998b).

nancy, erythromycin or amoxicillin is recommended for pregnant women with uncomplicated gonorrhea (CDC, 1998b).

Pregnant women who are diagnosed with gonorrhea should be evaluated by history and pelvic examination to rule out the possibility of upper genital tract infection. Moreover, pregnant women with lower abdominal, adnexal, and cervical motion tenderness meet the minimum criteria for PID and should be hospitalized for parenteral therapy, even if their culture results are unavailable or negative (CDC, 1998b).

Suspected or confirmed disseminated gonococcal infection is an absolute indication for the patient's hospitalization. The initial treatment regimen should be ceftriaxone (1 g intramuscularly or intravenously every 24 h) (CDC, 1998b). The regimen may be changed to cefixime (400 mg orally twice a day) 24 to 48 h after the patient shows signs of improvement.

Treatment of Infants with Gonococcal Infection

Infants who are born to mothers who have untreated gonorrhea are at very high risk of infection, even if ocular prophylaxis is applied (Table 3). Such infants should be carefully evaluated with orogastric and rectal cultures, and blood cultures should be performed if there are signs suggestive of sepsis (Wilfert and Gutman, 1987; Glaser et al., 1966). In the absence of any evidence of gonococcal infection, such infants should be treated with ceftriaxone (25 to 50 mg/kg intravenously or intramuscularly, not to exceed 125 mg in a single dose) (CDC, 1998b).

Infants who present with conjunctivitis should have specimens taken from the conjunctivae (including exudate) for Gram stain and culture (for *N. gonorrhoeae* and for *Chlamydia* infection) (Israel et al., 1975). Culture is essential to confirm susceptibility to the antimicrobial agents used, and the laboratory should be asked to perform confirmatory testing to differentiate *N. gonorrhoeae* from *Moraxella catarrhalis* and other *Neisseria* species that can mimic *N. gonorrhoeae* on Gram staining. Infants for whom treatment for gonococcal ophthalmia is contemplated should be hospitalized and carefully evaluated for disseminated infection, particularly bloodstream infection, arthritis, and meningitis (CDC, 1998b; Israel et al., 1975).

Gonococcal conjunctivitis has been the source of nosocomial transmission of gonorrhea to other infants and may be a source of occupational transmission to staff (Garner, 1996). Newborns with suspected or confirmed gonococcal conjunctivitis should be placed in a private room, if possible, for 24 h after initiation of effective therapy. The purulent exudate from their eyes should be considered infective, and health care workers should not handle it without gloves.

Patients who present with corneal involvement should have specimens for cultures and Gram stains obtained from the cornea in consultation with an expert. Ophthalmologic consultation to confirm a full response to treatment and to rule out sequelae should be considered for all infants diagnosed with gonococcal ophthalmia. One dose of ceftriaxone (25 to 50 mg/kg intravenously not intramuscularly, not to exceed 125 mg in a single dose) is probably adequate to treat gonococcal ophthalmia, but many pediatricians prefer to continue treatment until cultures are negative (CDC, 1998b).

Infants with sepsis, arthritis, meningitis, or scalp abscesses should be checked for evidence of gonorrhea by cultures of blood, cerebrospinal fluid, and joint aspirate on chocolate agar (CDC, 1998b; Israel et al., 1975). Repeated blood cultures and physical examinations are needed to rule out endocarditis and other bacteremic infection; sometimes more than one joint aspiration is needed. Cultures of specimens from the conjunctivae, vagina, oropharynx, and rectum are useful to identify sites of primary infection and may be needed to confirm the diagnosis if blood and joint aspirates are not positive. Gram-stained smears of exudate, cerebrospinal fluid, or joint aspirate provide a presumptive basis for starting treatment for disseminated gonococcal infection, but these results should be confirmed by definitive tests on culture isolates.

Infants with a presumptive or confirmed diagnosis of disseminated gonococcal infection should be hospitalized and treated with ceftriaxone (25 to 50 mg/kg/day in a single dose) for 7 days, or for 10 to 14 days if meningitis is documented (CDC, 1998b). The infants should be tested for chlamydial infection, and consideration should be given to evaluation for other vertically acquired sexually transmitted infections. The mother and her sexual partner(s) should be evaluated and treated in accordance with recommendations for treatment of gonococcal infections among adults.

Research Priorities

N. gonorrhoeae develops resistance to antimicrobial agents readily, and surveillance for antimicrobial susceptibility is essential to the evaluation of prevention strategies. Decreasing susceptibility to recommended agents should prompt active surveillance for evidence of treatment failure. Moreover, since many antimicrobial agents are poorly tolerated by pregnant women and others are contraindicated during pregnancy, research should be aimed at the development and testing of agents that can be administered orally in one dose to pregnant women; clinical trials of therapeutic agents for gonorrhea should include pregnant women, so that this population may receive early access to new regimens.

The high rate of recurrence of infection in late pregnancy among women treated for gonorrhea suggests that research is needed to identify whether treatment failures are more common during pregnancy and/or whether partner notification and treatment is less effective during pregnancy. The problem of low utilization of prenatal care in populations with a high prevalence of gonorrhea must be promptly addressed, and strategies to reach high-risk women for diagnosis and treatment outside the context of prenatal care require exploration. Urine screening for sexually transmitted pathogens in facilities attended by underserved high-risk pregnant women is a promising alternative.

REFERENCES

Alexander, E. R., and H. R. Harrison. 1983. Role of *Chlamydia trachomatis* in perinatal infection. *Rev. Infect. Dis.* **5:**713–719.

Alger, L. A., J. C. Lovchik, J. R. Hebel, L. R. Blackmon, and M. C. Crenshaw. 1988. The association of *Chlamydia trachomatis, Neisseria gonorrhoeae,* and group B streptococci with preterm rupture of the membranes and pregnancy outcome. *Am. J. Obstet. Gynecol.* **159:**397–404.

Amstey, M. S., and K. T. Steadman. 1976. Asymptomatic gonorrhea and pregnancy. *J. Am. Vener. Dis. Assoc.* **1:**14–16.

Armstrong, J. H., F. Zacarias, and M. F. Rein. 1976. Ophthalmia neonatorum: a chart review. *Pediatrics* **57:**884–892.

Behets, F. M. T., J. Desormeaux, D. Joseph, M. Adrien, G. Coicou, G. Dallabetta, H. A. Hamilton, S. Moeng, H. Davis, M. S. Cohen, and R. Boulos. 1995. Control of sexually transmitted disease in Haiti: results and implications of a baseline study among pregnant women living in Cité Soleil shantytowns. *J. Infect. Dis.* **172:** 764–771.

Bessen, D., and E. C. Gotschlich. 1986. Interactions of gonococci with HeLa cells: attachment and role of protein II. *Infect. Immun.* **54:**154–160.

Beutler, B., and A. Cerami. 1986. Cachectin and tumor necrosis factor as two sides of the same biological coin. *Nature* **320:**584–588.

Blackwell, A. L., P. D. Thomas, K. Wareham, and S. J. Emery. 1993. Health gains from screening for infection of the lower genital tract in women attending for termination of pregnancy. *Lancet* **342:**206–210.

Blanchard, A. C., J. G. Pastorek, and T. Weeks. 1987. Pelvic inflammatory disease during pregnancy. *South. Med. J.* **80:**1363–1365.

Bradford, W. L., and H. W. Kelley. 1933. Gonococcal meningitis in a newborn infant with review of the literature. *Am. J. Dis. Child.* **46:**543–549.

Brunham, R. C., and J. E. Embree. 1992. Sexually transmitted diseases: current and future dimensions of the problem in the Third World, p. 35–58. *In* A. Germain et al. (ed.), *Reproductive Tract Infections.* Plenum Press, New York, N.Y.

Burkman, R. T., J. A. Tonascia, M. F. Atienza, and T. M. King. 1976. Untreated endocervical gonorrhea and endometritis following elective abortion. *Am. J. Obstet. Gynecol.* **126:**648–651.

Cacciapuoti, A. F., W. S. Wegner, and S. A. Morse. 1979. Phospholipid metabolism in *Neisseria gonorrhoeae*: phospholipid hydrolysis in nongrowing cells. *Lipids* **14:** 718–726.

Campos-Outcalt, D., and K. Ryan. 1995. Prevalence of sexually transmitted diseases in Mexican-American pregnant women by country of birth and length of time in the United States. *Sex. Transm. Dis.* **22:**78–82.

Casey, M. L., and P. C. MacDonald. 1988. Biomolecular processes in the initiation of parturition: decidual activation. *Clin. Obstet. Gynecol.* **31:**533–552.

Centers for Disease Control. 1983. Neonatal gonococcal ophthalmia—California. *Morbid. Mortal. Weekly Rep.* **39:**518–519.

Centers for Disease Control and Prevention. 1991. Premarital sexual experience among adolescent women—United States, 1970–1988. *Morbid. Mortal. Weekly Rep.* **39:**929–932.

Centers for Disease Control and Prevention. 1993. Recommendations for the prevention and management of *Chlamydia trachomatis* infections, 1993. *Morbid. Mortal. Weekly Rep.* **42:**28–29.

Centers for Disease Control and Prevention. 1994. Increasing incidence of low birthweight—United States, 1981–1991. *Morbid. Mortal. Weekly Rep.* **43:**335–339.

Centers for Disease Control and Prevention. 1995. Fluoroquinolone resistance in *Neisseria gonorrhoeae*—Colorado and Washington. *Morbid. Mortal. Weekly Rep.* **44:** 250–253.

Centers for Disease Control and Prevention. 1996. *Division of STD Prevention: Sexually Transmitted Disease Surveillance, 1995.* U.S. Department of Health and Human Services, Public Health Service. Centers for Disease Control and Prevention, Atlanta, Ga.

Centers for Disease Control and Prevention. 1997. *Division of STD Prevention: Sexually Transmitted Disease Surveillance, 1996.* U.S. Department of Health and Human Services, Public Health Service. Centers for Disease Control and Prevention, Atlanta, Ga.

Centers for Disease Control and Prevention. 1998a. Fluoroquinolone-resistant *Neisseria gonorrheae,* San Diego, California, 1997. *Morbid. Mortal. Weekly Rep.* **47:**405–408.

Centers for Disease Control and Prevention. 1998b. Sexually transmitted diseases treatment guidelines. *Morbid. Mortal. Weekly Rep.* **47:**59–70.

Charles, A. G., S. Cohen, M. B. Kass, and R. Richman. 1970. Asymptomatic gonorrhea in prenatal patients. *Am. J. Obstet. Gynecol.* **108:**595–598.

Chen, C.-Y. 1988. Membrane proteolipids and iron-regulated proteins of *Neisseria gonorrhoeae.* Ph.D. thesis. Oregon Health Sciences University, Portland.

Chow, W. H., J. R. Daling, W. Cates, Jr., and R. S. Greenberg. 1987. Epidemiology of ectopic pregnancy. *Epidemiol. Rev.* **9:**70–93.

Christmas, J. T., G. D. Wendel, R. E. Bawdon, R. Farris, G. Cartwright, and B. B. Little. 1989. Concomitant infection with *Neisseria gonorrhoeae* and *Chlamydia trachomatis* in pregnancy. *Obstet. Gynecol.* **74:**295–298.

Corman, L. C., M. E. Levison, R. Knight, E. R. Carington, and D. Kaye. 1974. The high frequency of pharyngeal gonococcal infection in a prenatal clinic population. *JAMA* **230:**568–570.

Coulaud, J. P. 1991. Epidemiologie et prevention de la transmission neonatale des gonocoques et de *Chlamydia. Bull. Soc. Pathol. Exp.* **84:**597–602.

D'Auria, A., L. Tan, M. Kreitzer, and V. Galdi. 1975. Gonococcal scalp wound infection. *Morbid. Mortal. Weekly Rep.* **24:**115–116.

Dekker, N. P., C. J. Lammel, R. E. Mandrell, and G. F. Brooks. 1990. Opa (protein II) influences gonococcal organization in colonies, surface appearance, size and attachment to human fallopian tube tissues. *Microb. Pathog.* **9:**19–31.

Desenclos, J. C. A., D. Garrity, M. Scaggs, and J. E. Wroten. 1992. Gonococcal infection of the newborn in Florida, 1984–1989. *Sex. Transm. Dis.* **19:**105–110.

Donders, G. G., J. Desmyter, D. H. De Wet, and F. A. Van Assche. 1993. The association of gonorrhoea and syphilis with premature birth and low birthweight. *Genitourin. Med.* **69:**98–101.

Donders, G. G., V. vanGerven, H. G. de Wet, A. M. van Straten, and F. de Boer. 1996. Rapid antigen tests for *Neisseria gonorrhoeae* and *Chlamydia trachomatis* are not accurate for screening women with disturbed vaginal lactobacillary flora. *Scand. J. Infect. Dis.* **28:**559–562.

Doraiswamy, B., M. R. Hammerschlag, G. F. Pringle, and L. du Bouchet. 1983. Ophthalmia neonatorum caused by β-lactamase-producing *Neisseria gonorrhoeae. JAMA* **250:**790–791.

Elliott, B., R. C. Brunham, M. Laga, P. Piot, J. O. Ndinya-Achola, G. Maitha, M. Cheang, and F. A. Plummer. 1990. Maternal gonococcal infection as a preventable risk factor for low birth weight. *J. Infect. Dis.* **161:**531–536.

Frau, L. M., and E. R. Alexander. 1985. Public health implications of sexually transmitted diseases in pediatric practice. *Pediatr. Infect. Dis.* **4:**453–467.

Frost, E., F. Yvert, J. Zue Ndong, and B. Ivanoff. 1987. Ophthalmia neonatorum in a semi-rural African community. *Trans. R. Soc. Trop. Med. Hyg.* **81:**378–380.

Garner, J. S. 1996. Guideline for isolation precautions in hospitals. *Infect. Control Hosp. Epidemiol.* **17:**53–80.

Gery, I., R. K. Gershon, and B. H. Waksman. 1972. Potentiation of cultured mouse thymocyte responses by factors released by peritoneal leucocytes. *J. Exp. Med.* **136:** 128–142.

Glaser, S., B. Boxerbaum, and J. H. Kennell. 1966. Gonococcal arthritis in the newborn: report of a case and review of the literature. *Am. J. Dis. Child.* **112:**185–188.

Goh, T. H., Y. F. Ngeow, and S. K. Teoh. 1981. Screening for gonorrhea in a prenatal clinic in southeast Asia. *J. Am. Vener. Dis. Assoc.* **8:**67–69.

Gorwitz, R. J., A. K. Nakashima, J. S. Moran, and J. S. Knapp. 1993. Sentinel surveillance for antimicrobial resistance in *Neisseria gonorrhoeae*—United States, 1988–1991. CDC surveillance summary SS-3, August 13, 1993. *Morbid. Mortal. Weekly Rep.* **42:**29–39.

Graber, W. J., III, J. P. Sanford, and M. Ziff. 1968. Sex incidence of gonococcal arthritis. *Arthritis Rheum.* **11:**569–578.

Gregg, C. R., M. A. Melly, C. G. Hellerquist, J. G. Coniglio, and Z. A. McGee. 1981. Toxic activity of purified lipopolysaccharide of *Neisseria gonorrhoeae* for human fallopian tube mucosa. *J. Infect. Dis.* **143:**432–439.

Hagblom, P., E. Segal, E. Billyard, and M. So. 1985. Intragenic recombination leads to pilus antigenic variation in *Neisseria gonorrhoeae. Nature* **315:**156–158.

Handsfield, H. H., W. A. Hodson, and K. K. Holmes. 1973. Neonatal gonococcal infection: orogastric contamination with *Neisseria gonorrhoeae. JAMA* **225:**697–701.

Harkness, A. H. 1948. The pathology of gonorrhoea. *Br. J. Vener. Dis.* **24:**137–147.

Heckels, J. E., B. Blackett, J. S. Everson, and M. E. Ward. 1976. The influence of surface charge on the attachment of *Neisseria gonorrhoeae* to human cells. *J. Gen. Microbiol.* **96:**359–364.

Holmes, K. K., G. W. Counts, and H. N. Beaty. 1971. Disseminated gonococcal infection. *Ann. Intern. Med.* **74:**979–993.

Israel, K. S., K. B. Rissing, and G. R. Brooks. 1975. Neonatal and childhood gonococcal infections. *Clin. Obstet. Gynecol.* **18:**142–151.

Joesoef, M. R., H. Sumampouw, M. Linnan, S. Schmid, A. Idajadi, and M. E. St. Louis. 1996. Douching and sexually transmitted diseases in pregnant women in Surabaya, Indonesia. *Am. J. Obstet. Gynecol.* **174:**115–119.

Jones, D. E. D., R. G. Brame, and C. P. Jones. 1976. Gonorrhea in obstetric patients. *J. Am. Vener. Dis. Assoc.* **2:**30–32.

Kamwendo, F., L. Forslin, L. Bodin, and D. Danielsson. 1996. Decreasing incidence of gonorrhea- and chlamydia-associated acute pelvic inflammatory disease. A 25-year study from an urban area of central Sweden. *Sex. Transm. Dis.* **23:**384–391.

Keiser, H., F. L. Ruben, E. Wolinsky, and I. Kushner. 1968. Clinical forms of gonococcal arthritis. *N. Engl. J. Med.* **279:**234–240.

Kiviat, N. B., J. A. Paavonen, P. Wolner-Hanssen, C. W. Critchlow, W. E. Stamm, J. Douglas, D. A. Eschenbach, L. A. Corey, and K. K. Holmes. 1990. Histopathology of endocervical infection caused by *Chlamydia trachomatis,* herpes simplex virus, *Trichomonas vaginalis,* and *Neisseria gonorrhoeae. Hum. Pathol.* **21:** 831–837.

Kupsch, E. M., B. Knepper, T. Kuroki, I. Heuer, and T. F. Meyer. 1993. Variable opacity (Opa) outer membrane proteins account for the cell tropisms displayed by *Neisseria gonorrhoeae* for human leukocytes and epithelial cells. *EMBO J.* **12:** 641–650.

Laga, M., F. A. Plummer, H. Nzanza, W. Namaara, R. C. Brunham, J. O. Ndinya-Achola, G. Naitha, A. R. Ronald, L. J. D. D'Costa, V. B. Bhullar, J. K. Mati, L. Fransen, M. Cheang, and P. Piot. 1986. Epidemiology of ophthalmia neonatorum in Kenya. *Lancet* **ii:**1145–1148.

Laga, M., F. Plummer, P. Piot, P. Datta, W. Namaara, J. O. Ndinya-Achola, H. Nzanza, G. Maitha, A. R. Ronald, H. O. Pamba, and R. C. Brunham. 1988. Prophylaxis of gonococcal and chlamydial ophthalmia neonatorum: a comparison of silver nitrate and tetracycline. *N. Engl. J. Med.* **318:**653–657.

Laga, M., A. Meheus, and P. Piot. 1989. Epidemiology and control of gonococcal ophthalmia neonatorum. *Bull. W. H. O.* **67:**471–478.

Limberger, R. J., R. Biega, A. Evancoe, L. McCarthy, L. Slivienski, and M. Kirkwood. 1992. Evaluation of culture and the Gen-Probe PACE 2 assay for detection of *Neisseria gonorrhoeae* and *Chlamydia trachomatis* in endocervical specimens transported to a state health laboratory. *J. Clin. Microbiol.* **30:**1162–1166.

Lind, I. 1997. Antimicrobial resistance in *Neisseria gonorrhoeae. Clin. Infect. Dis.* **24**(Suppl. 1):S93–S97.

Mabey, D., P. Hanlon, L. Hanlon, V. Marsh, and T. Forsey. 1987. Chlamydial and gonococcal ophthalmia neonatorum in The Gambia. *Ann. Trop. Pediatr.* **7:**177–180.

Makino, J., J. P. M. van Putten, and T. F. Meyer. 1991. Phase variation of the opacity outer membrane protein controls invasion by *Neisseria gonorrhoeae* into human epithelial cells. *EMBO J.* **10:**1307–1315.

Mayoud, P., H. Grosskurth, J. Changalucha, J. Todd, B. West, R. Gabone, K. Senkoro, M. Rusizoka, M. Laga, R. Hayes, and D. Mabey. 1995. Risk assessment and other screening options for gonorrhoea and chlamydial infection in women attending rural Tanzanian antenatal clinics. *Bull. W. H. O.* **73:**621–630.

McGee, Z. A., A. P. Johnson, and D. Taylor-Robinson. 1976. Human fallopian tubes in organ culture: preparation, maintenance, and quantitation of damage by pathogenic microorganisms. *Infect. Immun.* **13:**608–618.

McGee, Z. A., A. P. Johnson, and D. Taylor-Robinson. 1981. Pathogenic mechanisms of *Neisseria gonorrhoeae*: observations on damage to fallopian tubes in organ culture by gonococci of colony type 1 or type 4. *J. Infect. Dis.* **143:**413–422.

McGee, Z. A., G. L. Gorby, P. B. Wyrick, R. Hodinka, and L. H. Hoffman. 1988. Parasite-directed endocytosis. *Rev. Infect. Dis.* **10:**S311–S316.

McGee, Z. A., C. M. Clemens, R. L. Jensen, J. J. Klein, L. R. Barley, and G. L. Gorby. 1992. Local induction of tumor necrosis factor as a molecular mechanism of mucosal damage by gonococci. *Microb. Pathog.* **12:**333–341.

Melly, M. A., Z. A. McGee, and R. S. Rosenthal. 1984. Ability of monomeric peptidoglycan fragments from *Neisseria gonorrhoeae* to damage human fallopian tube mucosa. *J. Infect. Dis.* **149:**378–386.

Murphy, G. L., T. D. Connell, D. S. Barritt, M. Koomey, and J. G. Cannon. 1989. Phase variation of gonococcal protein II: regulation of gene expression by slipped-strand mispairing of a repetitive DNA sequence. *Cell* **56:**539–547.

Niles, J. H., and E. W. Lowe. 1966. Gonococcal arthritis in pregnancy. *Med. Ann. D.C.* **35:**69–74.

Owen, J., L. J. Groome, and J. C. Hauth. 1993. Randomized trial of prophylactic antibiotic therapy after preterm amnion rupture. *Am. J. Obstet. Gynecol.* **169:**976–981.

Paruchuri, D. K., H. S. Seifert, R. S. Ajioka, K. A. Karisson, and M. So. 1990. Identification and characterization of a *Neisseria gonorrhoeae* gene encoding a glycolipid-binding adhesin. *Proc. Natl. Acad. Sci. USA* **87:**333–337.

Plummer, F. A., M. Laga, R. C. Brunham, P. Piot, A. R. Ronald, V. Bhullar, J. Y. Mati, J. O. Ndinya-Achola, M. Cheang, and H. Nsanze. 1987. Postpartum upper genital tract infections in Nairobi, Kenya: epidemiology, etiology and risk factors. *J. Infect. Dis.* **156:**92–98.

Quinn, T. C. 1997. Nucleic acid amplification assays for sexually transmitted diseases, p. 201–232. *In* H. Lee, S. Morse, and Ø. Olsvik (ed.), *Nucleic Acid Amplification Technologies: Application to Disease Diagnosis.* Eaton Publishing Co., Natick, Mass.

Rolfs, R. T., E. I. Galaid, and A. A. Zaidi. 1992. Pelvic inflammatory disease: trends in hospitalizations and office visits, 1979 through 1988. *Am. J. Obstet. Gynecol.* **156:** 983–990.

Ross, J. D. 1996. Systemic gonococcal infection. *Genitourin. Med.* **72:**404–407.

Rothenberg, R. 1979. Ophthalmia neonatorum due to *Neisseria gonorrhoeae*: prevention and treatment. *Sex. Transm. Dis.* **6:**187–191.

Schachter, J., M. Grossman, R. L. Sweet, J. Holt, C. Jordan, and E. Bishop. 1986. Prospective study of perinatal transmission of *Chlamydia trachomatis. JAMA* **255:** 3374–3377.

Schulz, K. F., W. J. Cates, Jr., and P. R. O'Mara. 1987. Pregnancy loss, infant death and suffering: legacy of syphilis and gonorrhoea in Africa. *Genitourin. Med.* **63:** 320–325.

Schulz, K. F., J. M. Schutte, and S. M. Berman. 1992. Maternal health and child survival: opportunities to protect both women and children from the adverse consequences of reproductive tract infections, p. 145–182. *In* A. Germain, K. K. Holmes, P. Piot, and J. Wasserheit (ed.), *Reproductive Tract Infections: Global Impact and Priorities for Women's Reproductive Health.* Plenum Publishing Corp., New York, N.Y.

Simon, D., and R. F. Rest. 1992. *Escherichia coli* expressing a *Neisseria gonorrhoeae* opacity-associated outer membrane protein invade human cervical and endometrial cell lines. *Proc. Natl. Acad. Sci. USA* **89:**5512–5516.

So, M., E. Billyard, C. Deal, E. Getzoff, P. Hagblom, T. F. Meyer, E. Segal, and J. Tainer. 1985. Gonococcal pilus: genetics and structure. *Curr. Top. Microbiol. Immunol.* **118:**13 28.

Solberg, D. A., J. Butler, and N. N. Wagner. 1973. Sexual behavior in pregnancy. *N. Engl. J. Med.* **238:**1098–1108.

Stutz, D. R., M. R. Spence, and C. Duangmani. 1976. Oropharyngeal gonorrhea during pregnancy. *J. Am. Vener. Dis. Assoc.* **3:**65–67.

Swanson, J. 1973. Studies of gonococcus infection. IV. Pili: their role in attachment of gonococci to tissue culture cells. *J. Exp. Med.* **137:**571–589.

Taylor, H. A., S. A. Bradford, and S. P. Patterson. 1966. Gonococcal arthritis in pregnancy. *Obstet. Gynecol.* **27:**776–782.

van der Lugt, B., A. C. Dogendijk, and J. R. J. Banffer. 1980. Prevalence of cervical gonorrheae in women with unwanted pregnancies. *Br. J. Vener. Dis.* **56:**148–150.

Van Dyck, E., F. Crabbe, N. Nzila, J. Bogaerts, J.-P. Munyabikali, P. Ghys, M. Diallo, and M. Laga. 1997. Increasing resistance of *Neisseria gonorrhoeae* in West and Central Africa. Consequence on therapy of gonococcal infection. *Sex. Transm. Dis.* **24:**32–37.

Vuyllsteke, B., M. Laga, and M. Alary. 1993. Clinical algorithms for the screening of women for gonococcal and Chlamydial infection: evaluation of pregnant women and prostitutes in Zaire. *Clin. Infect. Dis.* **17:**82–88.

Ward, M. E., J. N. Robertson, P. M. Englefield, and P. J. Watt. 1975. Gonococcal infection: invasion of mucosal surfaces of the genital tract, p. 188–199. *In* D. Schlessinger (ed.), *Microbiology—1975.* American Society for Microbiology, Washington, D.C.

Webster, L. A., S. M. Berman, and J. R. Greenspan. 1993. Surveillance for gonorrhea and primary and secondary syphilis among adolescents—United States, 1981–1991. CDC surveillance summary SS-3, August 13, 1993. *Morbid. Mortal. Weekly Rep.* **42:**1–12.

Weel, J. F. L., C. T. P. Hopman, and J. P. M. van Putten. 1991. In situ expression and localization of *Neisseria gonorrhoeae* opacity proteins in infected epithelial cells. Apparent role of opa proteins in cellular invasion. *J. Exp. Med.* **6:**1395–1406.

Welgemoed, N. C., A. Mahaffey, and J. Van Den Ende. 1986. Prevalence of *Neisseria gonorrhoeae* infection in patients attending an antenatal clinic. *S. Afr. Med. J.* **69:** 32–34.

Wendel, P. J., and G. D. Wendel. 1993. Sexually transmitted diseases in pregnancy. *Semin. Perinatol.* 17:443–451.

Wilfert, C., and L. Gutman. 1987. Sexually transmitted diseases, p. 595–621. *In* R. D. Feigin and J. D. Cherry (ed.), *Textbook of Pediatric Infectious Diseases.* The W. B. Saunders Co., Philadelphia, Pa.

Yip, L., P. J. Sweeney, and B. F. Bock. 1993. Acute suppurative salpingities with concomitant intrauterine pregnancy. *Am. J. Emerg. Med.* **11:**476–479.

Yvert, F., E. Frost, P. Walter, R. Gass, and B. Ivanoff. 1985. Prepartal infection of the placenta with *Neisseria gonorrhoeae. Genitourin. Med.* **61:**103–105.

10
Ureaplasma Infection

Gail H. Cassell

The ubiquity and subtle pathogenicity of mycoplasmas often have concealed their etiologic significance. The history of practically every disease of proven mycoplasmal etiology has been plagued with controversy. The most noteworthy examples are the proof that *Mycoplasma pulmonis* is the etiologic agent of murine "chronic respiratory disease" and that *Ureaplasma urealyticum* is one of the causes of nongonococcal urethritis in humans. The former took almost half a century to resolve and ultimately required inoculation of germ-free animals (Cassell and Hill, 1979). The latter, finally resolved by experimental ureaplasmal inoculation of humans in 1977 (Taylor-Robinson et al., 1977), settled a debate initiated in the early 1950s.

The most controversial area in mycoplasmology today continues to be the potential role of *U. urealyticum* in adverse pregnancy outcome in humans. Advancement of knowledge in this area has been seriously impeded by the lack of a suitable animal model. The value of experimental animal models of human disease cannot be overestimated. However, the value of a naturally occurring disease in animals which closely parallels one in humans is far greater. With the ability to study an infectious agent in its natural host under defined microbiological and environmental conditions, one can most easily establish the critical determinants of disease and the role of individual organisms. We have attempted to define the etiology and pathogenesis of a naturally occurring, chronic genital tract disease in rats that results in adverse outcomes of pregnancy and diseases of the newborn. Koch's postulates have been fulfilled, and it is now clear that this genital disease in rats also is due to *M. pulmonis*. It is our findings in *M. pulmonis*

Gail H. Cassell, Drug Discovery Research and Clinical Investigation, Lilly Research Laboratories, Eli Lilly and Company, Indianapolis, IN 46285.

Sexually Transmitted Diseases and Adverse Outcomes of Pregnancy
Edited by P. J. Hitchcock, H. T. MacKay, J. N. Wasserheit, and R. Binder
©1999 American Society for Microbiology, Washington, D.C.

respiratory and genital disease that led us to examine the potential role of *U. urealyticum* in adverse outcomes of pregnancy in humans. Without exception, all of the studies we have performed to date in humans have been informed by the *M. pulmonis* infection in rats.

This chapter is not meant to be a comprehensive review of the literature or of our work. Reviews have been published relatively recently (Cassell et al., 1993, 1994; Simecka et al., 1992); this chapter is a personal perspective based upon my studies in animals and humans.

MYCOPLASMA PULMONIS: A CAUSE OF CHRONIC RESPIRATORY DISEASE AND ADVERSE PREGNANCY OUTCOMES IN LABORATORY RODENTS

Chronic Respiratory Disease

Chronic bronchopneumonia in rats first was described in 1915 when this species was brought into the laboratory for experimental purposes (Hektoen, 1915–1918). Around 1940, a *Mycoplasma* sp., later identified as *M. pulmonis*, was recognized as a possible cause of the respiratory disease (Nelson, 1940a, 1940b). However, the ubiquity of the organism and its frequent isolation from healthy as well as diseased rats and mice (even from the trachea and lungs) made it difficult to tell whether the organism was commensal or pathogenic. The failure of experimental inoculation to consistently produce disease of the lower respiratory tract also precluded its acceptance as the etiologic agent. It was not until the early 1970s that *M. pulmonis* alone was shown to consistently reproduce all of the characteristic clinical and pathological features of the natural respiratory disease when inoculated into germ-free animals (Cassell et al., 1979).

The respiratory disease caused by *M. pulmonis* is slow in onset and of long duration. Consequently, there are various stages of pathologic lesions and nonuniformity of lesions even among animals in the same cages. These features are due in part to the large number of variables which can affect lesion development and progression, including irritation caused by ammonia produced on soiled bedding, synergy with endogenous murine respiratory viruses and other bacteria, and nutritional factors (Cassell et al., 1979). However, comparison of animals matched for age, sex, and microbial and environmental factors indicates that the genetic background of the host is probably the most critical determinant of susceptibility and disease severity (Cassell et al., 1973; Davis et al., 1982, 1985; Cartner et al., 1996).

Intranasal inoculation of *M. pulmonis* produces markedly different lesions in F344 rats and in CD-1 mice, even when the dose is comparable on the basis of lung and body weight. In rats the lesions progress slowly from the upper respiratory tract, with alveolar involvement occurring days to months following inoculation. In mice, alveolar lesions develop within hours of inoculation and acute alveolar disease and death occur within 3 to 5 days. When LEW and F344 rats are matched for age, sex, and microbial and environmental factors, the respiratory tract lesions progress more rapidly and are more severe in the LEW rats than in the F344 rats (Davis et al., 1982). In contrast to findings observed in CD-1 mice, LEW rats do not develop acute disease.

Pulmonary lesions in F344 rats are generally limited to epithelial hyperplasia and proliferation of bronchial-associated lymphoid tissue (BALT). LEW rats not only develop more extensive BALT hyperplasia but also develop alveolar consolidation with mononuclear cells. In the absence of extrinsic factors, lung lesions in F344 rats tend to resolve 28 days after intranasal inoculation, whereas the lesions in LEW rats continue to progress for at least 120 days with infiltration of lymphoid cells and ultimate development of lesions similar to those in chronic obstructive lung disease of humans, including the development of bronchiectasis (Cassell et al., 1979; Davis et al., 1982). Differences in severity and progression of the lung lesions in LEW and F344 rats are related to differences in the degree of nonspecific lymphocyte activation in the two strains (Simecka et al., 1992). *M. pulmonis* possesses a potent B-cell mitogen, and in addition the organism is chemotactic for B cells.

M. pulmonis Genital Disease in Rats

Although *M. pulmonis* can be isolated from ovaries and uteri of rats in the absence of gross or microscopic lesions, the organism has been shown to cause naturally occurring, chronic genital disease. All lesions observed in the natural disease can also be produced by inoculating pure cultures of *M. pulmonis* into germ-free animals (Cassell et al., 1979). We know very little about disease pathogenesis, but the genital disease caused by *M. pulmonis*, like the respiratory disease, progresses slowly and host genetics may predispose to upper reproductive tract disease. The most impressive feature of the genital disease, like the respiratory disease, is the inconsistency of lesions and the inconsistency of the impact upon pregnancy outcome.

Naturally Occurring Genital Disease in Rats

The exact relationship between genital and respiratory disease is unknown; each has been detected independently. Females can acquire genital infection early in life, in some cases even prior to coitus. Since rats are coprophagic, females harboring mycoplasmas in the upper respiratory passages may, through grooming, transfer the infection to the vagina. von Juhr (1971) has demonstrated a septicemic phase in respiratory disease caused by *M. pulmonis*, and so it is possible that organisms reach the urogenital tract hematogenously.

Although infection of the lower reproductive tract (vagina and cervix) is common, ascension to the upper tract (uterus and fallopian tubes) occurs in only ~25% and <5% of infected female LEW rats and F344 rats, respectively. Infection may result in minimal or no microscopic changes; in some instances cervicitis, vaginitis, endometritis, salpingitis, and perioophoritis occur. Genital tracts that are grossly normal may have extensive histological changes. A uterus that appears histologically normal can be shown by immunofluorescence and electron microscopy to have numerous mycoplasmas attached to the epithelium (Cassell and Hill, 1979; Cassell et al., 1979).

Experimentally Induced Genital Disease in Rats

The entire spectrum of natural disease can be reproduced by intranasal, intravaginal, or intravenous inoculation of *M. pulmonis* into germ-free 2-month-old female LEW rats (Cassell et al., 1979). Animals inoculated intravaginally or intranasally first develop a mild vaginitis, cervicitis, and endometritis and eventually develop salpingitis and oophoritis. Intravenous inoculation results in inflammation of the oviducts and the ovarian bursae. Just as with *M. pulmonis* respiratory disease, differences in the pathogenesis of genital infection in LEW and F344 rats are dramatic. Regardless of the route of inoculation, development of gross and microscopic lesions progresses slowly in both LEW and F344 rats (in some cases requiring up to 8 months for development), but disease progression is faster and severity is greater in LEW than F344 rats. Not only are LEW rats easily infected by direct intravaginal inoculation of *M. pulmonis*, but also they develop severe, ascending genital disease after intranasal inoculation. This aspect of pathogenesis is not seen in F344 rats. The decreased susceptibility of F344 rats to cervicovaginal infection may explain why naturally occurring disease in the upper reproductive tract is not observed in this strain.

Maternal Infection and Outcome of Pregnancy in Rats

A 50% reduction in fertility has been observed in LEW rat colonies naturally infected with *M. pulmonis* (Cassell et al., 1979). Infection can result in complete infertility or significantly reduced litter sizes. However, the effects upon birth rate are erratic and unpredictable; normal rat pups can be born to mothers with uterine and oviductal infection. To further determine the effect of maternal infection on pregnancy outcome, 3-month-old LEW rats (previously shown to be fertile) were infected intravenously with 10^8 CFU of *M. pulmonis* and then, 49 days after inoculation, bred with fertile, uninfected male rats. Laparotomies were performed 10 days after breeding, and the corpora lutea and fetuses were counted. At term, the animals were euthanized. A 50% fetal loss between days 10 and 20, with ≥30% attributable to resorption, was observed in the infected animals. Reduced fertility was observed in half of the infected animals and ranged from complete infertility to a 66% fetal loss after implantation. Another group of rats were injected intravenously with 10^8 CFU on day 10 of pregnancy. Although fetal survival was unaffected in rats inoculated intravenously on day 10 of pregnancy, *M. pulmonis* was cultured from amniotic fluid and fetal tissues on day 20 in animals infected before and after conception. Immunofluorescence and light microscopy revealed acute inflammation of the placental disks; *M. pulmonis* was localized at the fetomaternal junction of the placenta. Fetal infection occurred at a higher frequency when mycoplasmas were present in maternal blood. Mycoplasma pneumonia and meningitis were observed in newborn pups.

The reduction in fertility was greatest in animals infected before mating. This finding is consistent with in vitro fertilization studies in mice, which suggest that embryonic development is not affected by infection with *M. pulmonis* after the blastocyst stage (Fraser and Taylor-Robinson, 1977).

In contemplating the potential role of *U. urealyticum* in reproductive disorders of humans, it is important to consider the genital disease caused by *M. pulmonis* in rats. Infertility and adverse pregnancy outcome occur in infection of the upper, not the lower, reproductive tract. Ascension of infection, even in the most susceptible rat strain, occurs in some but not all animals with lower tract infection. The upper reproductive tract remains colonized for months to years. Finally, variability in adverse pregnancy outcomes is tremendous even when the animals are matched for heredity, age, and microbial and environmental factors. Pregnancy outcome is highly dependent upon whether infection occurs pre- or postimplantation. While inflammation of the amnion and subchorion is common, the organism and an inflammatory response are less commonly found in fetal tissues. However, both pneumonia and meningitis due to *M. pulmonis* do occur in newborn pups.

UREAPLASMA UREALYTICUM: INVASION OF THE UPPER REPRODUCTIVE TRACT AND PERINATAL MORBIDITY AND MORTALITY IN HUMANS

U. urealyticum can be isolated from the cervix and vagina in 52 to 76% of postpubertal girls in the absence of symptoms (Cassell and Cole, 1981). This suggests that the organism is commensal. Since 1970, 13 studies involving approximately 12,000 patients have been conducted to evaluate the role of cervical ureaplasmal infection in premature birth. No consistent relationship has been delineated (Cassell et al., 1993). However, the *M. pulmonis* model would suggest that if *U. urealyticum* is involved in adverse outcome of pregnancy, it is likely to do so by invasion of the upper reproductive tract of only a subpopulation of those colonized in the lower tract. Furthermore, the model suggests that in order to cause adverse outcomes of pregnancy, the organism must be present prior to implantation and/or in the early stages of gestation. We thus designed studies to address these questions.

Ureaplasmal Colonization of the Endometrium in Nonpregnant Females and Presence in Amniotic Fluid at 12 to 20 Weeks Gestation

Endometrial biopsy specimens and peritoneal lavage fluid were collected at the time of diagnostic laparoscopy (for reasons other than pelvic inflammatory disease) from 319 women by methods shown to preclude cervical contamination (Cassell et al., 1983b). *U. urealyticum* was isolated in pure culture from the endometrium and peritoneal lavage fluid of 4% of those colonized in the cervix and vagina. In at least one individual, the organism was repeatedly isolated from the endometrium, suggesting that some individuals may be chronically infected in the upper reproductive tract.

Analysis of amniocentesis samples taken for prenatal diagnosis in the first or second trimester revealed *U. urealyticum* in the amniotic fluid, in the presence of intact membranes and in the absence of other microorganisms (Gray et al., 1992; Cassell et al., 1983). Our study, as well as other individual case reports (Cassell et al., 1983a; Gray et al., 1992; Foulon et al., 1986), indicates that *U. urealyticum* can persist in the amniotic fluid for as long as 7 weeks even when membranes are intact; although there is an inflammatory response, labor does not occur, and no other microorganisms are detected. Furthermore, in such cases, ureaplasmas can be demonstrated by immunofluoresence in the inflammatory infiltrates in the fetal membranes (Cassell et al., 1986). Taken together these findings provide a convincing argument that ureaplasmas alone can actually produce chorioamnionitis and can do so within the first trimester.

That ureaplasmas can be isolated in pure culture from endometria of nonpregnant females and from amniotic fluid in pregnant women between 12 and 20 weeks gestation indicates that these organisms may contribute to early fetal loss. Isolation of *U. urealyticum* from amniotic fluid in pure culture from women with intact membranes and subsequent fetal loss has now been reported in three studies (Foulon et al., 1986; Cassell et al., 1983a; Gray et al., 1992). Unlike previous reports (Cassell and Cole, 1981), it is clear in these later cases that the fetus was alive before the *U. urealyticum* infection and that there were no other apparent causes of abortion. This suggests that in some cases of spontaneous abortion and first-trimester intrauterine fetal death, *U. urealyticum* may be causal. Just as in the *M. pulmonis* model, repeated spontaneous abortions and stillbirths in the same individual may be associated with chronic *U. urealyticum* infection of the endometrium.

Ureaplasmal Infection of the Chorioamnion and Amniotic Fluid and Premature Birth

Two prospective studies were conducted to evaluate the presence of ureaplasmas at the time of genetic amniocentesis at 12 to 20 weeks gestation when membranes were intact and there was no labor (Cassell et al., 1983a; Gray et al., 1992). Women were age-matched and similar with respect to indication for amniocentesis; findings were similar with respect to the percentage of chromosomal anomalies and α-fetoprotein levels. In our amniocentesis study (Cassell et al., 1983a), the two infants from women with ureaplasmas isolated from amniotic fluid were delivered prematurely and subsequently died. *U. urealyticum* was isolated in pure culture at autopsy from both infants. In the study by Gray et al. (1992), 7 of 10 patients whose amniotic fluid contained ureaplasmas subsequently aborted within 4 to 7 weeks following amniocentesis and at less than 25 weeks gestation. Of the three remaining patients, all delivered prematurely and two of the neonates died. Histologic evidence of chorioamnionitis was present in all 10 placentas and histologic evidence of pneumonia was present in all 9 fetuses. Cultures were positive for *U. urealyticum* and negative for all other microorganisms in six of seven placentas evaluated at delivery and in four of six fetal lungs. Three other studies were conducted to evaluate the amniotic fluid of women admitted to the hospital with preterm labor and intact membranes. In these women, the presence of *U. urealyticum* was not positively correlated with premature birth (Gravett et al., 1986; Romero et al., 1989; Watts et al., 1992). However, it is difficult to interpret these studies because chorioamnion infection was not assessed. Another difference between the two groups of studies is that the mean week of gestation for the women in labor was 31 to 32 weeks. *U. urealyticum* is isolated from the chorioamnion almost three times more often in infants who weigh <1,500 g at birth and are born before 32 weeks gestation compared with larger and older infants (Hillier et al., 1988; Kundsin et al., 1984; Cassell et al., 1993).

Isolation of *U. urealyticum* from the chorioamnion, with or without other bacteria, is associated with chorioamnionitis and was a consistent finding in two studies (Cassell et al., 1993; Eschenbach, 1993). Furthermore, *U. urealyticum* in the absence of other microorganisms can be a cause of chorioamnionitis. Although numerous studies have shown a strong correlation between histologic chorioamnionitis and premature birth (Russell, 1979), only three of six prospective studies have shown a significant association between isolation of *U. urealyticum* from the chorioamnion and premature birth (Embree et al., 1980; Hillier et al., 1988, 1991; Kundsin et al., 1984; Naessens et al., 1989, Zlatnik et al., 1990). In contrast to amniotic fluid studies, these studies included a large number of patients and some specifically investigated infection related to birth before 34 weeks gestation. However, most patients had their membranes ruptured, which makes interpretation of microbiological findings difficult. In addition, these studies did not include a control group of women who delivered at similar preterm gestational ages but who did not have spontaneous onset of labor. Such a control group is essential to establish that microbial colonization of the chorioamnion is causally related to spontaneous preterm labor and not to preterm gestational age alone. As discussed above, prospective studies begun at 16 to 20 weeks gestation indicate that in at least some cases, *U. urealyticum* infection of the chorioamnion is associated with premature birth. If *U. urealyticum* is a significant cause of prematurity, one should be able to demonstrate that it precedes the onset of labor and rupture of membranes. Recent studies at the University of Alabama at Birmingham indicate that *U. urealyticum* is the single most common microorganism isolated from the chorioamnion of women with spontaneous labor delivered by cesarean section with intact membranes (Cassell et al., 1993). Furthermore, logistic regression analysis of demographic and obstetric variables indicates that *U. urealyticum* alone or in the presence of other bacteria in the chorioamnion is independently associated with birth earlier than 34 weeks regardless of the duration of labor. Isolation was three to five times more frequent in women with spontaneous labor than in women who had indicated deliveries. Isolation of the organism from women with indicated deliveries was not associated with premature birth, suggesting that subclinical chorioamnion infection with *U. urealyticum* may be causally associated with preterm labor. The isolation of organisms from the chorioamnion and/or amniotic fluid was associated with microscopic chorioamnionitis but not with clinical amnionitis. Furthermore, ureaplasmal infection of the amniotic fluid occurred in less than half of the individuals with ureaplasmal infection of the chorioamnion (Cassell, unpublished). The culture results from amniotic fluid were confirmed by analysis of the amniotic fluid by PCR (Blanchard et al., 1993). These results suggest that culture of amniotic fluid alone will greatly underestimate the role of ureaplasmal infection in adverse pregnancy outcome.

Risk factors for *U. urealyticum* colonization of the female lower genital tract include younger age, lower socioeconomic status, sexual activity with multiple partners, black ethnicity, and oral contraceptive use (Cassell and Cole, 1981). However, virtually nothing is known about risk factors associated with upper tract infection. Bacterial vaginosis (BV) may be a risk factor (Cassell et al., 1993). It is independently and significantly associated with birth earlier than 37 weeks gestation when cervical organisms and obstetrical and demographic factors are taken into consideration (Hillier et al., 1988). However, it has not been determined whether BV is associated with premature delivery independently of chorioamnion infection. Although *U. urealyticum* is not independently associated with BV, women with BV are twice as likely to be colonized by *U. urealyticum*; furthermore, the intravaginal concentrations of these organisms are increased 100-fold in patients with BV (Gravett and Eschenbach, 1986). It is possible that certain BV-associated microorganisms, like *U. urealyticum*, are more likely to invade the intact fetal membranes simply because they are present in larger numbers in the lower tract. However, this possibility cannot be the total explanation for the association of *U. urealyticum* with prematurity, since intravaginal concentrations of *Peptococcus* species are also increased in women with BV, but these organisms are found infrequently in the chorioamnion and amniotic fluid. Although *Mycoplasma hominis* and *Gardnerella vaginalis* were the next most common organisms isolated from women with intact membranes in the University of Alabama at Birmingham study described above, they were not independently associated with birth before 34 weeks gestation. A distinct possibility based on current evidence is that both BV and *U. urealyticum* are of etiologic significance independently of each other but are synergistic when present simultaneously.

U. urealyticum as a Cause of Pneumonia, Chronic Lung Disease, and Meningitis in the Newborn

Infection of the chorioamnion and/or amniotic fluid does not always result in infection of the amniotic fluid or fetus. Several studies have shown a significant association between isolation of *U. urealyticum* from the chorioamnion and perinatal morbidity and mortality (Kundsin et al., 1984; Quinn et al., 1985a; Madan et al., 1988, 1989). However, these investigators did not culture samples from the infants. Thus, it is unclear whether the morbidity and mortality resulted from the direct effect of fetal and neonatal infection due to *U. urealyticum* or whether it was the result of the complications associated with premature birth. Likewise, surface colonization alone (e.g., eyes, ears, nose, throat, gastric aspirates, vagina, and urine) is not indicative of invasive infection.

Pneumonia

Retrospective (Tafari et al., 1976) and prospective (Cassell et al., 1983a; Quinn et al., 1985a, 1985b; Gray et al., 1992) studies indicate an association of *U. urealyticum* with congenital pneumonia. Individual case reports from our laboratory and those of others also provide evidence that *U. urealyticum* is a cause of pneumonia in newborn infants (Waites et al., 1989; Gray et al., 1992; Brus et al., 1991). The organism has been isolated from lungs in the absence of chlamydiae, viruses, fungi, and bacteria and in the presence of chorioamnionitis and funisitis (Cassell et al., 1983a). It has also been detected in fetal membranes by immunofluorescence microscopy (Cassell et al., 1983a) and in lung lesions of newborns by electron and immunofluorescence microscopy (Quinn et al., 1985b). A specific immunoglobulin M response in the newborn has been demonstrated in some individuals with pneumonia; this is also consistent with in utero infection (Quinn et al., 1985a, 1985b).

U. urealyticum is the most common microorganism isolated from endotracheal aspirates of infants weighing ≤2,500 g who required oxygen within the first 24 h after birth (Cassell et al., 1988b). Infants weighing ≤1,000 g and from whom *U. urealyticum* is isolated from the endotracheal aspirate are twice as likely to die as uninfected infants of similar birth weight or infected infants who weigh >1,000 g. These findings support the hypothesis that only a select group of infants, i.e., those with very low birth weights, is at risk of mortality due to *U. urealyticum*. This fact may account for the seeming disparities in the conclusions about the role of *U. urealyticum* in neonatal respiratory disease reached in earlier prospective studies that failed to control for infant weight (Rudd and Carrington, 1985; Taylor-Robinson et al., 1984).

The evidence that the endotracheal isolation of *U. urealyticum* reflects true infection of the lower respiratory tract includes initial isolation of ureaplasmas in numbers exceeding 1,000 CFU and in some cases exceeding 10,000 CFU, as well as repeated isolations of the organism from tracheal aspirates of infants who require mechanical ventilation for extended periods. The tracheal isolates are unlikely to be contaminants of the nasopharynx, since this site is often culture negative. Furthermore, *U. urealyticum* is isolated in pure culture from endotracheal aspirates in over 85% of these infants (Cassell et al., 1988b). Concomitant recovery of the organism from blood is possible in 26% of infants with positive endotracheal aspirates; cerebrospinal fluid (CSF) isolates have also been recovered in some infants (Cassell et al., 1988b). Fourteen percent of the *U. urealyticum* endotracheal isolates were from infants delivered by cesarean section with intact membranes, indicating that in utero transmission may occur rather commonly, at least in premature infants.

In another study of 98 infants (Ollikainen et al., 1993a), respiratory distress syndrome, assisted ventilation, severe respiratory insufficiency, and death were significantly more common among premature infants (<34 weeks) from whom *U. urealyticum* was cultured from endotracheal aspirates than among uninfected premature infants. In the group of infected infants, *U. urealyticum* was also isolated in the blood (34%) and the CSF (66%) and from brain and lung autopsy specimens (66%). Eighty-two percent of the ureaplasma isolates were present in pure culture. In infants delivered by cesarean section with intact membranes, 48% had ureaplasmas isolated from one or more sites. Infants weighing ≤1,251 g at birth, from whom *U. urealyticum* was isolated from their endotracheal aspirate, had >2+ polymorphonuclear leukocytes/ml at 1 to 3 days of age compared to uninfected infants. Other investigators have observed an association between infection of the respiratory tract and neutrophilia (Ohlsson et al., 1993).

In organ culture models of the human fetal trachea, *U. urealyticum* induces ciliostasis and mucosal lesions (Quinn et al., 1985b). Furthermore, we have shown that ureaplasmas isolated from the lungs of human infants with congenital and neonatal pneumonia produce a histologically similar pneumonia in newborn mice (Rudd et al., 1989). In the mouse model of ureaplasma pneumonia, age is also a critical determinant of disease. Newborn mice are susceptible to infection of the respiratory tract and development of pneumonia, while 14-day-old mice are resistant.

We have also used the baboon model to study the association of *U. urealyticum* with pneumonia. At 140 days gestational age, the animals have the same physiologic and pathologic characteristics as human neonates of 30 to 32 weeks gestation. We have shown that experimental challenge of prematurely born baboons with *U. urealyticum* results in acute bronchiolitis with epithelial ulceration and polymorphonuclear infiltration that is distinguishable from hyaline membrane disease (Walsh et al., 1993). *U. urealyticum* can be isolated from blood, endotracheal aspirates, and pleural fluid and lung tissue from some of these animals up to 6 days postinoculation. Taken together, the available evidence suggests that *U. urealyticum* is causally associated with pneumonia in newborn infants, particularly those born before 34 weeks gestation.

Chronic Lung Disease of Prematurity

Some but not all studies show an association between isolation of *U. urealyticum* from the respiratory tract of newborn infants and the development of chronic lung disease (Cassell et al., 1994). Differing results can probably be explained by the fact that some studies do not limit culture to the lower respiratory tract, i.e., the affected site, and/or do not define the patient population by gestational age or birth weight of $<$1,000 g, and/or do not conduct microbiological sampling within 12 h of delivery. Dyke et al. (1993) found that *U. urealyticum* in the gastric aspirates of infants weighing $\leq$1,000 g was associated with a significantly increased risk of chronic lung disease in those infants delivered by cesarean section but not in those delivered vaginally. This could result from a longer exposure to *U. urealyticum*, as a result of in utero exposure, or it may be a reflection of differences in virulence.

Available evidence creates a cohesive argument that *U. urealyticum* infection of the lower respiratory tract is a risk factor for chronic lung disease. Isolation of *U. urealyticum* from endotracheal aspirates not only is a risk factor for development of pneumonia but also has been shown to be a risk factor for development of precocious dysplastic changes (Crouse et al., 1993). Walsh et al. (1991) isolated *U. urealyticum* directly from pleural fluid and tissue collected by open-lung biopsy in four of eight infants who had chronic lung disease. We (Cassell et al., 1988b) continued to recover ureaplasmas for months from endotracheal aspirates of infants with chronic lung disease.

There are several animal models that have demonstrated a causal role for respiratory pathogens in respiratory disease. *U. urealyticum* isolated from two sources, an endotracheal aspirate of an infant with chronic lung disease (Cassell et al., 1988b) and lung tissue of an infant with congenital pneumonia (Cassell et al., 1983b), caused pneumonia in two different strains of newborn germ-free mice (Rudd et al., 1989). Furthermore, infection with *U. urealyticum* and exposure to 80% oxygen caused more severe lung lesions and organism persistence and resulted in death more often than did either infection or oxygen exposure alone. These results suggest that the increased oxygen requirements of very-low-birth-weight infants might predispose them to lower respiratory tract infection or, alternatively, that *U. urealyticum* infection potentiates oxygen-induced injury. Exposure to oxidants is known to enhance respiratory disease and death due to *M. pulmonis* respiratory disease in mice (Parker et al., 1989). Hyperoxia-induced lung injury is thought to contribute to development of chronic lung disease via stimulation of the proinflammatory cytokine interleukin-6 (Stancombe et al., 1993). *U. urealyticum* may also contribute to development of chronic lung disease by stimulation of proinflammatory cytokines.

The available data provide very strong evidence that *U. urealyticum* can actually be a primary cause or a contributing cofactor in the development of chronic lung disease in newborns, but the data are not definitive. Although a randomized trial of antibiotic treatment might provide critical information related to patient management, it would not necessarily bring us closer to proving causality. Even if treatment is found to be efficacious, conclusions about causation will be limited by the fact that unrecognized microbes might also be susceptible to the antibiotic chosen. Nevertheless, a treatment trial might identify drugs that can reduce the morbidity and mortality associated with chronic lung disease.

Infection of the Central Nervous System

U. urealyticum is one of the most common microorganisms isolated from the CSF of infants with suspected sepsis and meningitis (Waites et al., 1988, 1990; Ollikainen et al., 1993a; McCormack, 1986; Valencia et al., 1993). CSF samples from 100 predominantly preterm infants undergoing lumbar puncture for suspected sepsis and/or meningitis or for treatment of posthemorrhagic hydrocephalus were cultured for conventional bacteria and mycoplasmas (Waites et al., 1988). *U. urealyticum* was isolated from eight infants, and *M. hominis* was isolated from five infants. Only one other CSF infection, in an infant with *Eschericia coli* meningitis, was identified in this group, making ureaplasmas the most common organisms isolated. CSF was cultured from an additional 318 infants born preterm in three suburban community hospitals in Birmingham, Ala. (Waites et al., 1990). *M. hominis* was isolated from the CSF of nine infants, and *U. urealyticum* was isolated from five infants. Of the 17 bacterial CSF isolates in this population, mycoplasmas were again the most common microorganisms recovered. In a recent study by Ollikainen et al. (1993a), *U. urealyticum* was isolated from the CSF of four of six infants of less than 34 weeks gestational age; cultures were taken within 30 min of birth. The same group of investigators reported isolation of *U. urealyticum* from the brain tissues of premature twins who died 1 and 3 days after birth; both had larger intraventricular hemorrhages. The organism was isolated from the endotracheal aspirate and from lung tissue at autopsy; however, blood samples of both infants were negative.

Findings from other studies have been inconsistent. Valencia et al. (1993) isolated *M. hominis* from CSF in 9 (13%) and *U. urealyticum* from CSF in 1 (1.5%) of 54 infants from whom samples were obtained for culture within the first 24 h of life and from 15 infants from whom samples were obtained 2 to 90 days after birth. In other prospective studies, Likitnukul et al. (1986) and Mardh (1983) failed to recover mycoplasmas from CSF of infants. The study by Likitnukul et al. involved primarily older term infants, all of whom had been discharged from the hospital and returned because of suspected sepsis or meningitis (Likitnukul et al., 1986, 1987). Mardh did not specify the ages and birth weights of the infants in his study (Mardh, 1983). No mycoplasmas were recovered from the CSF of 47 preterm infants from whom samples were obtained for culture within the first week of life by Izraeli et al. (1991).

Shaw et al. (1989) performed a prospective study of 135 preterm infants undergoing lumbar puncture and found only one isolate of *U. urealyticum*. The reason for the lumbar puncture was not stated. In some hospitals it has been common practice to evaluate the CSF of all infants weighing <2,500 g regardless of clinical evidence of sepsis or meningitis. If this were the case, the isolation rates for any microorganism would be significantly lower than that if only symptomatic infants were cultured.

The clinical findings in infants with *U. urealyticum* infection of the CSF are variable. Isolation of *U. urealyticum* may be concordant with CSF pleocytosis, with either polymorphonuclear or mononuclear cells predominating, or the inflammatory reaction in the CSF may be minimal or absent (Waites et al., 1988; Ollikainen et al., 1993a; Valencia et al., 1993). In some patients, the organisms are eradicated spontaneously from the CSF, while in others, the organisms persist in the CSF for weeks or even months, even with antibiotic treatment (Shaw et al., 1989; Waites et al., 1988; Garland and Murton, 1987)

Lack of inflammation in the CSF, when the presence of the *U. urealyticum* has been verified in the CSF on multiple occasions, may logically lead to some skepticism about the significance of mycoplasmal CSF infection. However, it should be noted that early in the course of infection with a number of other proven bacterial pathogens, inflammatory reactions may be scant or absent. Visser and Hal (1980) reported "normal" CSF (cell count, <25; protein level, <2,000 mg/dl) in 6 (29%) of 39 infants with culture-proven meningitis. Subsequent examination of CSF revealed increases in cell counts and protein levels. The magnitude of the inflammatory response depends upon the type of pathogen and may be related to differences in cell wall components. For example, the median number of cells in the CSF of 98 infants with gram-negative meningitis was more than 2,000/mm^3, whereas the median number of cells in 21 infants with group B streptococcal meningitis was less than 100/mm^3 (Sarff et al., 1976). The lack of a cell wall in mycoplasmas may be related to the reduced inflammatory response to these organisms. Glucose and protein values found in the normal infant may overlap those in the infant with bacterial meningitis. Severely ill infants with meningitis may in fact represent only a fraction of the total number of ureaplasma-infected infants, with the majority experiencing only a mild, often subclinical infection that may resolve spontaneously.

The prevalence, risk factors, typical manifestations, and long-term effects of mycoplasmal central nervous system infections in the newborn have remained an enigma until results were obtained from prospective studies. Until there is widespread awareness of and acceptance of how common mycoplasmal infections of the central nervous system can be, knowledge of what group is at risk for infection, and development of improved diagnostic capabilities, it is likely that the majority of cases will not be identified.

FUTURE CONSIDERATIONS

Based on current knowledge, ureaplasmal infection of the chorioamnion should be given serious consideration as a significant cause of adverse pregnancy outcome, with the major impact being premature birth, pneumonia, and meningitis in the newborn. When interpreting studies related to the etiologic significance of *U. urealyticum* or in designing future studies, the following facts must be taken into account.

1. *U. urealyticum* can be detected in the chorioamnion and amniotic fluid prior to 12 to 16 weeks gestation in the presence of intact membranes and in the absence of labor. Therefore, studies evaluating the role of ureaplasmas in spontaneous preterm labor and premature birth should focus on those women with intact membranes. It may be that pathogenesis of membrane rupture is different from that of induction of preterm labor.

2. Chorioamnion infection with *U. urealyticum* alone or with other bacteria in the presence of intact membranes is positively correlated with birth prior to 34 weeks gestation. Isolation of ureaplasmas from the chorioamnion is almost three times higher in infants whose birth weight is <1,500 g and who are born before 32 weeks gestation, compared with larger and older infants. Thus studies assessing the role of *U. urealyticum* in premature birth must enroll a sufficient number of infants of less than 32 weeks gestation.

3. Subclinical infection of *U. urealyticum*, in the absence of other detectable microorganisms, can elicit an inflammatory response in the chorioamnion and amniotic fluid. Thus those studies limited to women with

evidence of clinical amnionitis will lead to erroneous results related to ureaplasmas.

4. Of women who have ureaplasmas in chorioamnionic membranes, *U. urealyticum* can be isolated from the amniotic fluid 50% of the time. Thus studies to address the role of infection and premature birth and which are limited to culture of only amniotic fluid will greatly underestimate the presence of ureaplasmas.

5. Since *U. urealyticum* is the single most common microorganism isolated from the chorioamnion and amniotic fluid, studies designed to assess the role of infection and prematurity should include methods for detection of these organisms.

6. Furthermore, because of the discordance between amniotic fluid infection and chorioamnion infection, studies which use placental cultures without direct culture of the fetus/infant will likely result in erroneous interpretation of data.

REFERENCES

Blanchard, A., J. Hentschel, L. Duffy, K. Baldus, and G. H. Cassell. 1993. Detection of *Ureaplasma urealyticum* by polymerase chain reaction in the urogenital tract of adults, in amniotic fluid, and in the respiratory tract of newborns. *Clin. Infect. Dis.* **17:**S148–S153.

Brus, F., W. M. van Waarde, C. Schoots, and S. B. Oetomo. 1991. Fetal ureaplasmal pneumonia and sepsis in a newborn infant. *Eur. J. Pediatr.* **150:**782–783.

Cartner, S. C., J. W. Simecka, D. E. Briles, G. H. Cassell, and J. R. Lindsey. 1996. Resistance to mycoplasmal lung disease in mice is a complex genetic trait. *Infect. Immun.* **64:**5326–5331.

Cassell, G. H. Unpublished observation.

Cassell, G. H., and B. C. Cole. 1981. Mycoplasmas as agents of human disease. *N. Engl. J. Med.* **304:**80–89.

Cassell, G. H., and A. Hill. 1979. Murine and other small animal mycoplasmas, p. 235–273. *In* J. G. Tully and R. F. Whitcomb (ed.), *The Mycoplasmas*, vol. 2. *Human and Animal Mycoplasmas.* Academic Press, Inc., New York, N.Y.

Cassell, G. H., J. R. Lindsey, R. G. Overcash, and H. J. Baker. 1973. Murine *Mycoplasma* respiratory disease. *Ann. N. Y. Acad. Sci.* **225:**395–412.

Cassell, G. H., J. R. Lindsey, and H. J. Baker. 1979. Mycoplasmal and rickettsial disease, p. 243–269. *In* H. J. Baker, J. R. Lindsey, and S. H. Weisbroth (ed.), *The Laboratory Rat*, vol. I. Academic Press, Inc., New York, N.Y.

Cassell, G. H., R. O. Davis, K. B. Waites, M. B. Brown, P. A. Marriott, S. Stagno, and J. K. Davis. 1983a. Isolation of *Mycoplasma hominis* and *Ureaplasma urealyticum* from amniotic fluid at 16–20 weeks gestation: potential effect on outcome of pregnancy. *Sex. Transm. Dis.* **10**(4S)**:**294–302.

Cassell, G. H., J. B. Younger, M. B. Brown, R. E. Blackwell, J. K. Davis, P. Marriott, and S. Stagno. 1983b. Microbiologic study of infertile women at the time of diagnostic laparoscopy: association of *Ureaplasma urealyticum* with a defined subpopulation. *N. Engl. J. Med.* **308:**502–505.

Cassell, G. H., K. B. Waites, R. S. Gibbs, and J. K. Davis. 1986. The role of *Ureaplasma urealyticum* in amnionitis. *Pediatr. Infect. Dis. J.* **5:**S247–S252.

Cassell, G. H., D. T. Crouse, K. B. Waites, P. T. Rudd, and J. K. Davis. 1988a. Does *Ureaplasma urealyticum* cause respiratory disease in newborns? *Pediatr. Infect. Dis. J.* **7:**535–541.

Cassell, G. H., K. B. Waites, D. T. Crouse, P. T. Rudd, K. C. Canupp, S. Stagno, and G. Cutter. 1988b. Association of *Ureaplasma urealyticum* infection of the lower respiratory tract with chronic lung disease and death in very-low-birthweight infants. *Lancet* **ii:**240–245.

Cassell, G. H., K. B. Waites, H. L. Watson, D. T. Crouse, and R. Harasawa. 1993. *Ureaplasma urealyticum* intrauterine infection: role in prematurity and disease in the newborn. *Clin. Microbiol. Rev.* **6:**69–87.

Cassell, G. H., K. B. Waites, and D. T. Crouse. 1994. Mycoplasmal infections, p. 619–655. *In* J. S. Remington and J. O. Klein (ed.), *Infectious Disease of the Fetus and Newborn Infant.* The W. B. Saunders Co., Philadelphia, Pa.

Crouse, D. T., G. H. Cassell, K. B. Waites, J. M. Foster, and G. Cassady. 1990. Hyperoxia potentiates *Ureaplasma urealyticum* pneumonia in newborn mice. *Infect. Immun.* **58:**3487–3493.

Crouse, D. T., G. T. Odrezin, G. R. Cutter, J. M. Reese, W. B. Hamrick, K. B. Waites, and G. H. Cassell. 1993. Radiographic changes associated with tracheal isolation of *Ureaplasma urealyticum* from neonates. *Clin. Infect. Dis.* **17:**S122–S130.

Davis, J. K., R. B. Thorp, P. A. Maddox, M. B. Brown, and G. H. Cassell. 1982. Murine respiratory mycoplasmosis in F344 and LEW rats: evolution of lesions and lung lymphoid cell populations. *Infect. Immun.* **36:**720–729.

Davis, J. K., R. F. Parker, H. White, D. Dziedzic, G. Taylor, M. K. Davidson, N. R. Cox, and G. H. Cassell. 1985. Strain differences in susceptibility to murine respiratory mycoplasmosis in C57BL/6 and C3H/HeN mice. *Infect. Immun.* **50:**647–654.

Dyke, M. P., A. Grauaug, R. Kohan, K. Ott, and R. Andrews. 1993. *Ureaplasma urealyticum* in a neonatal intensive care population. *J. Paediatr. Child Health.* **29:** 295–297.

Embree, J. E., V. W. Krause, J. A. Embil, and S. McDonald. 1980. Placental infection with *Mycoplasma hominis* and *Ureaplasma urealyticum*: clinical correlation. *Obstet. Gynecol.* **56:**475–481.

Eschenbach, D. 1989. Bacterial vaginosis. *Obstet. Gynecol. Clin. North Am.* **16:**593.

Eschenbach, D. A. 1993. *Ureaplasma urealyticum* and premature birth. *Clin. Infect. Dis.* **17**(Suppl. 1)**:**S100–S106.

Foulon, W., A. Naessens, M. Dewaele, S. Lauwers, and J. J. Amy. 1986. Chronic *Ureaplasma urealyticum* amnionitis associated with abruptio placentae. *Obstet. Gynecol.* **68:**280.

Fraser, L. R., and D. Taylor-Robinson. 1977. The effect of *Mycoplasma pulmonis* on fertilization and preimplantation development in vitro of mouse eggs. *Fertil. Steril.* **28:**488–498.

Garland, S. M., and L. J. Murton. 1987. Neonatal meningitis caused by *Ureaplasma urealyticum. Pediatr. Infect. Dis. J.* **6:**868–870.

Gravett, M. G., and D. A. Eschenbach. 1986. Possible role of *Ureaplasma urealyticum* in preterm premature rupture of fetal membranes. *Pediatr. Infect. Dis. J.* **5:**S253–S257.

Gravett, M. G., D. Hummel, D. Eschenbach, and K. K. Holmes. 1986. Preterm labor associated with subclinical amniotic fluid infection and with bacterial vaginosis. *Obstet. Gynecol.* **67:**229–237.

Gray, D. J., H. B. Robinson, and J. Malone. 1992. Adverse outcome in pregnancy following amniotic fluid isolation of *Ureaplasma urealyticum. Prenatal Diagn.* **12:** 111–117.

Hektoen, L. 1915–1918. Observations on pulmonary infections in rats, 1915–1918. *Trans. Chicago Pathol. Soc.* **10:**105–108.

Hillier, S. L., J. Martius, M. Krohn, N. Kiviat, K. K. Holmes, and D. A. Eschenbach. 1988. A case-control study of chorioamnionic infection and histologic chorioamnionitis in prematurity. *N. Engl. J. Med.* **319:**972–978.

Hillier, S. L., M. A. Krohn, N. B. Kiviat, H. D. Watts, and D. A. Eschenbach. 1991. Microbiologic causes and neonatal outcomes associated with chorioamnion infection. *Am. J. Obstet. Gynecol.* **165:**955–961.

Izraeli, S., Z. Samra, L. Sirota, P. Merlob, and S. Davidson. 1991. Genital mycoplasmas in preterm infants: prevalence and clinical significance. *Eur. J. Pediatr.* **150:**804–807.

Kundsin, R. B., S. G. Driscoll, and R. R. Monson. 1984. Association of *Ureaplasma urealyticum* in the placenta with perinatal morbidity and mortality. *N. Engl. J. Med.* **310:**941–945.

Likitnukul, S., H. Kusmiesz, J. D. Nelson, and G. H. McCracken. 1986. Role of genital mycoplasmas in young infants with suspected sepsis. *J. Pediatr.* **109:**971–974.

Likitnukul, S., J. D. Nelson, G. H. McCracken, and H. Kusmiesz. 1987. Rarity of genital mycoplasma infection in young infants with aseptic meningitis. *J. Pediatr.* **110:**998.

Madan, E., M. P. Meyer, and A. J. Amortegui. 1988. Isolation of genital mycoplasmas and *Chlamydia trachomatis* in stillborn and neonatal autopsy material. *Arch. Pathol. Lab. Med.* **112:**749–751.

Madan, E., M. P. Meyer, and A. J. Amortegui. 1989. Histologic manifestations of perinatal genital mycoplasmal infection. *Arch. Pathol. Lab. Med.* **113:**465–469.

Mardh, P. A. 1983. *Mycoplasma hominis* infections of the central nervous system in newborn infants. *Sex. Transm. Dis.* **10:**331–334.

McCormack, W. M. 1986. *Ureaplasma urealyticum*: ecologic niche and epidemiologic considerations. *Pediatr. Infect. Dis. J.* **5:**S232–S233.

Naessens, A., W. Foulon, J. Breynaert, and S. Lauwers. 1989. Postpartum bacteremia and placental colonization with genital mycoplasmas and pregnancy outcome. *Am. J. Obstet. Gynecol.* **160:**647–650.

Nelson, J. B. 1940a. Infectious catarrh of the albino rat. I. Experimental transmission in relation to the role of *Actinobacillus muris. J. Exp. Med.* **72:**645–654.

Nelson, J. B. 1940b. Infectious catarrh of the albino rat. II. The causal relation of coccobacilliform bodies. *J. Exp. Med.* **72:**666–662.

Ohlsson, A., E. Want, and M. Vearncombe. 1993. Leukocyte counts and colonization with *Ureaplasma urealyticum* in prematerm neonates. *Clin. Infect. Dis.* **17**(Suppl. 1): S117–S121.

Ollikainen, J., H. Heikkaniemi, M. Korppi, H. Sarkkinen, and K. Heinonen. 1993a. *Ureaplasma urealyticum* infection associated with acute respiratory insufficiency and death in premature infants. *J. Pediatr.* **122:**756–760.

Ollikainen, J., H. Heikkaniemi, M. Korppi, M. L. Katila, and K. Heinonen. 1993b. *Ureaplasma urealyticum* cultured from brain tissue of preterm twin who died of intraventricular hemorrhage. *Scand. J. Infect. Dis.* **25:**529–531.

Parker, R. F., J. K. Davis, G. H. Cassell, H. White, D. Dziedzic, D. K. Blalock, R. B. Thorp, and J. W. Simecka. 1989. Short-term exposure to nitrogen dioxide enhances susceptibility to murine respiratory mycoplasmosis and decreases intrapulmonary killing of *Mycoplasma pulmonis. Am. Rev. Respir. Dis.* **140:**502–512.

Payne, N. R., S. Steinberg, P. Ackerman, B. A. Cheenka, S. M. Sane, K. T. Anderson, and J. J. Fangman. 1993. New prospective studies of the association of *Ureaplasma urealyticum* colonization and chronic lung disease. *Clin. Infect. Dis.* **178**(Suppl. 1)**:**S117–S121.

Quinn, P. A., J. Butany, M. Chipman, J. Taylor, and W. Hannah. 1985a. A prospective study of microbial infection in stillbirths and early neonatal death. *Am. J. Obstet. Gynecol.* **151:**238–249.

Quinn, P. A., J. E. Gillian, T. Markestad, M. A. St. John, A. Daneman, K. I. Lie, H. C. S. Li, E. Czegledy-Nagy, and A. M. Klein. 1985b. Intrauterine infection with *Ureaplasma urealyticum* as a cause of fatal neonatal pneumonia. *Pediatr. Infect. Dis. J.* **4:**538–543.

Romero, R., M. Sirtoir, E. Oyarzun, C. Avila, M. Mazor, R. Callahan, V. Sabo, A. P. Athanassiadis, and J. C. Hobbins. 1989. Infection and labor. V. Prevalence, microbiology, and clinical significance of intraamniotic infection in women with preterm labor and intact membranes. *Am. J. Obstet. Gynecol.* **161:**817–824.

Rudd, P. T., and D. Carrington. 1985. A prospective study of chlamydial, mycoplasmal and viral infections in a neonatal intensive care unit. *Arch. Dis. Child.* **59:** 120–125.

Rudd, P. T., G. H. Cassell, K. B. Waites, J. K. Davis, and L. B. Duffy. 1989. *Ureaplasma urealyticum* pneumonia: experimental production and demonstration of age-related susceptibility. *Infect. Immun.* **57:**918–925.

Russell, P. 1979. Inflammatory lesions of the human placenta. I. Clinical significance of acute chorioamnionitis. *Am. J. Diagn. Gynecol. Obstet.* **2:**127–137.

Sarff, L. D., L. H. Platt, and G. H. J. McCracken. 1976. Cerebrospinal fluid evaluation in neonates: comparison of high-risk infants with and without meningitis. *J. Pediatr.* **88:**473.

Saxen, H., K. Hakkarainen, M. Pohjavuori, and A. Miettinen. 1993. Chronic lung disease of preterm infants in Finland is not associated with *Ureaplasma urealyticum* colonization. *Acta Paediatr.* **82:**198–201.

Shaw, N. J., B. C. Pratt, and A. M. Weindling. 1989. Ureaplasma and mycoplasma infections of central nervous system in preterm infants. *Lancet* **ii:**1530–1531.

Sidiropoulos, D., U. Herrmann, A. Morell, F. P. Koontz, and L. F. Burmeister. 1986. Transplacental passage of intravenous immunoglobulin in the last trimester of pregnancy. *J. Pediatr.* **109:**505–508.

Simecka, J. W., J. K. Davis, M. K. Davidson, S. E. Ross, C. T. K.-H. Städtlaender, and G. H. Cassell. 1992. Mycoplasma disease of animals, p. 391–415. *In* J. Maniloff, R. McElhaney, L. Finch, and J. Baseman (ed.), *Mycoplasmas: Molecular Biology and Pathogenesis.* American Society for Microbiology, Washington, D.C.

Stancombe, B. B., W. F. Walsh, S. Derdak, P. Dixon, and D. Hensley. 1993. Induction of human neonatal pulmonary fibroblast cytokines by hyperoxia and *Ureaplasma urealyticum. Clin. Infect. Dis.* **17**(Suppl. 1)**:**S154–S157.

Tafari, N., S. Ross, and R. L. Naeye. 1976. Mycoplasma 'T' stains and perinatal death. *Lancet* **i:**108–109.

Taylor-Robinson, D., G. W. Csonka, and M. J. Prentice. 1977. Human intra-urethral inoculation of ureaplasmas. *Q. J. Med.* **46:**309–326.

Taylor-Robinson, D., P. M. Furr, and M. M. Liberman. 1984. The occurrence of genital mycoplasmas in babies with and without respiratory diseases. *Acta Paediatr. Scand.* **73:**383.

Valencia, G. B., F. Banzon, M. Cummings, W. M. McCormack, L. Glass, and M. R. Hammerschlag. 1993. *Mycoplasma hominis* and *Ureaplasma urealyticum* in neonates with suspected infections. *Pediatr. Infect. Dis. J.* **12:**571–573.

Visser, V. E., and R. T. Hall. 1980. Lumbar puncture in the evaluation of suspected neonatal sepsis. *J. Pediatr.* **96:**1063.

von Juhr, N.-C. 1971. Untersuchungen zur Chronischen Murinen Pneumonie. Vorkommen and Resistenz von Mycoplasma pulmonis in der Unweit. *Z. Versuchsteirkd.* **13:**217–223.

Waites, K. B., P. T. Rudd, D. T. Crouse, K. C. Canupp, K. G. Nelson, A. Ramsey, and G. H. Cassell. 1988. Chronic *Ureaplasma urealyticum* and *Mycoplasma hominis* infections of central nervous system in preterm infants. *Lancet* **ii:**17–21.

Waites, K. B., D. T. Crouse, J. B. Phillips III, K. C. Canupp, and G. H. Cassell. 1989. Ureaplasmal pneumonia and sepsis associated with persistent pulmonary hypertension of the newborn. *Pediatrics* **83:**79–85.

Waites, K. B., L. B. Duffy, D. T. Crouse, M. E. Dworsky, M. J. Strange, K. G. Nelson, and G. H. Cassell. 1990. Mycoplasmal infections of cerebrospinal fluid in newborn infants from a community hospital population. *Pediatr. Infect. Dis. J.* **9:**241–245.

Walsh, W. F., S. Stanley, K. P. Lally, R. E. Stribley, D. P. Greece, F. McClesky, and D. M. Null. 1991. *Ureaplasma urealyticum* demonstrated by open lung biopsy in newborns with chronic lung disease. *Pediatr. Infect. Dis. J.* **10:**823–827.

Walsh, W. F., J. Butler, J. Coalson, D. Hensley, G. H. Cassell, and R. A. Delemos. 1993. A primate model of *Ureaplasma urealyticum* infection in the premature infant with hyaline membrane disease. *Clin. Infect. Dis.* **17**(Suppl. 1)**:**S158–S162.

Watts, D. H., M. A. Krohn, S. L. Hillier, and D. A. Eschenbach. 1992. The association of occult amniotic fluid infection with gestational age and neonatal outcome among women in preterm labor. *Obstet. Gynecol.* **79:**351–357.

Zlatnik, F. J., T. M. Gellhaus, J. A. Benda, G. von Muralt, and S. Barandun. 1990. Histologic chorioamnionitis, microbial infection, and prematurity. *J. Obstet. Gynaecol.* **76:**355–359.

11
Chlamydial Infection

Robert B. Jones

PERINATAL TRANSMISSION

Perinatal transmission of *Chlamydia trachomatis* is a frequent occurrence and is the most clearly defined adverse outcome of chlamydial infections during pregnancy. Recent evidence obtained by survival analysis suggests that of infants born to infected women, as many as 76% delivered vaginally and 23% delivered by cesarean section are infected (Bell et al., 1994). Presumably, the majority of newborns acquire the infection during the birth process, although infection of infants born by cesarean section to women with intact membranes suggests that infection may occur in utero (Bell et al., 1994). Between 18 and 44% of exposed infants develop neonatal inclusion conjunctivitis and 8 to 22% develop infant pneumonia due to *Chlamydia trachomatis* (Harrison and Alexander, 1990). Significant morbidity is associated with neonatal infection, including predisposition to reactive airway disease later in life (Harrison et al., 1982; Weiss et al., 1986). Several excellent reviews of neonatal chlamydial infection are available (Alexander and Harrison, 1983; Bell et al., 1992; Harrison and Alexander, 1990), and the reader is referred to these for further information on this subject. The objective of this communication is to assess available information on other possible adverse outcomes of chlamydial infection in pregnancy.

EARLY PREGNANCY LOSS

C. trachomatis infection in women may be completely asymptomatic, with or without suggestive physical signs. It may cause urethritis, cervicitis, endometritis, or salpingitis, and these may be either clinically apparent or

Robert B. Jones, Department of Medicine, Indiana University School of Medicine, 545 Barnhill Dr., Emerson Hall 435, Indianapolis, IN 46202-5124.

Sexually Transmitted Diseases and Adverse Outcomes of Pregnancy
Edited by P. J. Hitchcock, H. T. MacKay, J. N. Wasserheit, and R. Binder
©1999 American Society for Microbiology, Washington, D.C.

subclinical (Jones et al., 1986; Paavonen et al., 1985; Wasserheit et al., 1986). Chlamydial endometritis has been characterized as a plasma cell endometritis because of infiltration of the endometrium with plasma cells (Paavonen et al., 1985). This association of chlamydial infection with inflammatory infiltrates in the endometrium raises the possibility that such infections are associated with failure of implantation or early pregnancy loss due to spontaneous abortion. Several investigators have attempted to address this question indirectly by measuring the levels of anti-chlamydial antibodies in the serum of women undergoing in vitro fertilization or embryo transfer. In one study such an association was found (Lunenfeld et al., 1989), while in others it was not (Lessing et al., 1991; Osser et al., 1990; Torode et al., 1995). Such discrepancies are not too surprising, since chlamydial serologic tests do not reliably distinguish active infection from past exposure with or without residual damage (Schachter et al., 1979; Wang and Grayston, 1982). Anti-chlamydial immunoglobulin G antibodies can persist for months and probably for years in the absence of an acute infection (Wang and Grayston, 1982). Perhaps more relevant are recent observations by using the more sensitive technique of PCR amplification to detect *C. trachomatis* DNA in women undergoing in vitro fertilization. A strong correlation was observed between a positive test indicating infection and both failure to become pregnant and the occurrence of spontaneous abortion (Witkin et al., 1995). In a separate study, the same investigators found a strong association between failure to achieve pregnancy after embryo transfer and the presence in endocervical secretions of immunoglobulin A antibodies directed against the 57-kDa chlamydial heat shock protein (also known as HSP60) (Witkin et al., 1994). Most of these women did not have other evidence of current infection, and it was postulated that other immune system stimuli might elicit a deleterious inflammatory response to this chlamydial heat shock protein in women previously sensitized by a *C. trachomatis* infection. Thus, it appears that either an unsuspected infection or reactivation of an immune system response impairs embryo implantation or facilitates rejection by the immune system after transfer of in vitro-fertilized embryos (Witkin et al., 1994), or both.

SPONTANEOUS ABORTION

Based on the above observations from in vitro fertilization, one might expect that *C. trachomatis* infections would play a role in recurrent spontaneous abortions. Quinn et al. (1987) evaluated 101 women who had undergone two previous spontaneous abortions and compared them with 63 pregnant controls. The seropositivity rate was 58% in the women who had the abortions as opposed to 34% in the controls. All of these women were cultured for *Chlamydia* and were negative.

Similarly, Witkin and Ledger (1992) evaluated 30 infertile women who had undergone three or more spontaneous abortions and had a seropositivity rate of 41%, as opposed to 13% in women who had undergone no spontaneous abortions ($P < 0.01$). However, they used a relatively high titer, of 3,128, to determine seropositivity, and they found no difference between women who had undergone fewer than three spontaneous abortions and women who had had none. In contrast, Rae et al. (1994) evaluated 106 women who had undergone three or more recurrent abortions and found no difference in the prevalence of anti-chlamydial antibodies at a titer of 316 from that in 3,890 unselected women attending a maternity clinic shortly after delivery. In a study of 349 women who had undergone a spontaneous abortion, Osser and Persson (1996) reported similar results. Thus, the putative role of *C. trachomatis* infections in spontaneous abortions, while seemingly logical, appears inconsistent and remains unproven at present.

ECTOPIC PREGNANCY

In contrast to the above findings in studies of early fetal loss, an association between *C. trachomatis* infection and ectopic pregnancy seems stronger. Multiple investigators have found a clear relationship between infection, as evidenced by antibody levels in serum, and occurrence of ectopic pregnancy (Brunham et al., 1986; Chow et al., 1990; Osser and Persson, 1992; Svensson et al., 1985; Ville et al., 1991; Walters et al., 1988), although one study (Phillips et al., 1992) of 69 women experiencing ectopic pregnancy and 101 pregnant controls found that after adjustment for cigarette smoking, the association disappeared. However, the sample was relatively small and the seroprevalence of *C. trachomatis* was low. Most investigators have not been able to demonstrate active fallopian tube infection with *C. trachomatis* at the time of the ectopic pregnancy either by culture (Brunham et al., 1986) or by nucleic acid amplification (Osser and Persson, 1992), and the presumption has been that past rather than current infection is responsible for the association with ectopic pregnancy. An exception is a study from Gabon (Ville et al., 1991) in which *C. trachomatis* was recovered from the fallopian tubes of 71% of women with ectopic pregnancy. Data even more convincing of an association between *C. trachomatis* infection and ectopic pregnancy come from a retrospective cohort study (Hillis et al., 1997) in which the risk of being hospitalized for ectopic pregnancy was determined for 11,000 women who had had one or more documented *C. trachomatis* infections. The relative risk increased from 3.8 in women with two infections to 10.8 in those with more than three infections.

The mechanism by which *C. trachomatis* infections cause ectopic pregnancy is presumably the same as that by which they cause tubal infertility. Tubal scarring is thought to result either from a persistent infection (Campbell et al., 1993; Shepard and Jones, 1989) or, more likely, from one or more infections which damage the tubes and then resolve before the ectopic pregnancy or discovery of infertility (Brunham et al., 1992; Lan et al., 1995; Wagar et al., 1990). Of particular interest are two studies which show an association between ectopic pregnancy and antibodies to chlamydial HSP60 (Brunham et al., 1992; Wagar et al., 1990). For women with tubal infertility, it has been postulated that a hypersensitivity response to the chlamydial HSP60 may play a role in the pathogenesis of disease (Brunham et al., 1985; Morrison, 1991). This is, of course, analogous to its postulated role in failure of in vitro fertilization (Witkin et al., 1994).

OTHER ADVERSE OUTCOMES

Adverse pregnancy outcomes are usually defined in terms of perinatal complications affecting either the mother or the fetus, with particular emphasis on parameters predictive of neonatal mortality and morbidity. Examples include preterm delivery, premature rupture of membranes (PROM), low birth weight, and stillbirth. The effect of maternal *C. trachomatis* infection on pregnancy outcome has been evaluated in several prospective studies; these findings are summarized in Table 1. The only consistent observation has been that the patients who have immunoglobulin M antibodies to *C. trachomatis* in serum appear to be at increased risk for premature rupture of the membranes or low birth weight, or both.

Limited data suggest that IgM antibody persists for only a short time after acquisition of a primary chlamydial infection or sometimes after a repeat infection with a different serovar (Wang and Grayston, 1982). Thus, it appears that a recently acquired infection may increase the likelihood of PROM, but an infection that has become chronic or is a reinfection with a serovar with which one has been previously infected does not appear to have the same consequences.

Other relevant information comes from evaluations of the effect of treatment of chlamydial infections during pregnancy. In a study by Cohen et al. (1990), samples from a population of predominantly African American urban women were cultured for *C. trachomatis* at the first prenatal visit and every 2 to 3 months during the remainder of their pregnancies. Women found to be infected were treated with erythromycin ethylsuccinate at 2.0 g daily for 7 days. Those who were culture negative after treatment were considered treatment successes (group 1, Table 2). Based on age, race, gravidity, marital status, socioeconomic status, and history of smoking or alcohol or other drug use, they were matched to a control group of 244 women who were culture negative during pregnancy (group 3). Another group (group 2) of 79 women were classified as treatment failures. This group consisted of 26 patients who had persistently positive cultures for *C. trachomatis* in spite of treatment, plus another 26 who were initially culture negative after treatment but became culture positive again, and 27 who

Table 1 Association of adverse pregnancy outcomes with maternal *C. trachomatis* infection

Study	No. culture positive/ no. tested	Associations
Martin et al. (1982)	18/26	Preterm birth, low birth weight, fetal demise[a]
Harrison et al. (1983)	97/1,365	Low birth weight, PROM, IgM positive (17/72 [24%])
Gravett et al. (1986)	47/534	Preterm birth, low birth weight, PROM[b]
Berman et al. (1987)	251/1,152	Low birth weight, IgM positive only[c]
Sweet et al. (1987)	270[d]	Preterm birth, and PROM in IgM positive only
Germain et al. (1994)	1,057/11,583	None[e]
Claman et al. (1995)	103[f]	Preterm birth, low birth weight, IgG positive

[a] This study was not controlled for coexisting infections but did control for age, socioeconomic status, marital status, and pregnancy order. Also, 12 *Chlamydia*-negative women with spontaneous abortions before 19 weeks gestation were excluded from the analysis.
[b] An independent association was observed between bacterial vaginosis and preterm labor, PROM, and low birth weight.
[c] IgM or recent seroconversion was present in only 16. An association between *M. hominis* and low birth weight and postpartum endometritis was also observed.
[d] Case control study with 270 culture-negative, pregnant controls matched for age, race, and socioeconomic status. IgM was found in 67 (40%) of the 270.
[e] Intrauterine growth retardation was the only dependent variable reported. Chlamydial serologic test results were not reported. An association between intrauterine growth retardation and recovery of selected anaerobes, *M. hominis*, *U. urealyticum*, and *T. vaginalis*, was reported.
[f] Case control study based on chlamydial serologic test results. Cultures not done.

were culture positive at their first antenatal visit but were not treated prior to delivery because their first antenatal visit was less than 1 week before delivery. Of the 323 women who were culture positive during pregnancy, 40 (12.4%) were negative on their initial visit but were found to be positive on a subsequent visit. The results are given in Table 2.

Compared to the treatment failure group, the treatment success group had a lower incidence of premature delivery, PROM, premature contractions, and low birth weight ($P < 0.0019$ for each category). The treatment success group was not different from the culture-negative controls except for the category of premature delivery, where the incidence was 12% in the

Table 2 Evaluation of treatment and adverse outcome[a]

Outcome	No. (%) with outcome in:		
	Group 1 (treatment success, $n = 244$)	Group 2 (treatment failure, $n = 79$)	Group 3 (control, $n = 244$)
Premature delivery	7 (2.9)	11 (13.9)	29 (11.9)
PROM	18 (7.4)	16 (20.2)	18 (7.4)
Premature contractions	10 (4.1)	19 (24.0)	4 (1.6)
Small for gestational age	32 (13.1)	20 (25.3)	29 (11.9)

[a] Adapted from Cohen et al. (1990) with permission.

controls and 2.9% in the treatment success group ($P = 0.0001$). The results of this study suggest that treatment of the *Chlamydia*-infected women reduced the incidence of all the complications listed. Of particular interest is the observation that the premature delivery was reduced relative to the control group as well as the treatment failure group. This raises the possibility either that treatment was affecting something else besides chlamydia or that the culture-negative group contained a number of *Chlamydia*-infected women. The latter is almost certainly true, since the sensitivity of culture is substantially lower than 100% in most settings (Jones et al., 1989; Viscidi et al., 1993). However, the extent to which this contributes to observations such as that noted above is unknown.

A treatment trial by Ryan et al. (1990) produced similar results, although it was conducted in a different manner (Table 3). The population

Table 3 Results of pregnancy treatment trial[a]

Outcome	% with outcome:		
	Infected treated	Infected untreated	Culture negative
PROM	2.9	5.2[b]	2.7
Birth weight <2,500 g	11	20[b]	12
Perinatal death	0.6[c]	2.4[c]	1.5[c]

[a] Adapted from Ryan et al. (1990) with permission.
[b] $P < 0.001$ for untreated infected versus either treated infected or culture-negative controls (univariate analysis).
[c] Infected untreated versus culture negative, $P < 0.05$; infected treated versus culture negative, $P < 0.01$; infected untreated versus infected treated, $P < 0.001$ (univariate analysis).

consisted of urban African American women. For 16 months, endocervical cultures for *C. trachomatis* were performed for all women presenting for their first prenatal visit. During this phase of the study, infected women were not treated and follow-up cultures were not obtained. Then, during the next 20 months of the study, all the women who were identified as infected at their first prenatal visit were treated with erythromycin at 500 mg, four times daily for 7 days. Those who could not tolerate this regimen were treated with erythromycin at 250 mg, four times daily for 14 days. A test-of-cure culture was performed after treatment, and if it was still positive the women were re-treated. The subjects were then divided into three groups: those who were infected but had not been treated (first 16 months of the study), those who were infected and had been treated (second 20 months of the study), and those who were presumed uninfected, i.e., were culture negative at their first prenatal visit (entire 36 months of the study).

Perinatal deaths were defined as stillborn infants, infants who died in the neonatal period, and infants who remained continuously hospitalized beyond 28 days from the time of birth to death. Newborn survival was significantly better in the treated group than in either the untreated group ($P < 0.08$) or the culture-negative group ($P < 0.01$), even after adjustments for race, age, PROM, birth weight, urinary tract infection, smoking, hypertension, and diabetes. The incidence of chorioamnionitis was not significantly different among the three groups. The overall prevalence of chlamydial infection was 21%. It did not change during the study period, nor did the demographics of the study population. In addition, there was a slight overall increase in perinatal mortality from the beginning of the study period, when no one was being treated, to the end of the study period, when all the infected women were being treated. This overall trend is the opposite direction from that seen in the treated as opposed to untreated groups. It strongly suggests that the observed treatment effect is, in fact, due to the treatment rather than to other unmeasured events in the population under study. Thus, in spite of the use of historical controls (the infected untreated group), the data are fairly convincing that treatment of *Chlamydia*-infected women with erythromycin reduces the incidence of the adverse outcomes listed.

In this study, as in the previous study, the culture-negative group had a higher incidence of perinatal deaths than the treated group, again raising the question whether there is something besides *Chlamydia* that affects perinatal mortality that is being treated by erythromycin or whether there are significant numbers of *Chlamydia*-infected patients who are not detected among the culture-negative group. Because such women would not be identified as infected, they would not be treated and therefore would contribute to the complication rate in the uninfected, untreated group. Parenthetically, an association between smoking and low birth weight also was observed.

In contrast to these two studies, in a large multicenter study on vaginal infection and prematurity, Germain et al. (1994) reported no difference in intrauterine growth retardation between women infected with *C. trachomatis* and those not infected. However, in a separate analysis of these data, an association with preterm delivery (odds ratio, 1.53; 95% confidence limit of 1.21 to 1.93) was observed even after adjustment for other organisms also found to be associated, i.e., *Mycoplasma hominis*, *Ureaplasma urealyticum*, and *Trichomonas vaginalis* (Nugent et al., 1990). *C. trachomatis*-infected women participating in this study also were potential candidates for enrollment in a placebo-controlled treatment trial with erythromycin base at 333 mg three times daily for 7 days (Martin et al., 1997). A total of 414 women were randomized to receive erythromycin (205 women) or placebo (209 women). Treatment was found not to affect pregnancy outcome when combined data from all study sites were analyzed. However, in three of the six centers a high proportion of both the placebo- and erythromycin-treated patients were culture negative at the follow-up examination. When the data were analyzed for just the sites that had a high persistence of *C. trachomatis* in placebo-treated women, the treatment was found to have a significant effect on the rate of low birth weight (8 and 17%, in treated and placebo-treated patients, respectively; $P < 0.04$) (Martin et al., 1997). Additional data suggest that chlamydial infections may interact with host factors such as a short cervix (Iams et al., 1996) or bacterial vaginosis due to other members of the microflora to facilitate preterm birth (Andrews, 1997).

TREATMENT

While the above-mentioned studies are not entirely conclusive, they strongly suggest that treatment of *C. trachomatis*-infected women in pregnancy has a favorable effect on pregnancy outcome. This could be due primarily to the effect of treatment on the *C. trachomatis* infection itself or to its effect on both the *C. trachomatis* and other, less well characterized, infections. In any case, treatment of *C. trachomatis*-infected women to prevent transmission to their infants is the current standard of care (CDC, 1993). However, Centers for Disease Control and Prevention recommendations on sexually transmitted diseases are that screening and treatment be done late rather than early in pregnancy to avoid reinfection or acquisition of new infections before delivery (CDC, 1993). Support for this position comes from studies such as that by Cohen et al. (1990), cited above, in which 40 chlamydia-infected women were initially culture negative. Similarly, in a study by Oh et al. (1993), adolescent girls were screened for chlamydial infection at their first prenatal visit and again in the third trimester. Of 267, 50 (18.7%) were infected at enrollment. However, in the third trimester, 14 of 178 (7.9%) were also found to be infected. Of these, 12 had initially been culture negative while 2 had been positive and had been treated. This presents an obvious dilemma, since treatment early in pregnancy presumably would not necessarily prevent adverse outcomes due to infections acquired later in pregnancy. The currently recommended treatment regimen is erythromycin or amoxicillin; many women have difficulty complying with erythromycin regimens because of gastrointestional side effects (Crombleholme et al., 1990; Turrentine and Newton, 1995). Amoxicillin renders women culture negative and prevents transmission to their infants (Crombleholme et al., 1990; Turrentine and Newton, 1995). Whether the amoxicillin cures infection or has effects on other microorganisms is unknown.

CONCLUSIONS AND FUTURE DIRECTIONS

In summary, *C. trachomatis* infections in women are clearly associated with tubal infertility and ectopic pregnancy. In addition, they may be associated with first-trimester spontaneous abortions and, in some instances, with PROM, prematurity, low birth weight, and, possibly, survival. Because of these associations and the risk of perinatal transmission, additional data are needed on the optimum time for screening and treatment during pregnancy. In addition, the optimum treatment regimen must be better defined. Compliance with multiple-dose regimens is problematic (Katz et al., 1992; Martin, 1990). Single-dose therapy with azithromycin is effective in the treatment of nonpregnant women and of men with *C. trachomatis* lower genital tract infections (Martin et al., 1992), although this agent has not been adequately evaluated in pregnant women. Finally, although some data suggesting that there may be differences between serovars in the degree of inflammation (Batteiger et al., 1989; Dean et al., 1995) and tissue tropism (Barnes et al., 1987) have been collected, there are no studies on the relationship between the infecting serovar and adverse pregnancy outcome. Similarly, there are no data on the role of the immune system response to chlamydial infections in patients with adverse outcomes. The immune response appears to play a significant role in the pathogenesis of ocular trachoma and in *Chlamydia*-associated tubal infertility and ectopic pregnancy (Taylor et al., 1990). Investigation of these questions could help clarify the relationship between chlamydial infections in women and adverse pregnancy outcomes and would lead to effective interventions to reduce pregnancy-associated morbidity and mortality.

REFERENCES

Alexander, E. R., and H. R. Harrison. 1983. Role of *Chlamydia trachomatis* in perinatal infection. *Rev. Infect. Dis.* **5:**713–719.

Andrews, W. W. 1997. The preterm predictions study: association of mid-trimester genital chlamydia infection and subsequent spontaneous preterm birth (SPTB). Proceedings of the 17th Annual Meeting of the Society of Perinatal Obstetricians,

Anaheim, California, January 20–25, 1997. *Am. J. Obstet. Gynecol.* **176:**abstr. no. 151.

Barnes, R. C., A. M. Rompalo, and W. E. Stamm. 1987. Comparison of *Chlamydia trachomatis* serovars causing rectal and cervical infections. *J. Infect. Dis.* **156:**953–958.

Batteiger, B. E., W. Lennington, W. J. Newhall, B. P. Katz, H. T. Morrison, and R. B. Jones. 1989. Correlation of infection serovar and local inflammation in genital chlamydial infections. *J. Infect. Dis.* **160:**332–336.

Bell, T. A., W. E. Stamm, S. P. Wang, C. C. Kuo, K. K. Holmes, and J. T. Grayston. 1992. Chronic *Chlamydia trachomatis* infections in infants. *JAMA* **267:**400–402. (Erratum, **267:**177.)

Bell, T. A., W. E. Stamm, C. C. Kuo, S. P. Wang, K. K. Holmes, and J. T. Grayston. 1994. Risk of perinatal transmission of *Chlamydia trachomatis* by mode of delivery. *J. Infect.* **29:**165–169.

Berman, S. M., H. R. Harrison, W. T. Boyce, W. J. Haffner, M. Lewis, and J. B. Arthur. 1987. Low birth weight, prematurity, and postpartum endometritis: association with prenatal cervical *Mycoplasma hominis* and *Chlamydia trachomatis* infections. *JAMA* **257:**1189–1194.

Brunham, R. C., I. W. Maclean, B. Binns, and R. W. Peeling. 1985. *Chlamydia trachomatis*: its role in tubal infertility. *J. Infect. Dis.* **152:**1275–1282.

Brunham, R. C., F. Binns, J. McDowell, and M. Paraskevas. 1986. *Chlamydia trachomatis* infection in women with ectopic pregnancy. *Obstet. Gynecol.* **67:**722–726.

Brunham, R. C., R. Peeling, I. Maclean, M. L. Kosseim, and M. Paraskevas. 1992. *Chlamydia trachomatis*-associated ectopic pregnancy: serologic and histologic correlates. *J. Infect. Dis.* **165:**1076–1081.

Campbell, L. A., D. L. Patton, D. E. Moore, A. L. Cappuccio, B. A. Mueller, and S. Wang. 1993. Detection of *Chlamydia trachomatis* deoxyribonucleic acid in women with tubal infertility. *Fertil. Steril.* **59:**45–50.

Centers for Disease Control and Prevention. 1993. Sexually transmitted diseases treatment guidelines. *Morbid. Mortal. Weekly Rep.* **42:**1–56.

Chow, J. M., L. Yonekura, G. A. Richwald, S. Greenland, R. L. Sweet, and J. Schachter. 1990. The association between *Chlamydia trachomatis* and ectopic pregnancy: a matched-pair, case-control study. *JAMA* **263:**3164–3167.

Claman, P., B. Toye, R. W. Peeling, P. Jessamine, and J. Belcher. 1995. Serologic evidence of *Chlamydia trachomatis* infection and risk of preterm birth. *Can. Med. Assoc. J.* **153:**259–262.

Cohen, I., J. C. Veille, and B. M. Calkins. 1990. Improved pregnancy outcome following successful treatment of chlamydial infection. *JAMA* **263:**3160–3163. (Comments, **263:**3191–3192.)

Crombleholme, W. R., J. Schachter, M. Grossman, D. V. Landers, and R. L. Sweet. 1990. Amoxicillin therapy for *Chlamydia trachomatis* in pregnancy. *Obstet. Gynecol.* **75:**752–756.

Dean, D., E. Oudens, G. Bolan, N. Padian, and J. Schachter. 1995. Major outer membrane protein variants of *Chlamydia trachomatis* are associated with severe upper genital tract infections and histopathology in San Francisco. *J. Infect. Dis.* **172:**1013–1022.

Germain, M., M. A. Krohn, S. L. Hillier, and D. A. Eschenbach. 1994. Genital flora in pregnancy and its association with intrauterine growth retardation. *J. Clin. Microbiol.* **32:**2162–2168.

Gravett, M. G., H. P. Nelson, T. DeRouen, C. Critchlow, D. Eschenbach, and K. K. Holmes. 1986. Independent associations of bacterial vaginosis and *Chlamydia trachomatis* infection with adverse pregnancy outcome. *JAMA* **256:**1899–1903.

Harrison, H. R., and E. R. Alexander. 1990. Chlamydial infections in infants and children, p. 811–820. *In* K. K. Holmes, P.-A. Mardh, P. F. Sparling, and P. J. Wiesner (ed.), *Sexually Transmitted Diseases,* 2nd ed. McGraw-Hill, Inc., New York, N.Y.

Harrison, H. R., D. Phil, L. M. Taussig, and V. A. Fulginiti. 1982. *Chlamydia trachomatis* and chronic respiratory disease in childhood. *Pediatr. Infect. Dis. J.* **1:**29–33.

Harrison, H. R., E. R. Alexander, L. Weinstein, M. Lewis, M. Nash, and D. A. Sim. 1983. Cervical *Chlamydia trachomatis* and mycoplasmal infections in pregnancy. *JAMA* **250:**1721–1727.

Hillis, S. D., B. S. Owens, P. A. Marchbanks, L. E. Amsterdam, and W. R. MacKenzie. 1997. Recurrent chlamydial infections increase the risks of hospitalization for ectopic pregnancy and pelvic inflammatory disease. *Am. J. Obstet. Gynecol.* **176:**103–107.

Iams, J. D., R. L. Goldenberg, P. J. Meis, B. M. Mercer, A. Moawad, A. Das, E. Thom, D. McNellis, R. L. Copper, F. Johnson, and J. M. Roberts. 1996. The length of the cervix and the risk of spontaneous premature delivery. *N. Engl. J. Med.* **334:**567–572.

Jones, R. B., J. B. Mammel, M. K. Shepard, and R. R. Fisher. 1986. Recovery of *Chlamydia trachomatis* from the endometrium of women at risk for chlamydial infection. *Am. J. Obstet. Gynecol.* **155:**35–39.

Jones, R. B., B. Van Der Pol, and B. P. Katz. 1989. Effect of differences in specimen processing and passage technique on recovery of *Chlamydia trachomatis. J. Clin. Microbiol.* **27:**894–898.

Katz, B. P., B. W. Zwickl, V. A. Caine, and R. B. Jones. 1992. Compliance with antibiotic therapy for *Chlamydia trachomatis* and *Neisseria gonorrhoeae. Sex. Transm. Dis.* **19:**351–354.

Lan, J., A. J. van den Brule, D. J. Hemrika, E. K. Risse, J. M. Walboomers, M. E. Schipper, and C. J. Meijer. 1995. *Chlamydia trachomatis* and ectopic pregnancy: retrospective analysis of salpingectomy specimens, endometrial biopsies, and cervical smears. *J. Clin. Pathol.* **48:**815–819.

Lessing, J. B., Y. Kletter, R. Amster, A. Amit, M. R. Peyser, and S. Berger. 1991. Success rates in in vitro fertilization treatment and its correlation with high titer antibodies for *Chlamydia trachomatis. Isr. J. Med. Sci.* **27:**546–549.

Lunenfeld, E., B. S. Shapiro, B. Sarov, I. Sarov, V. Insler, and A. H. Decherney. 1989. The association between chlamydial-specific IgG and IgA antibodies and pregnancy outcome in an in vitro fertilization program. *J. In Vitro Fert. Embryo Transfer* **6:**222–227.

Martin, D. H. 1990. Erythromycin (E) treatment of *Chlamydia trachomatis* (Ct) infections during pregnancy, abstr. 693. *In Program and Abstracts of the 30th Interscience*

Conference on Antimicrobial Agents and Chemotherapy. American Society for Microbiology, Washington, D.C.

Martin, D. H., L. Koutsky, D. A. Eschenbach, J. R. Daling, E. R. Alexander, J. K. Benedetti, and K. K. Holmes. 1982. Prematurity and perinatal mortality in pregnancies complicated by maternal *Chlamydia trachomatis* infections. *JAMA* **247:**1584–1588.

Martin, D. H., T. F. Mrochzkowski, Z. A. Dalu, J. McCarty, R. B. Jones, S. J. Hopkins, and R. B. Johnson. 1992. A controlled trial of a single dose of azithromycin for the treatment of chlamydial urethritis and cervicitis. The Azithromycin for Chlamydial Infections Study Group. *N. Engl. J. Med.* **327:**921–925.

Martin, D. H., D. A. Eschenbach, M. F. Cotch, R. P. Nugent, A. V. Rao, M. A. Klebanoff, Y. Lou, P. J. Rettig, R. S. Gibbs, J. G. Pastorek, J. A. Regan, and R. A. Kaslow. 1997. Double-blind placebo-controlled treatment trial of *Chlamydia trachomatis* endocervical infections in pregnant women. *Infect. Dis. Obstet Gynecol.* **5:**10–17.

Morrison, R. P. 1991. Chlamydial hsp60 and the immunopathogenesis of chlamydial disease. *Semin. Immunol.* **3:**25–33.

Nugent, R., D. Martin, M. F. Cotch, and P. Rettig. 1990. Chlamydial infection and adverse pregnancy outcome: interim results from a multicenter prospective study, p. 344–347. *In* W. R. Bowie, H. D. Caldwell, R. B. Jones, P.-A. Mardh, G. L. Ridgway, J. Schachter, W. E. Stamm, and M. E. Ward (ed.), *Chlamydial Infections: Proceedings of the Seventh International Symposium on Human Chlamydial Infections.* Cambridge University Press, Cambridge, United Kingdom.

Oh, M. K., G. A. Cloud, S. L. Baker, M. A. Pass, K. Mulchahey, and R. F. Pass. 1993. Chlamydial infection and sexual behavior in young pregnant teenagers. *Sex. Transm. Dis.* **20:**45–50.

Osser, S., and K. Persson. 1992. Chlamydial antibodies and deoxyribonucleic acid in patients with ectopic pregnancy. *Fertil. Steril.* **57:**578–582.

Osser, S., and K. Persson. 1996. Chlamydial antibodies in women who suffer miscarriage. *Br. J. Obstet. Gynaecol.* **103:**137–141.

Osser, S., K. Persson, H. Wramsby, and P. Liedholm. 1990. Does previous *Chlamydia trachomatis* infection influence the pregnancy rate of in vitro fertilization and embryo replacement? *Am. J. Obstet. Gynecol.* **162:**40–44.

Paavonen, J., N. Kiviat, R. C. Brunham, C. E. Stevens, C. C. Kuo, W. E. Stamm, A. Miettinen, M. Soules, D. A. Eschenbach, and K. K. Holmes. 1985. Prevalence and manifestations of endometritis among women with cervicitis. *Am. J. Obstet. Gynecol.* **152:**280–286.

Phillips, R. S., R. E. Tuomala, P. J. Feldblum, J. Schachter, M. J. Rosenberg, and M. D. Aronso. 1992. The effect of cigarette smoking, *Chlamydia trachomatis* infection, and vaginal douching on ectopic pregnancy. *Obstet. Gynecol.* **79:**85–90.

Quinn, P. A., M. Petric, M. Barkin, J. Butany, C. Derzko, M. Gysler, K. I. Lie, A. B. Shewchuck, J. Shuber, E. Ryan, and M. L. Chipman. 1987. Prevalence of antibody to *Chlamydia trachomatis* in spontaneous abortion and infertility. *Am. J. Obstet. Gynecol.* **156:**291–296.

Rae, R., I. W. Smith, W. A. Liston, and D. C. Kilpatrick. 1994. Chlamydial serologic studies and recurrent spontaneous abortion. *Am. J. Obstet. Gynecol.* **170:**782–785.

Ryan, G. M., Jr., T. N. Abdella, S. G. McNeeley, V. S. Baselski, and D. E. Drummond. 1990. *Chlamydia trachomatis* infection in pregnancy and effect of treatment on outcome. *Am. J. Obstet. Gynecol.* **162:**34–39. (Comments, **164:**234, 1991.)

Schachter, J., L. Cles, R. Ray, and P. A. Hines. 1979. Failure of serology in diagnosing chlamydial infections of the female genital tract. *J. Clin. Microbiol.* **10:**647–649.

Shepard, M. K., and R. B. Jones. 1989. Recovery of *Chlamydia trachomatis* from endometrial and fallopian tube biopsies in women with infertility of tubal origin. *Fertil. Steril.* **52:**232–238.

Svensson, L., P.-A. Märdh, M. Ahlgren, and F. Nordenskjöld. 1985. Ectopic pregnancy and antibodies to *Chlamydia trachomatis. Fertil. Steril.* **44:**313–317.

Sweet, R. L., D. V. Landers, C. Walker, and J. Schachter. 1987. *Chlamydia trachomatis* infection and pregnancy outcome. *Am. J. Obstet. Gynecol.* **156:**824–833.

Taylor, H. R., I. W. Maclean, R. C. Brunham, S. Pal, and J. Whittum-Hudson. 1990. *Chlamydia* heat shock proteins and trachoma. *Infect. Immun.* **58:**3061–3063.

Torode, H. W., P. A. Wheeler, D. M. Saunders, R. A. McPetrie, S. C. Medcalf, and V. P. Ackerman. 1987. The role of chlamydial antibodies in an in vitro fertilization program. *Fertil. Steril.* **48:**987–990.

Turrentine, M. A., and E. R. Newton. 1995. Amoxicillin or erythromycin for the treatment of antenatal chlamydial infection: a meta-analysis. *Obstet. Gynecol.* **86:** 1021–1025.

Ville, Y., M. Leruez, E. Glowaczower, J. N. Robertson, and M. E. Ward. 1991. The role of *Chlamydia trachomatis* and *Neisseria gonorrhoeae* in the aetiology of ectopic pregnancy in Gabon. *Br. J. Obstet. Gynaecol.* **98:**1260–1266.

Viscidi, R. P., L. Bobo, E. W. Hook, and T. C. Quinn. 1993. Transmission of *Chlamydia trachomatis* among sex partners assessed by polymerase chain reaction. *J. Infect. Dis.* **168:**488–492.

Wagar, E. A., J. Schachter, P. Bavoil, and R. S. Stephens. 1990. Differential human serologic response to two 60,000 molecular weight *Chlamydia trachomatis* antigens. *J. Infect. Dis.* **162:**922–927.

Walters, M. D., C. A. Eddy, R. S. Gibbs, J. Schachter, M. A. Holden, and C. J. Pauerstein. 1988. Antibodies to *Chlamydia trachomatis* and risk for tubal pregnancy. *Am. J. Obstet. Gynecol.* **159:**942–946.

Wang, S. P., and J. T. Grayston. 1982. Microimmunofluorescence antibody responses in *Chlamydia trachomatis* infection, a review, p. 301–316. *In* P. A. Mårdh, K. K. Holmes, J. D. Oriel, P. Piot, and J. Schachter (ed.), *Chlamydial Infections. Proceedings of the Fifth International Symposium on Human Chlamydial Infections.* Elsevier Biomedical Press, Amsterdam, The Netherlands.

Wasserheit, J. N., T. A. Bell, N. B. Kiviat, P. Wolner-Hanssen, V. Zabriskie, B. D. Kirby, E. C. Prince, K. K. Holmes, W. E. Stamm, and D. A. Eschenbach. 1986. Microbial causes of proven pelvic inflammatory disease and efficacy of clindamycin and tobramycin. *Ann. Intern. Med.* **104:**187–193.

Weiss, S. G., R. W. Newcomb, and M. O. Beem. 1986. Pulmonary assessment of children after chlamydial pneumonia of infancy. *J. Pediatr.* **108:**659–664.

Witkin, S. S., and W. J. Ledger. 1992. Antibodies to *Chlamydia trachomatis* in sera of women with recurrent spontaneous abortions. *Am. J. Obstet. Gynecol.* **167:**135–139.

Witkin, S. S., K. M. Sultan, G. S. Neal, J. Jeremias, J. A. Grifo, and Z. Rosenwaks. 1994. Unsuspected *Chlamydia trachomatis* infection and in vitro fertilization outcome. *Am. J. Obstet. Gynecol.* **171:**1208–1214.

Witkin, S. S., I. Kligman, J. A. Grifo, and Z. Rosenwaks. 1995. *Chlamydia trachomatis* detected by polymerase chain reaction in cervices of culture-negative women correlates with adverse in vitro fertilization outcome. *J. Infect. Dis.* **171:**1657–1659.

12
Trichomoniasis

Pål Wölner-Hanssen

Trichomoniasis is the most common nonviral sexually transmitted disease worldwide. It has been estimated that more than 180 million people are infected with *Trichomonas vaginalis* (Brown, 1972). The estimated incidence of the infection in the United States has declined during recent years. According to the National Disease and Therapeutic Index survey, the number of physician visits for trichomonal vaginitis declined from a high of 1.3 million in 1974 to less than 600,000 in 1987 (Kent, 1991).

Infection with *T. vaginalis* can be asymptomatic or can be associated with acute vaginitis. Some of the unresolved issues of trichomoniasis that are relevant to adverse outcomes of pregnancy include understanding the pathogenesis of vaginal infection, determining whether and how the protozoon can cause premature rupture of the membranes and premature delivery, determining the best screening plan for asymptomatic cases, and choosing the best treatment for infection early in pregnancy. These and related topics are discussed in this chapter.

MICROBIOLOGY

Anatomy

T. vaginalis is a protozoon of variable size and shape. Its size varies from 10 to 20 μm. Its shape tends to be ellipsoidal in axenic cultures and ameboid in vivo. The microorganism is mobile by way of four anterior flagella and one posterior flagellum, which is attached to an undulating membrane. The undulating membrane extends for about one-half to two-thirds of the length of the cell. The organism moves with jerky movements by the flagella and

Pål Wölner-Hanssen, Department of Obstetrics and Gynecology, University Hospital of Lund, Lund, Sweden.

Sexually Transmitted Diseases and Adverse Outcomes of Pregnancy
Edited by P. J. Hitchcock, H. T. MacKay, J. N. Wasserheit, and R. Binder
©1999 American Society for Microbiology, Washington, D.C.

the undulating membrane. Mitochondria, energy-producing cellular organelles, are lacking in trichomonads. Relatively large, unique dense granules called hydrogenosomes probably confer tolerance for a low-oxygen environment. Hydrogenosomes are characteristic of trichomonads.

PATHOGENESIS

T. vaginalis infects the squamous epithelium of the lower genital tract almost exclusively, in both women and men. In women, the vagina, exocervix, urethra, and Skene's glands are the main sites of infection. In men, the infection is urethral and usually without symptoms.

It is unclear why some infected women have severe local symptoms while others remain asymptomatic. This may be related to trichomonas virulence factors or to host factors. Factors that may influence the virulence of *T. vaginalis* include antigenic heterogeneity, phenotypic variation, cytotoxins, proteinases, and release of cell membrane components (Lehker and Alderete, 1990). Cytotoxicity is composed of both contact-dependent and contact-independent components. In contact-dependent cytotoxicity, specific trichomonad surface proteins (adhesins) mediate the interaction of *T. vaginalis* with epithelial cells (Arroyo et al., 1992). Scanning electron microscopy and transmission electron microscopy of the interaction between trichomonads and the epithelial-cell layer of human amniotic membranes have demonstrated damaged and desquamated cells in areas where parasites were in direct contact with the target cells (Mirhaghani and Warton, 1996). Secreted soluble factors causing contact-independent cytotoxicity may include free lactic acid or acetic acid (Pindak et al., 1993) and cell-detaching factor (Garber et al., 1989). Cell-detaching factor is a 200-kDa glycoprotein that causes detachment of monolayer cells in culture. Production of cell-detaching factor correlates with symptomatic trichomoniasis (Garber et al., 1989). The ability of *T. vaginalis* isolates to produce subcutaneous abscesses in mice, hemolytic activity, and adherence to HeLa cells have also been regarded as a surrogate marker of *T. vaginalis* pathogenicity. However, the clinical manifestations most strongly associated with trichomoniasis (colpitis macularis and purulent vaginal discharge) do not seem to correlate with these features (Krieger et al., 1990a). The observation that wet mounts are more often positive in women with symptomatic than with asymptomatic trichomoniasis suggests a relationship between the concentration of *T. vaginalis* in vaginal fluid and the severity of inflammation (Krieger et al., 1990a).

T. VAGINALIS AND CHORIOAMNIONITIS

Some investigators have found an association between *T. vaginalis* infection and prematurity. It is believed that the organism causes premature rupture of membranes and thereby reduces gestational age at delivery and increases the frequency of cervical low birth weight in infants. In a study of women enrolled during the second trimester of pregnancy, Minkoff et al. (1984) investigated the associations between the vaginal flora and prematurity/ premature rupture of the membranes. Infection with *T. vaginalis* (relative risk [RR] = 1.4) and infection with *Staphylococcus epidermidis* (RR = 1.57) were each significantly associated with premature rupture of the membranes. The association between infection and premature rupture of the membranes was stronger in coinfected women (RR = 2.1). Cotch et al. (1997) reported, in the Vaginal Infections and Prematurity Study (VIP study), that *T. vaginalis* carriage at midpregnancy was associated with premature delivery (adjusted odds ratio [OR] = 1.3), low birth weight (adjusted OR = 1.3), and preterm delivery of a low-birth-weight infant (adjusted OR = 1.4). McGregor et al. (1995) suggested a possible synergistic effect of combined reproductive tract infections on the risk of prematurity. The risk of preterm birth was 17.8% among women with bacterial vaginosis (BV) but not trichomoniasis, 9.1% among those with trichomoniasis but not BV, and 27.8% among those with both BV and trichomoniasis. In contrast, several studies could not find a connection between adverse pregnancy outcomes and trichomoniasis. For example, Mason and Brown (1980) found no association between trichomoniasis and low birth weight. In a placebo-controlled trial, treatment of trichomoniasis was not associated with increased birth weight or reduced prematurity rate (Ross and Middelkoop, 1983). In a study by Hillier et al. (1988) *T. vaginalis* was not recovered from the placentas of any of 38 women who delivered prematurely. In another study, of more than 200 culture specimens obtained from between the membranes after premature delivery, none were positive for *T. vaginalis* (Cassell, personal communication). However, the investigators did not examine vaginal fluid for *T. vaginalis*. In a more recent multicenter study, 2,929 pregnant women were examined at gestational weeks 24 and 28 to identify vaginal pathogens (Meis et al., 1995). Detection of *T. vaginalis* had no significant association with preterm birth in that study. A Lithuanian study of 212 women in preterm labor and 62 women in term labor failed to show any association between preterm labor and *T. vaginalis* in the endocervix (Nadisauskiene et al., 1995).

In an analysis of the VIP study, Read et al. (1993) identified *T. vaginalis* infection of the vagina at 23 to 26 weeks as a significant risk factor for prematurity only among women having frequent intercourse (more than once a week). In contrast, among women having infrequent intercourse (less than once a week), *T. vaginalis* infection was not associated with prematurity. A hypothesis that intercourse helps microorganisms ascend to the upper genital tract is supported by studies of pelvic inflammatory disease (PID) among nonpregnant women. Lee et al. (1991) found a threefold-increased risk of PID among monogamous women having intercourse six or more times a week compared with those having intercourse once a week or less. Preliminary analyses of the results of PID studies in Seattle showed a significant association between PID and frequency of intercourse among women with nongonococcal, nonchlamydial PID (Wölner-Hanssen, unpublished). This association remained significant after adjusting for potentially confounding variables.

In summary, the available data suggest that *T. vaginalis* can cause rupture of the membranes and/or prematurity in some women. The protozoan probably acts in the lower genital tract, i.e., the vagina and cervix, or at the lower pole of the chorioamnion. Pathogenic mechanisms involved might include contact-dependent cytotoxicity (this is mediated by lysing of membranes) (Mirhaghani and Warton, 1996) or production of metabolites that can stimulate prostaglandin synthesis (e.g., phospholipase A_2) (McGregor et al., 1992) or erode the fetal membranes (e.g., cystein proteases) (Alderete et al., 1991c). The organism is most probably sexually transmitted. Infection of the vagina and the resulting metabolic products impact on the intact membranes.

Future studies should focus on host factors, including vaginal douching and frequent intercourse, which might help *T. vaginalis* and/or its products ascend through the cervix. Moreover, the possible effects of soluble *Trichomonas* products on fetal membranes should be investigated by using in vitro systems.

IMMUNITY TO *T. VAGINALIS*

After successful therapy, recurrent vaginal infection may occur. However, *T. vaginalis* almost never spreads outside the human genitourinary system. Therefore, while host defense mechanisms efficiently control the infection, it is not eliminated in women. The nature of the host defense against *T. vaginalis* is poorly characterized.

Immunoglobulin G antibodies in serum to *T. vaginalis* cysteine proteases are present in patients with trichomoniasis (Alderete et al., 1991b). These antibodies are not found in uninfected or treated women. Antibodies to trichomonad cysteine proteases are also detected in vaginal wash specimens from some infected women (Alderete et al., 1991c). IgG and IgA that are reactive with trichomonad surface immunogens have also been detected in vaginal wash specimens (Alderete, 1984; Street et al., 1982). Vaginal wash antibodies among women with trichomoniasis are highly specific and are directed primarily against a 230-kDa *Trichomonas* immunogen called P230 (Alderete et al., 1991a). These antibodies can also be detected several weeks after treatment but are not found in uninfected controls (Alderete et al., 1991). Vaginal antibodies against P230 are not cytolytic (Alderete et al., 1991). However, some noncytolytic antibodies may inhibit the motility and adherence of trichomonads (Krieger et al., 1990b). The P230 protein appears to undergo phase variation; the accessibility of antibodies to P230 and other surface immunogens seems variable among protozoa within the same culture. Only trichomonads with certain high-molecular-weight proteins exposed on their surface induce an antibody response (Alderete et al., 1986; Alderete, 1988). This property has been termed epitope phenotypic variation (Alderete et al., 1986) and may be important as an immune system evasion strategy (Alderete et al., 1991).

Infection with *T. vaginalis* may elicit an inflammation characterized by discharge. Neutrophils are the predominant inflammatory cell type in trichomoniasis (Buchvald et al., 1992). It has been suggested that trichomonads activate the alternative complement pathway and attract neutrophils (Rein et al., 1980). An uncharacterized polypeptide produced by *T. vaginalis* is also chemotactic for neutrophils (Mason and Forman, 1982). Groups of neutrophils kill and then ingest the fragmented protozoa (Rein et al., 1980). The activity of the neutrophils against *T. vaginalis* relies on the presence of oxygen. Macrophage-mediated spontaneous cytotoxicity has also been observed (Mantovani et al., 1981). The relatively strong local immune reaction to trichomonads in some women probably results in release of cytokines into the vaginal fluid. In fact, monocytes react to *T. vaginalis* membrane components by producing large amounts of interleukin-8 (IL-8) (Shaio et al., 1995). The cytokine profile in the vaginal fluid in trichomoniasis and the role for cytokines in premature rupture of the membranes or premature uterine contractions deserve further study.

CLINICAL FINDINGS

Symptoms of vaginal trichomoniasis include abnormal frothy discharge and genital irritation. However, of 131 infected women attending a sexually transmitted disease (STD) clinic, only 12% had frothy vaginal discharge (Fouts and Kraus, 1980). Nevertheless, frothy discharge was the only manifestation studied that was significantly associated with trichomoniasis. Dysuria and the presence of other types of abnormal discharge were not related to trichomoniasis. Later, McLellan et al. (1982) studied 226 consecutive women attending an inner-city STD clinic. Women with trichomoniasis were more likely to have signs of abnormal vaginal discharge, but the infection was not related to symptoms of abnormal discharge or pruritus.

In a more recent study, we studied 779 randomly selected women attending an inner-city STD clinic; 118 had proven trichomoniasis (Wölner-Hanssen et al., 1989). Symptoms of yellow discharge and vulvar itching and signs of cervical red spots (colpitis macularis), purulent discharge, frothy discharge, and vaginal redness (erythema) were independently and significantly associated with trichomoniasis. Colposcopic evidence of colpitis macularis showed the strongest association with trichomoniasis (OR, 241.4; positive predictive value, 90%). Frothy discharge was significantly associated with trichomoniasis, but only 8% of infected women had this sign. Trichomoniasis was not related to abdominal pain ($P = 0.2$) or adnexal tenderness ($P = 0.5$).

DIAGNOSTIC PROCEDURES

Wet Mount

Observation of live protozoa in specimens from the vagina or urethra is definitive evidence of genital trichomoniasis. During microscopy, trichomonads are recognized among other cellular matter in the specimen by the jerky motion of the flagella.

About 50 to 80% of men and women with proven trichomoniasis will have organisms detected by wet mount examination. For 570 pregnant women, of whom 10.2% were infected with *T. vaginalis*, wet mount examination had a sensitivity of 55.8% and a positive predictive value of 78.4% compared to culture (Pastorek et al., 1996). The sensitivity of direct microscopy is related to several factors, including the concentration of protozoa, the expertise of the readers (Mason and Forman, 1982), and recent vaginal douching (Lossick, 1988). In some women, particularly those with few symptoms, the concentration of protozoa in the genital specimen may be too low for diagnosis by microscopy. For example, the sensitivity of wet mount examination for diagnosis of trichomoniasis was much lower for examination of nonpurulent vaginal fluid (30%) than it was for examination of purulent vaginal fluid (81%) (Wölner-Hanssen et al., 1989). In a study of 2,000 women with trichomoniasis, Lossick (1988) reported a 64% sensitivity of wet mounts in asymptomatic women, 75% in women with clinical vaginitis, and 80% in those with "characteristic" symptoms.

The habit of vaginal douching is common among African American women, particularly in the southeastern United States. Women of the same ethnic group are also more likely to be infected with *T. vaginalis*. The sensitivity of wet mounts is reduced from 57% to 22% ($P < 0.001$) if vaginal douching has been performed within 24 h prior to examination (Fouts and Kraus, 1980).

Culture

T. vaginalis culture is 100% specific and is therefore considered a "gold standard" for trichomoniasis diagnosis. *Trichomonas* culture is the most sensitive diagnostic procedure but will miss up to 15% of infected cases (Lossick, 1988). Detailed aspects of *T. vaginalis* cultivation were reviewed by Linstead (1989). A number of different media have been studied. Modified Diamond's medium (tryptose-yeast extract maltose medium [TYM]; [Müller et al., 1988]) and Feinberg-Whittington medium (Feinberg and Whittington, 1957) are commonly used for *T. vaginalis* cultures. Both seem to be equally effective for the isolation of *T. vaginalis* (Krieger et al., 1988). Diamond's medium and modified Diamond's medium can detect 97 and 90% of isolates from vaginal secretions, respectively. A modified thioglycolate medium, supplemented with yeast extract, horse serum, and antimicrobial agents, was as reliable as the more expensive Diamond's medium according to one recent study (Poch et al., 1996). Disadvantages of culturing trichomonas include the need to maintain viability during transport of specimens to the laboratory, the long incubation time involved (2 to 7 days), the requirement for examination of three wet mount preparations by technical staff, and the relatively high costs of the procedure.

The InPouch (BioMed Diagnostics Inc., Santa Clara, Calif.) is a new culture method for *T. vaginalis*, and it resolves some disadvantages of traditional culture technique. The pouch, which can be used for both specimen transport and culture, can maintain trichomonad viability for periods from 41 to 131 days (Borchardt and Smith, 1991). Specimens may be sent by regular mail to the laboratory and examined under the microscope after a 24-h incubation. The test has a sensitivity of 4 organisms per ml (Borchardt et al., 1992), but requires up to 3 days of incubation to detect organisms by microscopic evaluation.

Antigen Detection

Monoclonal antibodies to *T. vaginalis* have been used to identify vaginal trichomoniasis. Broadly reactive, fluorescein isothiocyanate-conjugated monoclonal antibodies to *T. vaginalis* are used for this test. In one study, the direct fluorescent antibody test was 86% sensitive and 99% specific and had a positive predictive value of 96% (prevalence, 15%) (Yule et al., 1987). The sensitivity of this test is also related to the concentration of protozoa in the vaginal fluid. In women with positive wet mounts, more than 90% of cases are detected by the antibody test. However, in women with negative wet mounts, the antibody test has a sensitivity of only 69 to 77% (Yule et al., 1987).

An immunoassay developed for the detection of *T. vaginalis* in vaginal swabs had a sensitivity of 93%, a specificity of 97.5%, and a positive predictive value of 82% (prevalence, 9%) when culture based on modified Diamond's medium was used as reference (Krieger et al., 1988).

Nucleic Acid-Based Tests

Recently, DNA hybridization and gene amplification have also been used for the diagnosis of *T. vaginalis*. The commercial test, Affirm VP Microbial Identification Test (MicroProbe Corp., Bothell, Wash.), is based on synthetic oligonucleotide probes; it was evaluated by Briselden and Hillier (1994). The test system, designed for use in the physician's office, had a sensitivity of 83%, a positive predictive value of 100%, and a negative predictive value of 98% in a population with a 9% prevalence of *T. vaginalis*. DeMeo et al.

(1996) also compared the Affirm VP test with microscopy of vaginal "wet mounts" and with cultures in Diamond's medium; in that study of 615 women with signs or symptoms of vaginitis, the DNA test had a sensitivity of 90% and a specificity of 99.8%. PCR analysis is sensitive enough to be used on vaginal specimens. Witkin et al. (1996) used PCR to compare vaginal specimens with endocervical specimens and posterior vaginal vault specimens in 219 pregnant women and found that vaginal testing had a sensitivity of 95.5% and a specificity of 100%.

Screening

If *T. vaginalis* infection is a risk factor for prematurity and premature rupture of the membranes, intervention studies are needed to see whether treatment can reduce this risk. To identify patients infected with *T. vaginalis*, pregnant women must be screened for the infection. It is not established which of the above-mentioned diagnostic methods is most cost-effective for trichomoniasis screening. Moreover, it is not clear which patients should be selected for screening. Obviously, women with vaginal discomfort should be examined. Regarding wet mount examinations, the yield of screening among symptomatic patients depends on which symptoms or signs are used as criteria. For example, among nonpregnant women attending an STD clinic who had symptoms of yellow vaginal discharge or itching but no signs of purulent vaginal discharge, the yield of wet mount examination for trichomoniasis was only 3.4% (Wölner-Hanssen et al., 1989). The yield was 9.5 times greater among women with purulent vaginal discharge (25% yield) than among those without this sign (2.5% yield). For women with vaginal erythema, the yield of wet mount was 31%, whereas for those without this finding, it was 7%. Asymptomatic women have smaller numbers of protozoa in the vagina than symptomatic women do (Krieger et al., 1990a). Therefore, wet mount screening of asymptomatic women may be a time-consuming procedure with a low yield. These data suggest that it might be worthwhile to screen for trichomoniasis among women in high-risk groups with purulent vaginal discharge and/or vaginal erythema.

Women in high-risk groups were characterized by Cotch et al. (1991). The authors identified risk factors and risk markers for trichomoniasis by using the data from the VIP study. As in many studies of nonpregnant women, the prevalence of *T. vaginalis* was higher in African American women than in Caucasian women. Smokers had double the infection rate of nonsmokers. Women who lack these risk factors are unlikely to be infected (<10% chance). However, signs and symptoms of vaginitis were poor predictors of infection. A more recent report from the same group concluded that there are no sensitive clinical parameters or combination of parameters that would successfully identify pregnant women needing further testing (Pastorek et al., 1996).

Given that a new improved culture method is available as a gold standard, improved algorithms for screening need to be developed. The cost-effectiveness of different screening methods could then be established.

THERAPY

It is now 30 years since metronidazole was introduced for the treatment of *T. vaginalis* infections. This drug revolutionized trichomonas therapy. Despite widespread use, metronidazole and other 5-nitroimidazoles remain highly effective against most *T. vaginalis* strains. Lossick (1989) has comprehensively reviewed trichomonas therapy.

Metronidazole can produce chromosomal alterations in bacteria (Legator et al., 1975) and may increase the incidence of tumors in susceptible animals (Rust, 1976). The drug must therefore be considered a weak carcinogen. Metronidazole crosses the placental barrier in small quantities (Amon et al., 1972). Because of concerns about prenatal susceptibility to DNA damage, physicians have been cautious about metronidazole treatment during the first trimester of pregnancy. However, its use is not restricted in the United States; furthermore, studies of pregnant women at all stages of gestation given oral metronidazole have not revealed an increased incidence of malformation, low birth weight, prematurity, or fetal death (Piper et al., 1993).

In the United States, there are no satisfactory alternatives to metronidazole for the treatment of trichomoniasis. Trinidazole, another 5-nitroimidazole available in Europe but not in the United States, may be an alternative to metronidazole in patients with metronidazole-resistant strains. According to one study, tinidazole was effective against 4 of 12 metronidazole-resistant strains (Narcisi and Secor, 1996). However, furazolindone, a nitrofuran used to treat giardiasis, was effective at a low minimum lethal concentration against all 12 strains. Topical metronidazole therapy is an alternative to oral treatment. In one study, oral dosing and vaginal dosing were compared; the concentrations of metronidazole in plasma were measured after application of 500 mg of the drug per os or per vaginam (Alper et al., 1985). The mean peak concentrations in plasma were much lower after vaginal application than after oral dosing (15.6 and 1.9 μg/ml, respectively). Importantly, topical therapy has been associated with high recurrence rates, probably due to coinfection of the urethra and periurethral glands. With respect to premature rupture of the membranes, it is possible that the reduction in numbers of protozoa in the vagina after local treatment is enough to reduce or eliminate any increased risk of adverse outcome in pregnancy associated with the protozoan.

In summary, *T. vaginalis* is likely to be an important factor in prematurity. Better diagnostic tests (amenable to screening use), better therapy, and the appropriate clinical trials are needed to determine whether screening and treatment should be used to prevent prematurity.

REFERENCES

Alderete, J. F. 1984. Enzyme-linked immunosorbent assay for detection of antibody to *Trichomonas vaginalis*: use of whole cells and aqueous extract as antigen. *Br. J. Vener. Dis.* **60:**160–170.

Alderete, J. F. 1988. Alternating phenotypic expression of two classes of *Trichomonas vaginalis* surface markers. *Rev. Infect. Dis.* **10:**408.

Alderete, J. F., L. Kasmala, E. Metcalfe, and G. E. Garza. 1986. Phenotypic variation and diversity among *Trichomonas vaginalis* isolates and correlation of phenotype with trichomonal virulence determinants. *Infect. Immun.* **53:**285–293.

Alderete, J. F., E. Newton, C. Dennis, J. Engbring, and K. A. Neale. 1991a. Vaginal antibody of patients with trichomoniasis is to a prominent surface immunogen of *Trichomonas vaginalis. Genitourin. Med.* **67:**220–225.

Alderete, J. F., E. Newton, C. Dennis, and K. A. Neale. 1991b. Antibody in sera of patients infected with *Trichomonas vaginalis* to trichomonad proteinases. *Genitourin. Med.* **67:**331–334.

Alderete, J. F., E. Newton, C. Dennis, and K. A. Neale. 1991c. The vagina of women infected with *Trichomonas vaginalis* has numerous proteinases and antibody to trichomonad proteinases. *Genitourin. Med.* **67:**469–474.

Alper, M. M., B. N. Barwin, W. M. McLean, I. J. McGilverary, and S. Sved. 1985. Systemic absorption of metronidazole by the vaginal route. *Obstet. Gynecol.* **65:** 781–784.

Amon, K., I. Amon, and H. Müller. 1972. Maternal-fetal passage of metronidazole, p. 113–115. *In* M. Hejzlar, M. Semonsky, and S. Masak (ed.), *Advances in Antimicrobial Antineoplastic Chemotherapy.* University Park Press, Baltimore, Md.

Arroyo, R., J. Engbring, and J. F. Alderete. 1992. Molecular basis of host cell recognition by *Trichomonas vaginalis. Mol. Microbiol.* **6:**853–862.

Borchardt, K. A., and R. F. Smith. 1991. An evaluation of an InPouch TV culture method for diagnosing *Trichomonas vaginalis* infection. *Genitourin. Med.* **67:**149–152.

Borchardt, K. A., V. Hernandez, S. Miller, et al. 1992. A clinical evaluation of trichomoniasis in San Jose, Costa Rica, using the InPouch TV test. *Genitourin. Med.* **68:** 328–330.

Briselden, A. M., and S. L. Hillier. 1994. Evaluation of Affirm VP Microbial Identification Test for *Gardnerella vaginalis* and *Trichomonas vaginalis. J. Clin. Microbiol.* **32:**148–152.

Brown, M. T. 1972. Trichomoniasis. *Practitioner* **209:**639.

Buchvald, D., P. Demes, A. Gombošová, P. Mráz, M. Valent, and J. Stefanovič. 1992. Vaginal leukocyte characteristics in urogenital trichomoniasis. *APMIS* **100:** 393–400.

Cassell, G. Personal communication.

Cotch, M. F., J. G. Pastorek II, R. P. Nugent, D. E. Yerg, D. H. Martin, and D. A. Eschenbach. 1991. Demographic and behavioral predictors of *Trichomonas vaginalis* infection among pregnant women. *Obstet. Gynecol.* **78:**1087–1092.

Cotch, M. F., J. G. Pastorek II, R. P. Nugent, S. L. Hillier, R. S. Gibbs, D. H. Martin, D. A. Eschenbach, R. Edelman, J. C. Carey, J. A. Regan, M. A. Krohn, M. A. Klebanoff, A. V. Rao, and G. G. Rhoads. 1997. *Trichomonas vaginalis* associated with low birth weight and preterm delivery. The Vaginal Infection and Prematurity Study Group. *Sex. Transm. Dis.* **24:**361–362.

DeMeo, L. R., D. L. Draper, J. A. McGregor, D. F. Moore, C. R. Peter, P. S. Kapernick, and W. M. McCormack. 1996. Evaluation of a deoxyribonucleic acid probe for the detection of *Trichomonas vaginalis* in vaginal secretions. *Am. J. Obstet. Gynecol.* **174:**1339–1342.

Feinberg, J. G., and M. J. A. Whittington. 1957. A culture medium for *Trichomonas vaginalis* Donne and species of *Candida. J. Clin. Pathol.* **10:**327–329.

Fouts, A. C., and S. J. Kraus. 1980. *Trichomonas vaginalis*: reevaluation of its clinical presentation and laboratory diagnosis. *J. Infect. Dis.* **141:**137–143.

Garber, G. E., L. T. Lemchuk-Favel, and W. R. Bowie. 1989. Isolation of a cell-detaching factor of *Trichomonas vaginalis. J. Clin. Microbiol.* **27:**1548–1553.

Hardy, P. H., J. B. Hardy, E. E. Nell, D. A. Graham, M. R. Spence, and R. C. Rosenbaum. 1984. Prevalence of six sexually transmitted agents among pregnant inner-city adolescents and pregnancy outcome. *Lancet* **ii:**333–337.

Hillier, S. L., J. Martius, M. Krohn, N. Kiviat, K. K. Holmes, and D. A. Eschenbach. 1988. A case-control study of chorioaminiotic infection and histologic chorioamnionitis in prematurity. *N. Engl. J. Med.* **319:**972–978.

Honigberg, B. M., and G. Brugerolle. 1989. Structure, p. 5–35. *In* B. M. Honigberg (ed.), *Trichomonads Parasitic in Humans.* Springer-Verlag, New York, N.Y.

Kent, H. L. 1991. Epidemiology of vaginitis. *Am. J. Obstet. Gynecol.* **165:**1168–1176.

Krieger, J. N., M. R. Tam, C. E. Stevens, I. O. Nielsen, J. Hale, N. B. Kiviat, and K. K. Holmes. 1988. Diagnosis of trichomoniasis: comparison of conventional wet-mount examination with cytologic studies, cultures, and monoclonal antibody staining of direct specimen. *JAMA* **259:**1223–1227.

Krieger, J. N., P. Wölner-Hanssen, C. Stevens, and K. K. Holmes. 1990a. Characteristics of *Trichomonas vaginalis* isolates from women with and without colpitis macularis. *J. Infect. Dis.* **161:**307–311.

Krieger, J. N., B. E. Torian, J. Hom, and M. R. Tam. 1990b. Inhibition of *Trichomonas vaginalis* motility by monoclonal antibodies is associated with reduced adherence to HeLa cell monolayers. *Infect. Immun.* **58:**1634–1639.

Lee, N. C., G. L. Rubin, and D. A. Grimes. 1991. Measures of sexual behavior and the risk of pelvic inflammatory disease. *Obstet. Gynecol.* **77:**425–430.

Legator, M. S., T. H. Connor, and M. Stoekel. 1975. Detection of mutagenic activity of metronidazole and niridazole in body fluid of humans and mice. *Science* **188:** 1118–1119.

Lehker, M. W., and J. F. Alderete. 1990. Properties of *Trichomonas vaginalis* grown under chemostat controlled growth conditions. *Genitourin Med.* **66:**193–199.

Linstead, D. 1989. Cultivation, p. 91–111. *In* B. M. Honigberg (ed.), *Trichomonads Parasitic in Humans.* Springer-Verlag, New York, N.Y.

Lossick, J. G. 1988. The diagnosis of vaginal trichomoniasis. *JAMA* **259:**1230.

Lossick, J. G. 1989. Therapy of urogenital trichomoniasis, p. 324–341. *In* B. M. Honigberg (ed.), *Trichomonads Parasitic in Humans.* Springer-Verlag, New York, N.Y.

Mantovani, A., N. Polentarutti, G. Peri, G. Martinotti, and F. Landolfo. 1981. Cytotoxicity of human peripheral blood monocytes against *Trichomonas vaginalis*. *Clin. Exp. Immunol.* **46:**391–396.

Mason, P. R., and M. T. Brown. 1980. Trichomonas in pregnancy. *Lancet* **ii:**1025.

Mason, P. R., and L. Forman. 1982. Polymorphonuclear cell chemotaxis to secretions of pathogenic and nonpathogenic *Trichomonas vaginalis*. *J. Parasitol.* **68:**457–462.

McGregor, J. A., J. I. French, W. Jones, R. Parker, E. Patterson, and D. Draper. 1992. Association of cervicovaginal infections with increased vaginal fluid phospholipase A_2 activity. *Am. J. Obstet. Gynecol.* **167:**1588–1594.

McGregor, J. A., J. I. French, R. Parker, D. Draper, E. Patterson, W. Jones, K. Thorsgard, and J. McFee. 1995. Prevention of premature birth by screening and treatment for common genital tract infections: results of a prospective controlled evaluation. *Am. J. Obstet. Gynecol.* **173:**157–167.

McLellan, R., M. R. Spence, M. Brockman, L. Raffel, and J. L. Smith. 1982. The clinical diagnosis of trichomoniasis. *Obstet. Gynecol.* **60:**30–34.

Meis, P. J., R. L. Goldenberg, B. Mercer, A. Moawad, A. Das, D. McNellis, F. Johnson, J. D. Iams, E. Thom, and W. W. Andrews. 1995. The preterm prediction study: significance of vaginal infections. National Institute of Child Health and Human Development Maternal-Fetal Units Network. *Am. J. Obstet. Gynecol.* **173:** 1231–1235.

Minkoff, H., A. N. Grunebaum, R. H. Schwarz, J. Feldman, M. Cummings, W. Crombleholme, L. Clark, G. Pringle, and W. M. McCormack. 1984. Risk factors for prematurity and premature rupture of membranes: a prospective study of the vaginal flora in pregnancy. *Am. J. Obstet. Gynecol.* **150:**965–972.

Mirhaghani, A., and A. Warton. 1996. An electron microscope study of the interaction between *Trichomonas vaginalis* and epithelial cells of the human amnion membrane. *Parasitol. Res.* **82:**43–47.

Müller, M., J. G. Lossick, and T. E. Gorrell. 1988. *In vitro* susceptibility of *Trichomonas vaginalis* to metronidazole and treatment outcome in vaginal trichomoniasis. *Sex. Transm. Dis.* **15:**17–24.

Nadisauskiene, R., S. Bergström, I. Stankeviciene, and T. Spukaite. 1995. Endocervical pathogens in women with preterm and term labour. *Gynecol. Obstet. Invest.* **40:**179–182.

Narcisi, E. M., and W. E. Secor. 1996. In vitro effect of tinidazole and furazolidone on metronidazole-resistant *Trichomonas vaginalis*. *Antimicrob. Agents Chemother.* **40:** 1121–1125.

Pastorek, J. G., II, M. F. Cotch, D. H. Martin, and D. A. Eschenbach for the Vaginal Infection and Prematurity Study Group. 1996. Clinical and microbiological correlates of vaginal trichomoniasis during pregnancy. *Clin. Infect. Dis.* **23:**1075–1080.

Pindak, F. F., N. Mora de Pindak, and W. A. Gardner. 1993. Contact-independent cytotoxocity of *Trichomonas vaginalis*. *Genitourin. Med.* **69:**35–40.

Piper, J. M., E. F. Mitchel, and W. A. Ray. 1993. Prenatal use of metronidazole and birth defects: no association. *Obstet. Gynecol.* **82:**348–352.

Poch, F., D. Levin, S. Levin, and M. Dan. 1996. Modified thioglycolate medium: a simple and reliable means for detection of *Trichomonas vaginalis*. *J. Clin. Microbiol.* **34:**2630–2631.

Read, J. S., and M. A. Klebanoff for the Vaginal Infections and Prematurity Study Group. 1993. Sexual intercourse during pregnancy and preterm delivery: effects of vaginal microorganisms. *Am. J. Obstet. Gynecol.* **168:**514–519.

Rein, M. F., J. A. Sullivan, and G. L. Mandell. 1980. Trichomonacidal activity of human polymorphonuclear neutrophils: killing by disruption. *J. Infect. Dis.* **142:** 575–585.

Ross, S. M., and A. V. Middelkoop. 1983. Trichomonas infection in pregnancy—does it affect perinatal outcome? *S. Afr. Med. J.* **63:**566.

Rust, J. H. 1976. An assessment of metronidazole tumorigenicity: studies in mouse and rat, p. 138–144. *In* S. Finegold (ed.), *Metronidazole. Proceedings of the International Metronidazole Conference.* Excerpta Medica, Princeton, N.J.

Shaio, M. F., P. R. Lin, J. Y. Liu, and K. D. Yang. 1995. Generation of interleukin-8 from human monocytes in response to *Trichomonas vaginalis* stimulation. *Infect. Immun.* **63:**3864–3870.

Street, D. A., D. Taylor-Robinson, J. P. Ackers, N. F. Hanna, and A. McMillan. 1982. Evaluation of an enzyme-linked immunosorbent assay for the detection of antibody to *Trichomonas vaginalis* in sera and vaginal secretions. *Br. J. Vener. Dis.* **58:**330–333.

Witkin, S. S., S. R. Inglis, and M. Polaneczky. 1996. Detection of *Chlamydia trachomatis* and *Trichomonas vaginalis* by polymerase chain reaction in introital specimens from pregnant women. *Am J. Obstet. Gynecol.* **175:**165–167.

Wölner-Hanssen, P., J. N. Krieger, C. E. Stevens, N. B. Kiviat, L. Koutsky, C. Critchlow, T. De Rouen, S. Hillier, and K. K. Holmes. 1989. Clinical manifestations of vaginal trichomoniasis. *JAMA* **261:**571–576.

Wölner-Hanssen, P. Unpublished data.

Yule, A., M. C. A. Gelan, J. D. Oriel, and J. P. Ackers. 1987. Detection of *Trichomonas vaginalis* antigen in women by enzyme immunoassay. *J. Clin. Pathol.* **40:**566–568.

VIRAL DISEASE

13
Human Immunodeficiency Virus Infection and Pregnancy

Howard Minkoff

It is estimated that ten million children will be infected with human immunodeficiency virus (HIV) by the end of the decade (Chin, 1991). The overwhelming majority of those HIV infections will be acquired from HIV-infected mothers. In the coming years, it will be the responsibility of clinicians to try to prevent these infections and other adverse outcomes of pregnancy as well as to care for the infected women. Although the ideal approach to the prevention of pediatric infections would be the elimination of maternal infections, it is unlikely that either a "cure" for HIV or an effective vaccine will be universally available in the near future. For that reason, the attention of researchers has turned to the prevention of vertical transmission of HIV.

Attempts to prevent mother-to-child HIV transmission have included a recently completed trial of an antiretroviral drug (zidovudine [ZDV]) given during pregnancy and in the peripartum period to prevent the reverse transcription of HIV in fetal and neonatal target cells (ACTG protocol 076; Connor et al., 1994). The finding that zidovudine prevented a substantial percentage of transmissions raises a host of new issues including clinical (who are appropriate candidates for therapy), research (which component[s] of therapy is necessary), policy (what prenatal testing standards should derive from these findings), and ethical (how can a relatively expensive therapy be made widely available). Evidence suggesting that obstetrical interventions may have some utility in reducing the rate of mother-to-child transmission of HIV has also been presented (Minkoff and Mofenson, 1994).

Howard Minkoff, Department of Obstetrics and Gynecology, State University of New York, 450 Clarkson Ave., Box 24, Brooklyn, NY 11203-2098.

Sexually Transmitted Diseases and Adverse Outcomes of Pregnancy
Edited by P. J. Hitchcock, H. T. MacKay, J. N. Wasserheit, and R. Binder
©1999 American Society for Microbiology, Washington, D.C.

This chapter will familiarize clinicians with the literature regarding outcomes of pregnancies of HIV-infected women and describes strategies to minimize transmission and to reduce the frequency of adverse perinatal outcomes.

PRENATAL TRANSMISSION

Although mother-to-child HIV transmission is now accepted as the most common route of infection of neonates, the rate and determinants of such transmission remain uncertain. Reported transmission rates, prior to the advent of pharmaceutical interventions, showed wide geographic variation. The lowest published rates come from the European collaborative study that reported that only 14% of children born to infected mothers were eventually found to be HIV infected (European Collaborative Study, 1992). In Africa, conversely, transmission rates of approximately 40% have been reported (Lallemant et al., 1994a; Ryder et al., 1989). American authors have generally reported intermediate rates (Goedert et al., 1989; Mayers et al., 1991).

Some of the variation in reported rates may reflect different study methods. Clearly, however, there are also differences in the individuals under study. Lower CD4 counts and evidence of viremia, including p24 antigenemia, for example, have been related to higher rates of transmission (Dickover et al., 1996). Recent seroconversion of the mother and advanced clinical illness have also been linked to high transmission rates. D'Arminio et al. (1991) observed increased rates of vertical transmission in women with more advanced disease stages (100% in patients with Centers for Disease Control and Prevention [CDC] class IV disease compared with 13% in patients with CDC class II or III disease), and Hague et al. (1991) observed increased rates of HIV vertical transmission in women who had AIDS during pregnancy or whose cases were diagnosed after the birth of the child.

Risk Factors

Pregnant women with a high viral load, revealed by high titers of HIV or p24 antigenemia, apparently are a group at particularly high risk of transmission. Researchers in the European Collaborative Study found that transmission was associated with maternal p24 antigenemia and a CD4 count of less than 700/mm^3. Acute viremia associated with maternal seroconversion in the year prior to pregnancy or during breast-feeding appears to be associated with increased rates of vertical transmission (Hague et al., 1991; Kreiss et al., 1991). Kreiss et al. (1991) observed a vertical transmission rate of 72% associated with a proviral load of >10/100,000 lymphocytes within 6 months of delivery, compared with vertical transmission of 27% in patients with a proviral load of <10/100,000 lymphocytes. Boue et al. (1990) observed vertical transmission rates of 78% associated with high viral replication levels and 26% in patients without p24 antigenemia. In their cohort of 66 HIV-positive pregnant women, D'Arminio et al. (1991) observed transmission rates of 100% in seven p24 antigen-positive women compared with 10 of 59 (17%) p24 antigen-negative women. The viral load data from the ACTG 076 trial indicated that a high concentration of virus in maternal plasma is a risk factor for the transmission of HIV-1 from an untreated mother to her infant (Sperling et al., 1996). It was also found that the reduction in transmission associated with ZDV use could be explained only partially by the reduction in the levels of HIV RNA in plasma. Transmission was also reported to occur at all levels of HIV RNA in plasma, including undetectable levels. Recently, several groups have suggested that in addition to a correlation between maternal viral load and rates of mother-to-child HIV transmission, a clinically relevant threshold may exist (Fang et al., 1995; Dickover et al., 1996). Other researchers disagree (Landesman and Burns, 1996). Differences in study populations and techniques used for storing and assaying samples may explain some of the conflicting results.

The presence and amount of virus in the genital tract could affect transmission risk. Free virus and infected cells have been identified in cervicovaginal secretions of HIV-1-infected women (Mofenson, 1997). In a study of HIV-infected pregnant women from Nairobi, HIV-1 DNA was detected in 32% of cervical samples and in 10% of vaginal samples (John et al., 1997). The presence of HIV-1-infected cells in genital secretions was associated with immunosuppression, anemia, abnormal cervical or vaginal discharge, and severe vitamin A deficiency. The local genital tract viral burden was not directly correlated with systemic viral load or with $CD4^+$ count. In one study, 17% of women with high HIV-1 RNA levels in plasma did not have detectable HIV-1 RNA in cervicovaginal secretions and 26% of women without detectable RNA in plasma had significant levels of cell-free virus in genital secretions (Rasheed et al., 1996).

Routes of Transmission

Intensive exposure of the infant's thin skin or mucosal surfaces to maternal blood and secretions during the birth process could provide a significant route for virus transmission (Mofenson, 1997). Langerhans cells in the skin and gastrointestinal tract express CD4 and are infected by HIV-1. Primate studies have demonstrated that fetal skin and mucous membranes may provide a route for HIV-1 infection. In a rhesus monkey model, simian immunodeficiency virus (SIV) was injected into the amniotic fluid of uninfected mothers during late gestation; six of seven newborns were infected (Fazely et al., 1993). Additionally, transmission via the oral route has been demonstrated in newborn animals; four of four monkeys who were born by cesarean delivery to uninfected mothers and to whom SIV was administered orally immediately after birth became infected (Baba et al., 1994).

This indicates that swallowing infectious maternal fluids during birth may be another mechanism of transmission. By 7 days after oral exposure, SIV was identified by in situ hybridization in lymphoid follicles in the ileum and mesenteric lymph nodes but not in the peripheral lymph nodes of these animals. This suggests that mucosal Langerhans cells within the small bowel may play a major role in initial infection by this route in newborn animals. Consistent with a possible route of HIV-1 transmission by oral exposure in humans, in one study HIV-1 was detected in gastric aspirates from two of four newborns who were subsequently shown to be infected (Nielsen et al., 1996).

The importance of mucosal HIV-1 antibody in genital secretions in reducing the infection risk during the birth process is unknown. In a mouse model of genital herpes simplex virus (HSV) infection, vaginal application of HSV antibody protected mice against vaginal inoculation with HSV-2 (Whaley et al., 1994). However, intermittent cervicovaginal shedding of HIV-1 occurs despite the presence of mucosal HIV-1-specific immunoglobulin A (IgA) antibodies, suggesting that the antibody is not neutralizing the virus (Nielsen et al., 1996). In one study, anti-HIV-1 secretory IgA in maternal genital secretions was associated with an increased risk of transmission (Miotti et al., 1993); however, increased local antibody levels may be a reflection of higher levels of local viral replication (Belec et al., 1995).

Invasive procedures that breach an infant's skin could provide another mechanism for viral entry. In a large French cohort, invasive procedures (particularly amniocentesis and amnioscopy) were associated with increased transmission risk; other obstetric procedure-related risk factors were premature membrane rupture, hemorrhage in labor, and bloody amniotic fluid (Mandelbrot et al., 1996). As noted below, prolonged duration of membrane rupture could permit increased exposure to HIV-1 in secretions.

Immunologic Factors

Advanced immunologic deterioration, as demonstrated by decreased numbers of circulating $CD4^+$ lymphocytes, also has been associated with an increased risk of vertical transmission. St. Louis et al. (1993) observed an inverse relationship between the number of $CD4^+$ cells as a percentage of total lymphocytes and rates of vertical transmission (for >30, 20 to 29, 10 to 19, and <10% $CD4^+$ cells, the transmission rates were 23, 49, 63, and 77%, respectively). Similarly, Burns et al. (1994), in a study of a cohort of 162 pregnant women in New York City, observed that women whose lowest prepartum $CD4^+$ levels were ≤20% were at greater risk of transmitting HIV to their children. Tibaldi et al. (1991) reported vertical transmission rates of 71% in those with $CD4^+$ lymphocyte counts of <400/mm^3 or p24 antigenemia, or both, compared with rates of 6% in those without antigenemia and with $CD4^+$ counts of >400/cm^3. Boue et al. (1990) noted a vertical transmission rate of 66% in those with $CD4^+$ lymphocyte counts of <150/mm^3 compared with a rate of 26% in those with $CD4^+$ counts of >150/mm^3. Similar findings also were reported by Lindgren et al. (1991), who found that "mothers of infected children had longer durations of HIV infection and were symptomatic and/or had low CD4 cell counts to a significantly greater extent at follow-up than mothers of uninfected children."

Some researchers have suggested that the amount and type of maternal antibodies play roles in determining transmission. HIV-infected pregnant women with high antibody titers to certain epitopes of the gp120 envelope protein, particularly the third hypervariable loop (V3), may have a lower rate of HIV transmission to their infants. The absence of antibody to two epitopes of the gp120 envelope of HTLV-IIIB located near the base of the V3 loop was correlated with vertical transmission (Rossi et al., 1989; Broliden et al., 1989).

Goedert et al. (1989), in a prospective study of 51 HIV-infected pregnant women, reported a higher transmission rate from women who lacked antibodies to native gp120 when evaluated during the third trimester; 28 (80%) of 35 nontransmitting women had antibody compared to 6 (38%) of 16 transmitting women. In infants born prematurely (≤37 weeks), the amount of maternal antibody was not correlated with transmission, but in full-term infants (≥38 weeks) a high maternal reactivity against gp120 was associated with protection from transmission. In both this work and that of the European Collaborative Study, infection rates were higher in preterm infants (Kreiss et al., 1991).

Devash et al. (1990) reported that women with high-affinity or high-avidity antibodies directed toward a peptide they termed the principal neutralizing domain of gp120 (derived from the top of the V3 loop) were less likely to transmit HIV vertically. In a prospective study of 15 HIV-infected women and their infants, they reported that sera from all 11 transmitting women had reactivity below cutoff, demonstrating the presence of only low-affinity or low-avidity antibody, whereas sera from three of four nontransmitting women had high-affinity or high-avidity antibody.

These associations have not been confirmed by other investigators (Allain et al., 1991). Lallemant et al. (1994b) observed the opposite correlation between antibody titers and maternal transmission: high maternal antibody titers to the V3 region and to the immunodominant domain of gp41 were correlated with a higher rate of transmission. It is unclear whether this discrepancy is due to minor differences in technique, variations in the HIV strains studied by the various groups, or other factors. Important viral neutralizing activity may also be associated with antibody regions outside the V3 loop, such as to the gp41 peptide (Goedert et al., 1989), or to a conformational epitope of gp120.

Timing of Transmission

Over the last several years, a great deal has been learned about the timing of transmission. There are no data to support antepartum, intrapartum, and neonatal (breast-feeding) transmission of HIV. Some of the earliest work supporting antepartum transmission involved evaluations of abortuses and preterm deliveries (Lapointe et al., 1985). The HIV genome was identified by PCR as early as week 12 of pregnancy by Courgnaud et al. (1989). Soeiro et al. (1991) studied human abortus tissue and suggested that up to 30% of HIV transmissions may occur by the second trimester of pregnancy. However, the possibility of contamination from maternal sources is difficult to exclude definitively in any study of aborted fetal tissues. Given the exquisite sensitivity of certain virologic techniques (e.g., PCR), it is possible that even virus which is found in fetal tissues represents surface contamination that is carried into the viscera on dissecting instruments.

Invasive diagnostic procedures (amniocentesis, percutaneous umbilical blood sampling) have been used to detect evidence of fetal infection before the intrapartum period. Viscarello et al. (1992) found p24 antigen in the amniotic fluid of five of 13 HIV-infected women and in the serum of three of their fetuses. These findings are also subject to error related to maternal viral contamination that could be detected by extremely sensitive virologic techniques. Needles or catheters placed transcutaneously or transvaginally into the amniotic cavity or into the fetal circulation are theoretically capable of inoculating the fetus with sufficient virus to be detectable by PCR.

The presence of p24 antigen in newborn serum or a positive HIV culture shortly after birth has been taken to suggest that the infant was infected during pregnancy (Courpotin et al., 1988; Borkowski et al., 1989), although it is possible that positive viral cultures in the neonatal period are due to intensive exposure to virus present in maternal blood and genital tract secretions at the time of birth. Miles et al. (1993) used a rapid serologic test with immune-complex-dissociated HIV p24 antigen for early detection of HIV infection in neonates. Of eight cord samples from neonates with subsequently proven HIV infection, five were positive for immune-complex-dissociated p24 antigen and two of the neonates with negative cord samples tested positive on days 12 and 18. These findings and rapidly rising titers of the antigen in the neonatal period are compatible with antepartum transmission (Miles et al., 1993).

Alternatively, the inability to detect evidence of HIV infection before 4 months of age in 50 to 70% of exposed infants ultimately proven to be infected suggests that the timing of transmission may be peripartum in the majority of cases. Ehrnst et al. (1991), in a prospective evaluation of 47 pregnancies in 44 HIV-infected women, found no consistent transplacental spread of HIV during maternal viremia. Maternal viremia, in either peripheral blood mononuclear cells or plasma, was detected during pregnancy in

83% of women; however, HIV was isolated in 0 of 27 newborns, of whom 26% (5 of 19 for whom follow-up was available) were subsequently proven infected by 6 months. Viral genome was detected in only 2 of 12 abortuses. These investigators concluded that "The findings . . . indicate in most cases transmission occurs close to or at delivery."

Many of these studies are subject to misclassification bias. A child with a negative cord blood sample, for example, may have been infected the day before delivery and hence could not benefit from intrapartum interventions, but in these schemata his or her infection would be classified as an intrapartum event. Conversely, a sizable maternal-fetal bleed, in conjunction with the leukocytosis of labor, could theoretically result in a positive cord blood sample in the setting of intrapartum transmission. Such errors detract from the utility of schemata proposed for the classification of infection as ante- or intrapartum (Bryson et al., 1992). Although these errors make estimates of the percentage of transmission occurring in the intrapartum period inexact, they are probably infrequent and do not negate the general conclusion drawn from cord blood studies, i.e., that transmission can occur in both the intrapartum and antepartum periods.

Extensions of the cord blood studies are studies of the subsequent serologic course of the neonate. When focusing on exposed infants who were ultimately determined to be HIV infected, various investigators found that there was a significant increase in the number of children producing detectable levels of IgA between birth and 6 months of age. Landesman et al. (1991) reported that of 22 infants eventually demonstrated to be HIV infected, only 1 of 17 with evaluable serum had IgA at 1 month of age compared to 10 of 16 asymptomatic infants at 3 months and 5 of 5 at 6 months. Quinn et al. (1991) reported similar findings. Although these findings are compatible with the thesis that infection occurred peripartum with the subsequent production of IgA, it is also possible that in utero infection occurred but that fetal production of IgA was delayed until the postpartum period.

Perhaps the most provocative evidence for an intrapartum influence on vertical transmission is studies of twin births to HIV-infected women. Goedert et al. (1991) reported on 22 sets of twins who were ultimately found to have discordant HIV status (Blanche et al., 1994). In 18 of the 22 cases, twin A (the presenting twin) was the infected sibling. It was found that 50% of first-born twins delivered vaginally and 38% of first-born twins delivered by cesarean section were infected compared to 19% of second-born twins delivered by either method. Since twin A is also exposed more directly to maternal blood and secretions in the vagina and is at greater risk of having a scalp electrode placed transcutaneously, it is reasonable to hypothesize that peripartum events contributed to the discrepancy between siblings and HIV infection rates. The continued accrual of twins into the registry from which the original data were derived has substantiated the initial findings.

The greater infection rate of first-born twins has, as noted above, been linked to exposure to maternal secretions. Other evidence also suggests that such contact carries risk. Several studies have now been published that suggest a link between the duration of ruptured membranes and the transmission of HIV primarily in women with low CD4 levels (Minkoff et al., 1995; Landesman et al., 1996). These preliminary analyses have demonstrated a substantial increase in transmission after the membranes have been ruptured for more than 4 h (Minkoff et al., 1995; Landesman et al., 1996). As a consequence of these findings, some authors have suggested that there may be a role for operative delivery as a strategy for preventing intrapartum transmission. The fact that this association was limited to women with low CD4 levels in some studies is compatible with the hypothesis that increased viral load in maternal blood and perhaps other secretions may be found in conjunction with more advanced illness and may exacerbate the risk of neonatal exposure to the maternal vagina after membrane rupture. Although other authors have not found an association with duration of ruptured membranes, they have not assessed the effect of CD4 counts or examined a variety of durations of membrane rupture (Burns et al., 1994).

NEONATAL TRANSMISSION

While perinatal acquisition of HIV seems to be the major route of pediatric infection, there are many reports of infection acquired by ingestion of infected breast milk (Friedland et al., 1986; Ziegler et al., 1988; Lepage et al., 1987; Van de Perre et al., 1991). In most of these studies, the mothers were infected postnatally by blood transfusions from donors who subsequently went on to develop HIV disease. Although pretransfusion serostatus was generally undocumented, no other source of maternal infection was suspected and no other family members were known to be infected. These pediatric infections, along with reports of the isolation of free virus from the breast milk of healthy carriers of HIV, make it probable that HIV infection can be acquired by breast-feeding.

However, there is doubt about the efficiency of transmission of HIV through infected breast milk. Ziegler et al. (1988) reported that for breast-fed children, breast milk was a source of infection only when breast-feeding took place around the time when seroconversion was documented. For mothers who were HIV antibody positive, the incidence of infection in their children was the same whether or not the children were breast-fed. Others have suggested that as many as one-third of transmission in some African cohorts can be attributed to long-term breast-feeding. It is possible that maternal infectivity is maximal at the time of initial acquisition of infection, when a viral antigenemia occurs.

Finally, the clinical course of children with pediatric HIV infection also is consistent with two different times of infection. Some children become sick within the first months of life and generally follow a fulminant downhill course resulting in death before the first birthday. Many children, however, survive and are asymptomatic for many years (Shearer et al., 1997). These data have been offered as evidence of transmission at different times. It is also possible that the virulence of the transmitted virus or other factors contribute to these different natural histories. Blanche et al. (1994), for example, found that women with more advanced clinical illness gave birth to children whose course of pediatric HIV infection was much more fulminant that that in children born to healthier HIV-infected women.

OBSTETRICAL MORBIDITY

Most reports from developed countries suggest that, other than transmission of HIV infection, pregnancy outcomes are not affected by serostatus, at least in asymptomatic patients. Birth weight and gestational age did not differ between HIV-infected drug-using women and seronegative controls in reports from Britain (Blanche et al., 1994) or between seropositive and seronegative women in the United States, whether they had used drugs or not (Minkoff et al., 1990). However, studies that have included more symptomatic women have reported higher prematurity rates and lower birth weights of the infants of seropositive women (Ryder et al., 1989). Temmerman et al. (1994) reported on a cohort of women in Kenya, of whom 4% had AIDS, 43% had HIV-related symptoms, and 66% had a CD4 count less than 30%. They found that seropositive women had infants with significantly lower birth weights (2,913 and 3,072 g for seropositive and seronegative women, respectively) and had higher prematurity rates (21.1 and 9.4%, respectively). For seropositive women, lower CD4 counts correlated with prematurity. Many factors unique to populations in that area (extremely high rates of ulcerative diseases) may have contributed to the findings. While some investigators have concurred (e.g., Ryder et al. [1989] reported infants of seropositive mothers with birth weights 219 g lower than those of seronegative mothers in a cohort in which 18% of the women had AIDS), other investigators in Africa, reporting on asymptomatic cohorts, have not found the same results (Lepage et al., 1991).

PREVENTION OF PERINATAL TRANSMISSION

HIV Testing

There are several possible approaches to the prevention of perinatal transmission of HIV. All are contingent on women having access to HIV tests so that they can, if they desire, learn their HIV status. Current testing programs in the United States are cumbersome and "exceptional" in comparison to all other prenatal tests. Although the social stigma attached to HIV status is unique, the recent report of benefit from ZDV (Cotton, 1994) justifies a reconsideration of the relative benefits and burdens of testing. Rapid screening tests have recently become available (Irwin et al., 1996). These tests may eventually be shown to have clinical utility in settings such as labor and delivery suites, where they could be used to help identify HIV infection in patients who received no prenatal care.

Universal access to family planning services would be an additional step toward reducing perinatal HIV transmission by minimizing the number of unwanted pregnancies. Such services are not immediately available to many HIV-infected women (DeFasio et al., 1992). HIV-infected women who conceive should have the same opportunity as all other women to choose whether they wish to carry the pregnancy to term. Therefore, access to abortion service must also be provided.

Pretest counseling should be provided to all patients, regardless of their decision to be tested. Such counseling provides an opportunity to inform patients about behaviors that may put them at risk for HIV infection or any other sexually transmitted disease and to discuss risk reduction practices. This information can be imparted through clinician-patient discussion, the use of written materials or videotapes, or some combination of these methods. The particular mix will depend upon the clinical setting and the prevalence of HIV in the community. Patients should be counseled about HIV and offered the antibody test as early in their pregnancy as possible. Pretest counseling and patients' decisions about testing should be documented in the medical record.

HIV Treatment

Women who choose to maintain their pregnancy should be aware that certain interventions may reduce the risk of perinatal HIV transmission and that several other approaches are under study to determine whether they will have additional benefit (Minkoff and Moreno, 1990). Women whose CD4 counts are over 200/mm^3 and who are ZDV-naive have a reduced transmission of HIV compared to placebo-treated controls when ZDV is initiated prior to 34 weeks gestation and is given in the intrapartum and neonatal periods as well. In the ACTG 076 trial, such women had a transmission rate of 8.3% compared to placebo-treated controls, whose transmission rate was 25.5% (Connor et al., 1994). The results of ACTG 185 suggest that similar benefits will be seen in women with counts below 200/mm^3 and in ZDV-experienced women (Mofenson et al., 1997). Although protocols for antiretroviral therapy are not uniformly agreed upon, several references are available to guide the clinician in the management of the HIV-infected pregnant women (Minkoff and Augenbraun, 1997). CD4 counts and viral loads should be monitored at regular intervals, since they predict the course of disease and allow rational decisions regarding therapeutic interventions. If the CD4 count stays over 500/mm^3 and the viral load stays below 5,000, the obstetrician can anticipate an unremarkable course. ZDV would be required as part of a regimen to prevent the transmission of HIV, but additional therapy can be deferred. If these conditions are not met, multidrug antiretroviral therapy should be instituted. For the pregnant women whose CD4 count falls below 500/mm^3, as for all individuals with similar counts, consideration should be given to the use of combination therapy. If monotherapy has limited clinical or virologic effects and hastens the development of resistance, it would be inappropriate to continue such substandard care solely because a woman is pregnant. Whichever regimen is eventually shown to provide optimal care should be considered for use in pregnancy as well. Only in rare circumstances should considerations related to pregnancy lead clinicians to choose one approach over another. One such consideration could be differences in reported side effects. For example, while ritonavir is associated with gastrointestinal side effects, which may be particularly problematic in early gestation, indinavir is associated with hyperbilirubinemia and nephrolithiasis, potentially more serious perinatal events. Thus, in pregnancy, ritonavir (or nelfinavir) might be a more appropriate first choice from among the protease inhibitors. Although definitive evidence of the safety of the newer antiretroviral agents when used during pregnancy is lacking, no greater reassurance regarding the safety of ZDV was available at the time clinicians first used it in pregnancy (Sperling et al., 1992).

Other Factors

Other factors, such as duration of ruptured membranes, breast-feeding, and cesarean delivery, should be taken into consideration when trying to avoid perinatal transmission. Given preliminary evidence of a relationship between duration of ruptured membranes and transmission rate (Blanche et al., 1994), it would be reasonable to try to minimize exposure to vaginal secretions by avoiding amniotomy and by using conservative management of ruptured membranes when feasible. Since there is evidence to suggest that breast-feeding can be a source of HIV transmission, the Centers for Disease Control and Prevention has recommended that mothers with HIV disease avoid breast-feeding. Unfortunately, while these recommendations may make sense in countries where safe alternatives to breast-feeding are readily available, they are not appropriate in areas where breast-feeding is the only realistic source of nutrients. Finally, although there is some evidence to suggest a protective role for cesarean delivery, its inherent risks and the absence of documented benefit in the setting of ZDV therapy would make it seem prudent to await the results of continuing trials before recommending routine cesarean delivery.

The relationship of cesarean delivery to perinatal transmission of HIV has been examined by a number of investigators. Many of the papers that addressed this issue were summarized in a meta-analysis performed by Villari et al. (1993). Their publication focused on seven reports (primarily from Europe) which met their criteria for accuracy of pediatric diagnosis (HIV status) and mode of delivery (Rossi et al., 1989; Blanche et al., 1989; Hutto et al., 1991; European Collaborative Study, 1991; Gabiano et al., 1992; Goedert et al., 1991; Kind et al., 1992). While no study individually demonstrated significant protection due to cesarean delivery, statistical significance was achieved (odds ratio, 0.65; 95% confidence interval, 0.43 to 0.99; $P = 0.04$) when more than 900 evaluable cases were evaluated in combination, suggesting a protective effect of operative delivery.

A critical flaw in the meta-analysis was the failure of most individual studies to control for potential confounding factors by randomization or multivariate analysis. Clinicians caring for HIV-infected women may perform cesarean delivery differently based on maternal immune status, being quite liberal with surgery in the face of an immunocompetent woman and avoiding surgery except in dire circumstance when faced with a severely immunocompromised woman. Because the maternal immune status has been associated with transmission risk by a number of investigators, different rates of transmission owing to immune status may be falsely attributed to the mode of delivery (Burns et al., 1994; Tibaldi et al., 1991).

An additional shortcoming of the meta-analysis is that most studies did not separately analyze elective and emergent cesarean delivery. In contrast to emergency cesarean delivery, elective section takes place before labor and membrane rupture. Because elective section would prevent maternal-fetal blood transfusions from occurring during labor and hence would prevent exposure to infectious maternal genital secretions, it might be expected to be more effective in preventing transmission. However, one of the larger studies included in the meta-analysis made the seemingly contradictory observation that infection rates were lower only in women who had undergone emergency sections, while those who had had elective operative delivery had rates similar to women who had had a vaginal delivery.

Summary

In conclusion, the first step toward preventing HIV-associated perinatal morbidity is providing universal and convenient access to HIV testing. Women who are aware of their HIV-positive status could then take advantage of family planning or abortion services as outlined above. Beyond that, it would appear that the most productive means of avoiding adverse outcomes is meticulous prenatal and HIV care. Many of the adverse outcomes reported (prematurity, low birth weight) have occurred in populations with more advanced HIV disease and often with high rates of such important covariate risks as syphilis. Unfortunately, biological risks are often coupled with social barriers that circumscribe the access of pregnant women to standard treatments and research therapies (Minkoff and Moreno, 1990; Minkoff et al., 1992). The standard of care is often subject to modification based on serostatus. Scalp clips, scalp pH measurements, and invasive diagnostic procedures may be avoided. Although the balance between the benefits derived from such procedures and the risks of perinatal transmission might necessitate such modifications of standards, other changes in clinical behavior are not as easily justified. Delays in performing surgery or instituting therapy are seldom warranted on medical grounds. Rigorous adherence to obstetrical and medical standards with ready access to HIV medications and obstetrical interventions would seem to be the best safeguard against obstetrical morbidity. The single most important step in prenatal care today is the use of ZDV in the antepartum, intrapartum, and neonatal periods.

RESEARCH AGENDA

Despite significant progress in attempts to prevent perinatal transmission of HIV, a great deal remains to be learned about HIV during pregnancy. First, a further understanding of the timing of transmission as well as the relationship between transmission and severity of disease is required to facilitate an intelligent choice of proposed interventions. Clearly, transmission will not occur exclusively in any one period (antepartum, intrapartum, or postpartum), and intervention strategies should be predicated on the likelihood and mechanism of transmission at each point and the relative contribution of each time frame to the overall burden of transmission. Second, a greater understanding of the role of breast-feeding is needed to reduce mother-to-infant transmission even after successful peripartum interventions are developed. Some authors have suggested that up to one-third of transmissions may be related to long-term breast-feeding (Dunn et al., 1992). Strategies to reduce that occurrence require research on the mechanisms of breast milk transmission and modifiers of the rate of breast milk transmission. Third, interruption of antepartum transmission requires more research on the pharmacology of prevention: the identity of the essential component of the 076 protocol; whether HIV immune globulin will reduce transmission when given in conjunction with ZDV to those in low CD4 groups or to those previously treated with antiviral agents; when multidrug therapy is appropriate, etc. Fourth and finally, obstetrical interventions may be an important focus of research, particularly in parts of the world where access to pharmaceutical interventions may not be a practicable option for many infected women. Evidence that intrapartum transmission does occur is fairly strong. Although evidence that obstetrical interventions can influence that rate is not as compelling, there is reason to believe that they may prove useful. The intrinsic biases present in the observational studies of the protective benefits of cesarean delivery prohibit any definitive conclusions, leaving this subject as an appropriate focus of research.

The vast majority of perinatal HIV-1 infections occur in the developing world. Unfortunately, the ACTG 076 ZDV regimen is too costly and logistically complex for many nonindustrialized countries to implement on a widespread scale, and its efficacy in a breast-feeding population is unknown. An ideal preventive intervention would be cheap, nontoxic to the mother and fetus, and easy to administer; would need to be given only once or for a limited time; and would have utility in preventing postpartum transmission. The results of ACTG 076 have spurred the worldwide evaluation of numerous other modalities to reduce transmission.

Potential interventions to reduce transmission have focused on reduction of the maternal viral load, enhancement of the maternal and infant HIV-1-specific immune response, prophylaxis of the newborn, and attempts to reduce peripartum and postpartum exposure to the virus (Mofenson et al., 1997). At present, only ZDV has been proven to significantly reduce the rate of mother-to-child transmission of HIV. The future challenge for researchers is to use the increasing understanding of the pathogenesis of perinatal HIV-1 transmission to design preventive regimens that will be applicable on a global basis.

REFERENCES

Allain, J. P., T. Matthew, R. Coombs, et al. 1991. Antibody to V3 loop does not predict vertical transmission of HIV, abstr. W. C. 2263. *In Proceedings of the VII International Conference on AIDS.*

Baba, T. W., J. Koch, E., S. Mittler, M. Greene, M. Wyand, D. Pennick, and R. M. Rupect. 1994. Mucosal infection of neonatal rhesus monkeys with cell-free SIV. *AIDS Res. Hum. Retroviruses* **10:**351–357.

Belec, L., D. Meillet, O. Gaillard, T. Prazuck, E. Michel, J. Ngondi Ekome, and J. Pillot. 1995. Decreased cervicovaginal production of both IgA1 and IgA2 subclasses in women with AIDS. *Clin. Exp. Immunol.* **101:**100–106.

Blanche, S., C. Rouzioux, M.-L. Guihart Moscato, F. Veber, M. J. Mayaux, C. Jacomet, J. Tricoire, A. Deville, M. Vial, and G. Firtion. 1989. A prospective study of infants born to women seropositive for human immunodeficiency virus type 1. *N. Engl. J. Med.* **320:**1643–1648.

Blanche, S., M. J. Mayaux, C. Rouzioux, J. P. Teglas, G. Firtion, F. Monpoux, N. Ciraru-Vigneron, F. Meier, J. Tricoire, and C. Courpotin. 1994. Relation of the course of HIV infection in children to the severity of the disease in their mothers at delivery. *N. Engl. J. Med.* **330:**308–312.

Borkowski, W., K. Drazinski, D. Paul, R. Holzman, T. Moore, P. Bebenroth, R. Lawrence, and S. Chandwani. 1989. Human immunodeficiency virus type 1 antigenemia in children. *J. Pediatr.* **114:**940–945.

Boue, F., J. C. Pons, L. Keros, et al. 1990. Risk for HIV-1 perinatal transmission vary with the mother's stage of HIV infection, abstr. Th. C44. *In Proceedings of the VI International Conference on AIDS.*

Broliden, P. A., V. Moschese, K. Ljungren, J. Rosen, C. Fundaro, A. Plebani, M. Jondal, P. Ross, and B. Wahren. 1989. Diagnostic implications of specific immunoglobulin G patterns born to HIV infected women. *AIDS* **3:**577–582.

Bryson, E., K. Luzuriaga, J. L. Sullivan, and D. Ware. 1992. Proposed definition for in-utero versus intrapartum transmission of HIV-1. *N. Engl. J. Med.* **327:**1246–1247.

Burns, D. N., S. Landesman, L. R. Muenz, R. P. Nugent, J. J. Goedert, H. Minkoff, J. H. Walsh, H. Mendez, A. Rubinstein, and A. Willoughby. 1994. Cigarette smoking, premature rupture of membranes and vertical transmission of HIV-1 among women with low CD4$^+$ levels. *J. Acquired Immune Defic. Syndr.* **7:**718–726.

Chin, J. 1991. Current and future dimension of the HIV/AIDS pandemic in women and children. *Lancet* **336:**221–224.

Connor, E. M., R. S. Sperling, R. Gelber, P. Kiselev, G. Scott, M. J. O'Sullivan, R. Van Dyke, M. Bey, W. Shearer, and R. L. Jacobsen. 1994. Reduction of maternal-infant transmission of human immunodeficiency virus type 1 with zidovudine treatment. *N. Engl. J. Med.* **331:**1173–1180.

Cotton, P. 1994. Trial halted after drug cuts maternal HIV transmission rate by two thirds. *JAMA* **271:**807.

Courgnaud, V., F. Laure, F. Barin, et al. 1989. In utero HIV-1 transmission identified through PCR, abstr. MBP-1. *In Proceedings of the V International Conference on AIDS.*

Courpotin, C., G. Israel, D. Dubeaux, G. Vogt, H. di Maria, F. Bricout, and D. Dormont. 1988. Predictive value of HIV replication in cell culture in babies born to seropositive mothers. *Lancet* **ii:**1074–1074.

D'Arminio, M. A., M. Ravizza, M. L. Muggiasca, et al. 1991. HIV-infected pregnant women: possible predictors of vertical transmission, abstr. W.C. 49. *In Proceedings of the VII International Conference on AIDS.*

DeFasio, K., J. J. Kelly, J. Beuhler, B. M. Whyte, E. D. Mokotoff, C. E. Bell, W. Brandon, B. L. Nahlen, A. F. Phelps, J. H. Stephens, A. J. Davidson, and H. L. Minkoff. 1992. Provision of gynecologic care at outpatient medical facilities serving HIV infected persons. *Am. J. Women's Health* **1:**193–196.

Devash, Y., T. Calvelli, D. G. Wood, R. J. Reagen, and A. Rubinstein. 1990. Vertical transmission of HIV is correlated with absence of high affinity/avidity maternal antibodies to the gp120 principal neutralizing domain. *Proc. Natl. Acad. Sci. USA* **87:**345–349.

Dickover, R. E., E. M. Garraty, S. A. Hermann, M. S. Sim, S. Plaeger, P. J. Boyer, M. Keller, A. Deveikis, E. R. Steihm, and Y. J. Bryson. 1996. Identification of levels of HIV-1 RNA associated with risk of perinatal transmission: effect of maternal zidovudine treatment on viral load. *JAMA* **275:**599–605.

Dunn, D. T., N. L. Newell, A. E. Ades, and C. S. Peckham. 1992. Risk of human immunodeficiency virus type 1 transmission through breastfeeding. *Lancet* **340:** 585–588.

Ehrnst, A., S. Lindgren, M. Dictor, B. Johansson, A. Sonnerborg, J. Cjakowski, G. Sundin, and A. B. Bohlin. 1991. HIV in pregnant women and their offspring: evidence for late transmission. *Lancet* **338:**203–207.

European Collaborative Study. 1991. Children born to women with HIV-1 infection: natural history and risk of transmission. *Lancet* **337:**253–260.

European Collaborative Study. 1992. Risk factors for mother to child transmission of HIV-1. *Lancet* **339:**1007–1012.

Fang, G., H. Burger, R. Grimson, P. Tropper, S. Nachman, D. Mayers, O. Weislow, R. Moore, C. Reyelt, and N. Hutcheon. 1995. Maternal plasma human immunodeficiency virus type 1 RNA level: a determinant and projected threshold for mother-to-child transmission. *Proc. Natl. Acad. Sci. USA* **92:**12100–12104.

Fazely, F., P. L. Sharma, C. Fratazzi, M. F. Greene, M. S. Wyand, M. A. Mermon, D. Pennick, and R. M. Ruprect. 1993. Simian immunodeficiency virus infection via amniotic fluid: a model to study fetal immunopathogenesis and prophylaxis. *J. Acquired Immune Defic. Syndr.* **6:**107–114.

Friedland, G. H., B. R. Saltzman, M. F. Rogers, P. A. Kahl, M. L. Leser, M. M. Mayers, and R. S. Klein. 1986. Lack of transmission of HTLV111/LAV infection to household contacts of patients with AIDS or ARC with oral candidiasis. *N. Engl. J. Med.* **314:**3444.

Gabiano, C., P. Tovo, M. de Martino, L. Galli, C. Giaquinto, A. Loy, M. C. Schoeller, M. Giovannini, G. Ferranti, and L. Rancilo. 1992. Mother to child transmission of HIV 1: risk of infection and correlates of transmission. *Pediatrics* **90:**362–374.

Goedert, J. J., H. Mendez, J. E. Drummond, M. Robert-Guroff, H. L. Minkoff, S. Holman, S. Stevens, A. Rubinstein, W. A. Blattner, and A. Willoughby. 1989. Mother-to-infant transmission of HIV type 1: association with prematurity or low anti-gp120. *Lancet* **iii:**1351–1354.

Goedert, J. J., A. M. Duliege, C. I. Amos, S. Felton, and R. J. Biggar. 1991. High risk of HIV-1 infection for first born twins. *Lancet* **338:**1471–1475.

Hague, R. A., J. Y. Q. Mok, L. MacCallum, et al. 1991. Do maternal factors influence the risk of HIV?, abstr. W.C. 3237. *In Proceedings of the VII International Conference on AIDS.*

Hutto, C., W. P. Parks, S. Lai, M. C. Mastrucci, C. Mitchell, J. Munoz, E. Tropida, I. M. Master, and G. B. Scott. 1991. A hospital-based prospective study of perinatal infection with human immunodeficiency virus type 1. *J. Pediatr.* **118:**347–353.

Irwin, K., N. Olivo, C. A. Schable, J. T. Weber, R. Janssen, and J. Ernst. 1996. Performance characteristics of a rapid HIV antibody assay in a hospital with a high prevalence of HIV infection. *Ann. Intern. Med.* **125:**471–475.

John, G. C., R. W. Nduati, D. Mbori-Ngacha, J. Overbaugh, M. Welch, B. A. Richardson, J. Ndinya-Achola, J. Bwayo, J. Krieger, F. Onyango, and J. Kreiss. 1997. Genital shedding of human immunodeficiency virus type 1 DNA during pregnancy: association with immunosuppression, abnormal cervical or vaginal discharge, and severe vitamin A deficiency. *J. Infect. Dis.* **175:**57–62.

Kind, C., B. Brändle, C. A. Wyler, A. Calame, C. Rudin, U. B. Schaad, J. Schüpbach, H. P. Senn, L. Perrin, and L. Matter. 1992. Epidemiology of vertically transmitted HIV 1 infection in Switzerland: results of a nationwide prospective study. *Eur. J. Pediatr.* **151:**442–448.

Kreiss, J., P. Datta, D. Willerford, et al. 1991. Vertical transmission of HIV in Nairobi: correlation with maternal viral burden, abstr. W.C. 3062. *In Proceedings of the VII International Conference on AIDS.*

Lallemant, M., S. Le Coeur, L. Samba, D. Cheynier, P. M'Pelé, S. Nzingoula, and M. Essex. 1994a. Mother-child transmission of HIV-1 and infant survival in Brazzaville, Congo. *AIDS* **3:**643–646.

Lallemant, M., A. Baillou, S. Lallemant-Le Coeur, S. Nzingoula, M. Mampaka, P. M'Pelé, F. Barin, and M. Essex. 1994b. Maternal antibody response at delivery and perinatal transmission of human immunodeficiency virus type-1 in African women. *Lancet* **343:**1001–1005.

Landesman, S., and D. Burns. 1996. Quantifying HIV. *JAMA* **275:**640–641.

Landesman, S., H. Minkoff, S. Holman, S. McCalla, and O. Sijin. 1987. Serosurvey of human immunodeficiency virus infection in parturients. *JAMA* **258:**2701.

Landesman, S., B. Weiblem, H. Mendez, A. Willoughby, J. J. Goedert, A. Rubenstein, H. Minkoff, G. Moroso, and R. Hoff. 1991. Clinical utility of HIV-IgA assay in the early diagnosis of perinatal HIV infection. *JAMA* **266:**3443–3446.

Landesman, S. H., L. A. Kalish, D. N. Burns, H. Minkoff, H. E. Fox, C. Zorrilla, P. Garcia, M. G. Fowler, L. Mofenson, and R. Tuomala. 1996. The relationship of obstetrical factors to the mother-to-child transmission of HIV-1. *N. Engl. J. Med.* **334:**1617–1623.

Lapointe, N., J. Michaud, D. Pekovic, J. P. Chausseau, and J. P. Dupuy. 1985. Transplacental transmission of HTLV-III virus. *N. Engl. J. Med.* **312:**1325.

Lepage, P., P. Van de Perre, M. Caraël, F. Nsengumuremyi, J. Nkurunziza, J. P. Butzler, and S. Sprecher. 1987. Postnatal transmission of HIV mother to child. *Lancet* **ii:**400.

Lepage, P., F. Dabis, D. G. Hitimana, P. Msellati, C. Van Goethem, A. M. Stevens, F. Nsengumuremyi, A. Bazubagira, A. Serufilira, and A. De Clercq. 1991. Perinatal transmission of HIV-1: lack of impact of maternal HIV infection on characteristics of live births and neonatal mortality in Kigali, Rwanda. *AIDS* **5:**295–300.

Lindgren, S., B. Anzen, A. Bohlin, and K. Lidman. 1991. HIV and childbearing: clinical outcome and aspects of mother-to-infant transmission. *AIDS* **5:**1111–1116.

Mandelbrot, L., M. J. Mayaux, A. Bongain, A. Berrebi, Y. Moudoub-Jeanpetit, J. L. Bénifla, N. Ciraru-Vigneron, J. Le Chenadec, S. Blanche, and J. F. Delfraissy. 1996. Obstetric factors and mother-to-child transmission of human immunodeficiency virus type 1: the French perinatal cohorts. *Am. J. Obstet. Gynecol.* **175:**661–667.

Mayers, M. M., K. Davenny, E. E. Schoenbaum, A. R. Feingold, P. A. Selwyn, V. Robertson, C. Y. Ou, M. F. Rogers, and M. Naccarato. 1991. A prospective study of infants of human immunodeficiency virus seropositive and seronegative women with a history of intravenous drug-using partners in the Bronx, New York City. *Pediatrics* **88:**1248–1256.

Miles, S. A., E. Balden, L. Magpantay, L. Wei, A. Leiblein, D. Hofheinz, G. Toedter, E. R. Steihm, and Y. Bryson. 1993. Rapid serologic testing with immune-complex-dissociated HIV p24 antigen for early detection of HIV infection in neonates. *N. Engl. J. Med.* **328:**297–302.

Minkoff, H., and M. Augenbraun. 1997. Antiretroviral therapy of the pregnant women. *Am. J. Obstet. Gynecol.* **176:**478–489.

Minkoff, H., and M. Mofenson. 1994. The role of obstetrical interventions in the prevention of pediatric human immunodeficiency virus infection. *Am. J. Obstet. Gynecol.* **171:**1167–1175.

Minkoff, H., and J. Moreno. 1990. Drug prophylaxis for human immunodeficiency virus infected pregnant women: ethical considerations. *Am. J. Obstet. Gynecol.* **163:** 1111–1113.

Minkoff, H. L., C. Henderson, H. Mendez, M. H. Gail, S. Holman, A. Willoughby, J. J. Goedett, A. Rubinstein, P. Stratton, and J. H. Walsh. 1990. Pregnancy outcomes among women infected with HIV and matched controls. *Am. J. Obstet. Gynecol.* **163:**1598–1603.

Minkoff, H., J. Moreno, and K. Powderly. 1992. Fetal protection and women's access to clinical trials. *Am. J. Women's Health* **1:**137–140.

Minkoff, H., D. Burns, S. Landesman, J. Youchah, J. J. Goedert, R. P. Nugent, L. R. Muenz, and A. D. Willoughby. 1995. The relationship of the duration of ruptured membranes to vertical transmission of HIV. *Am. J. Obstet. Gynecol.* **173:**585–589.

Miotti, P., R. Yolken, J. Canner, et al. 1993. Mucosal factors and transmission of HIV from mother to infant, abstr. 673. *In Proceedings of the First National Conference on Human and Other Related Retroviruses.*

Mofenson, L. M. 1997. Mother-child HIV-1 transmission: timing and determinants. *Obstet. Gynecol. Clin. North Am.* **24:**759–784.

Mofenson, L. M., E. R. Stiehm, J. Lambert, et al. 1997. Efficacy of zidovudine (ZDV) in reducing perinatal HIV-1 transmission in HIV-1 infected women with advanced disease, abstr. I-117. *In Program and Abstracts of the 37th Interscience Conference on Antimicrobial Agents and Chemotherapy.* American Society for Microbiology, Washington, D.C.

Nielsen, K., P. Boyer, M. Dillion, D. Wafer, L. S. Wei, E. Garratty, R. E. Dickover, and Y. J. Bryson. 1996. Presence of human immunodeficiency virus (HIV) type 1 and HIV-1-specific antibodies in cervicovaginal secretions of infected mothers and in the gastric aspirates of their infants. *J. Infect. Dis.* **173:**1001–1004.

Quinn, T. C., R. L. Kline, N. Halsey, N. Hutton, A. Ruff, A. Butz, R. Boulos, and J. Modlin. 1991. Early diagnosis of perinatal HIV infection by detection of viral specific IgA antibodies. *JAMA* **266:**3439–3442.

Rasheed, S., Z. Li, D. Xu, and A. Kovacs. 1996. Presence of cell-free human immunodeficiency virus in cervicovaginal secretions is independent of viral load in the blood of human immunodeficiency virus-infected women. *Am. J. Obstet. Gynecol.* **175:**122–130.

Rossi, P., V. Moschese, P. A. Broliden, C. Fundaró, I. Quinti, A. Plebani, C. Giaquinto, P. A. Tovo, K. Ljunggren, and J. Rosen. 1989. Presence of maternal antibodies to human immunodeficiency virus 1 envelope glycoprotein gp120 epitopes correlates with the noninfective status of children born to seropositive mothers. *Proc. Natl. Acad. Sci. USA* **86:**8055–8058.

Ryder, R. W., W. Nsa, S. E. Hassig, F. Behets, M. Rayfield, B. Ekungola, A. M. Nelson, U. Mulenda, H. Francis, and K. Mwandagalirwa. 1989. Perinatal transmission of the human immunodeficiency virus type 1 to infants of seropositive women in Zaire. *N. Engl. J. Med.* **320:**1637–1642.

Shearer, W. T., T. C. Quinn, P. LaRussa, J. F. Lew, L. Mofenson, S. Almy, K. Rich, E. Handelsman, C. Diaz, M. Pagano, V. Smeriglio, and L. A. Kalish. 1997. Viral load and disease progression in infants infected with human immunodeficiency virus type 1. *N. Engl. J. Med.* **336:**1337–1342.

Soeiro, R., W. F. Rashburn, A. Rubenstein, and W. D. Lyman. 1991. The incidence of human fetal HIV-1 infection as determined by the presence of HIV-1 DNA in abortus tissues, abstr. W.C. 3250. *In Proceedings of the VII International Conference on AIDS.*

Sperling, R. S., P. Stratton, J. O'Sullivan, B. Boyer, D. H. Watts, J. S. Lambert, H. Hammill, E. Livingston, D. J. Gloeb, H. L. Minkoff, and H. Fox. 1992. A survey of Zidovudine use in pregnant women with immunodeficiency virus infection. *N. Engl. J. Med.* **326:**857–861.

Sperling, R. S., D. E. Shapiro, R. W. Coombs, J. A. Todd, S. A. Herman, G. D. McSherry, M. J. O'Sullivan, R. B. Van Dyke, E. Jimenez, C. Rouzioux, P. M. Flynn, and J. L. Sullivan. 1996. Maternal viral load, zidovudine treatment and the risk of transmission of human immunodeficiency virus type 1 from mother to infant. *N. Engl. J. Med.* **335:**1621–1629.

St. Louis, M. E., M. Kamenga, C. Brown, A. M. Nelson, T. Manzila, V. Batter, F. Behets, U. Kabagabo, R. W. Ryder, and M. Oxtoby. 1993. Risk for perinatal HIV-1 transmission according to maternal immunologic, virologic and placental factors. *JAMA* **269:**2853–2859.

Temmerman, M., E. N. Chomba, J. Ndinya-Achola, F. A. Plummer, M. Coppens, and P. Piot. 1994. Maternal HIV-1 infection and pregnancy outcome. *Obstet. Gynecol.* **83:**495–501.

Tibaldi, C., E. Palomba, N. Ziarati, et al. 1991. Maternal factors influencing vertical HIV transmission, abstr. W. C. 3277. *In Proceedings of the VII International Conference on AIDS.*

Van de Perre, P., A. Simonon, P. Msellati, D. G. Hitimana, D. Vaira, A. Baxubagira, C. Van Goethem, A. M. Stevens, E. Karita, and D. Sondag-Thull. 1991. Postnatal transmission of HIV type 1 from mother to infant. *N. Engl. J. Med.* **325:**593.

Villari, P., C. Spino, T. C. Chalmer, J. Lau, and H. S. Sacks. 1993. Cesarean section to reduce prenatal transmission of human immunodeficiency virus: a meta-analysis online. *J. Curr. Clin. Trials* (document 74).

Viscarello, R., M. T. Cullen, N. J. DeGennaro, and J. C. Hobbins. 1992. Fetal blood sampling in human immunodeficiency-seropositive women before elective midtrimester termination of pregnancy. *Am. J. Obstet. Gynecol.* **167:**1075–1079.

Whaley, K. J., L. Zeitlin, R. A. Barratt, T. E. Hoen, and R. A. Cone. 1994. Passive immunization of the vagina protects mice against vaginal transmission of genital herpes infections. *J. Infect. Dis.* **169:**647–649.

Ziegler, J. B., D. A. Cooper, R. O. Johnson, and J. Gold. 1985. Postnatal transmission of AIDS-associated retrovirus from mother to infant. *Lancet* **i:**896.

Ziegler, J. B., G. J. Stewart, R. Penney, et al. 1988. Breast-feeding and transmission of HIV from mother to infant, abstr. 5100. *In Proceedings of the Fourth Annual International AIDS Conference.*

14
Genital Herpes and Pregnancy

Zane A. Brown

Genital herpes is the most common ulcerative sexually transmitted disease in North America. It is estimated that 30 to 45 million adults are infected, with approximately 500,000 new cases annually. The seroprevalence of herpes simplex virus type 2 (HSV-2) has increased in the United States by about 30% over the past decade. Currently about 25% of the reproductive-aged women in the United States (blacks, 55%; whites, 19%) are HSV-2 seropositive (Fleming et al., 1997). Of these, approximately one in four are able to identify their recurrences and report symptoms, most commonly localized recurrent itching and pain with a vesiculoulcerative eruption (Koutsky et al., 1992). The remaining patients are unaware of their infection but are probably experiencing mild, episodic genital symptoms that they do not attribute to genital herpes and for which they either do not seek medical consultation, or if they do, are frequently diagnosed incorrectly. Over the last several decades, there has also been an apparent increase in the incidence of genital HSV-1 infections which in some areas accounts for as many as 30% of new cases of genital herpes. It is not clear whether this increase is due to changes in patterns of sexual behavior or to other environmental societal changes. However, some experts feel that in this HIV-conscious era, this increase in genital HSV-1 is due to a perception by the lay public that oral sex is "safe" compared to vaginal intercourse.

Neonatal HSV infection is by far the most dreaded complication of maternal genital HSV infections and has increased in incidence in parallel to the prevalence of genital HSV infection in the adult population. The incidence varies greatly in different populations, ranging from approxi-

Zane A. Brown, Department of Obstetrics and Gynecology, University of Washington, Seattle, WA 98195.

Sexually Transmitted Diseases and Adverse Outcomes of Pregnancy
Edited by P. J. Hitchcock, H. T. MacKay, J. N. Wasserheit, and R. Binder
©1999 American Society for Microbiology, Washington, D.C.

mately 1/2,000 to 1/15,000 live births. Even with antiviral chemotherapy, the outcome is poor, with high rates of developmental disability and death (Whitley et al., 1991a). Over the past decade, we have learned that the mothers transmitting this infection to their newborns are almost always asymptomatically seroconverting at or near the time of labor and that reactivation of genital HSV-2 at the time of labor is a relatively infrequent cause of the newborn infection (Brown et al., 1998).

Since genital herpes is primarily subclinical, the only hope of slowing the spread of this "silent epidemic" between adults and from mother to newborn is by widespread screening of large populations with HSV type-specific serology, combined with educational programs regarding methods of preventing transmission and chronic suppression of infected individuals with antiviral chemotherapeutic agents.

The précis for this discussion is that universal HSV serologic testing should be performed at the first prenatal visit. As a corollary, type-specific HSV serologic tests should be commercially available, easily accessible, and inexpensive. At the time of this writing, rapid kit-based, type-specific serologic tests have recently become available in the United States and Europe.

To discuss the rationale of HSV serologic testing in the prevention of neonatal herpes and other adverse consequences of genital herpes complicating pregnancy, it is necessary to review the classification of this infection. It is important to note that until recently, the classification of maternal HSV infection was based primarily upon the clinical presentation (Corey et al., 1983). For example, the diagnosis of a primary infection was thought to require bilateral, numerous lesions of long duration with considerable local reaction and pain, inguinal lymphadenopathy, and systemic signs and symptoms such as fever, headache, and myalgias. In contrast, recurrent genital herpes was thought to be characterized by a few unilateral lesions with localized discomfort of short duration without systemic signs and symptoms. However, recent studies have clearly demonstrated that genital herpes complicating pregnancy cannot be classified by the clinical presentation alone and that there is considerable overlap in the appearance of first primary and recurrent disease, with both types being primarily subclinical (Hensleigh et al., 1997; Brown et al., 1998). In fact, the use of a classification in pregnancy based on clinical presentation as a means of defining management strategies and patient counseling may be at best misleading and even possibly harmful.

It is evident from the above discussion that the appropriate classification of genital herpes during pregnancy depends upon accurate serotyping of the patient by type-specific serologic assays. Type-specific HSV serologic assays that detect antibodies directed against viral protein epitopes specific for each viral type have been developed (Ashley, 1993). This avoids the extensive cross-reactivity between HSV serotypes that renders the commonly used enzyme immunoassay and indirect immunofluorescence assay unreliable and therefore unusable in distinguishing HSV-1 from HSV-2 antibodies even though most proprietary laboratories report the results as "titers" to HSV-1 and HSV-2. Assays such as Western blot analysis, which use HSV type-specific antigens, are 98% sensitive and 100% specific for detecting the presence of HSV-2 antibodies even in the presence of HSV-1 antibodies and would enable the practitioner to detect HSV-2 seroconversion during pregnancy and identify the HSV-2-seropositive but asymptomatic or unaware patient. Recently, Diagnology has released a point-of-care, finger-stick-based HSV-2 serology in Europe that is type specific and extremely sensitive. It is in pre-marketing testing in the United States and should prove to be a reasonable alternative to the expensive, labor-intensive, and relatively unavailable Western blot assay.

SEROLOGIC CLASSIFICATION

Primary First Episode

The primary first episode is a first genital infection with either HSV-1 or HSV-2 in a woman who lacks antibodies to both HSV-1 and HSV-2. This infection is either subclinical or unrecognized in approximately 60% of cases (Brown et al., 1997). The remaining 40% of patients may have symptoms that range in severity from a very mild infection to a life-threatening, disseminated infection. However, the symptoms are most frequently attributed to some other infection such as "yeast" by the health care provider. Most importantly, the "classic" presentation of a primary infection, as described above, is unusual in pregnancy.

Nonprimary First Episode

The nonprimary first episode is an initial genital infection with HSV-2 in an individual who is HSV-1 seropositive. Rarely, an individual may have preexisting HSV-2 antibody and experience a first infection with HSV-1 (either orally or genitally). However, a recent study of HSV seroconversion during pregnancy failed to demonstrate any cases of an HSV-2-seropositive woman acquiring an HSV-1 infection during pregnancy, suggesting that antibody to HSV-2 protects against infection with HSV-1 but that preexisting HSV-1 antibody does not prevent the acquisition of HSV-2 (Brown et al., 1997). As with the primary infection, the majority of these infections are subclinical, and when symptoms occur, they range from mild to occasionally severe.

Recurrent Infection

An infection is defined as recurrent when the HSV type recovered from the patient's genital tract is the same as the serotype of HSV antibodies present in the serum. As with the first-episode infections, the recurrent (reactivation) infections are primarily subclinical, with approximately 25% of seropositive individuals recognizing or reporting symptoms of the infection. When symptoms occur, they are generally mild and of short duration. However, during pregnancy, symptoms can be severe, particularly during a first recurrence in late pregnancy.

Asymptomatic Shedding

Asymptomatic shedding is defined as the presence of infectious virus in the genital tract in the absence of symptoms perceived by the patient or lesions observed by a trained observer.

Recent studies have shown that as many as 60 to 75% of first episodes, whether primary or nonprimary, are asymptomatic or at least have symptoms that are unrecognized by the patient (Mertz et al., 1985; Boucher et al., 1990; Brown et al., 1991; Kulhanjian et al., 1992). The remaining 25% to 40% present with a spectrum of disease ranging from single, minimally painful genital lesions to severe disease with numerous bilateral genital lesions, moderate to severe local pain, dysuria, sacral paresthesia, tender regional lymph node enlargement, central nervous system symptoms, and the systemic symptoms of a viremia such as fever and malaise. Although considered to be "typical" of primary genital herpes, this may in fact be an uncommon presentation.

Similarly, approximately 60 to 75% of HSV-2 antibody-positive individuals do not report genital lesions or a history compatible with recurrent genital herpes (Koutsky et al., 1992). However, with education, more than 50% of these "asymptomatic" seropositive individuals can be taught to recognize and report their genital lesions (Langenberg et al., 1989). The frequency, duration, and severity of symptomatic recurrences increase as pregnancy progresses (Brown et al., 1985). Until recently, symptomatic recurrences in pregnancy were thought to be brief, typically lasting several days, usually unilateral, and infrequently associated with systemic signs and symptoms. However, with the declining immune competency of advancing gestation, asymptomatic HSV-2-seropositive women may experience a "first-ever" symptomatic recurrence in late pregnancy with a presentation ranging from a very mild to a more severe illness comparable to first-episode disease. In a recent study of 29 women presenting in pregnancy with a first episode, 50% had bilateral lesions, 40% had bilateral inguinal lymphadenopathy and malaise, 15% reported a headache, and 10% reported myalgias (Hensleigh et al., 1997). However, a type-specific HSV serologic assay showed that only 4 (14%) of the 29 women were experiencing first-episode disease (2 primary and 2 nonprimary); the remaining 25 women were HSV seropositive and experiencing a first-ever recurrence. This observation is of considerable social as well as medical importance. A woman experiencing a first-ever reactivation late in pregnancy who does not give a history of genital herpes antedating pregnancy would presume that her genital lesions represented newly acquired genital herpes, with the obvious social implications. Type-specific serologic testing demonstrating antibodies to the same viral type isolated from the genitalia would suggest that her infection probably antedated pregnancy.

Data from the University of Washington suggest that the rate of asymptomatic shedding at the time of labor in the general obstetrical population is 0.4%, or about 1.0% of the HSV-2-seropositive population (Brown et al., 1991). When the genital secretions of a subset of these women who were HSV-2 seropositive but HSV culture negative at the time of labor were examined by PCR, 20% showed evidence of HSV-2 DNA (Cone et al., 1994). None of the newborns were infected with HSV. Unpublished data from the University of Washington suggest that this HSV DNA represents infectious virus in a titer that is below the level of sensitivity of viral isolation techniques. From these data, it is apparent that asymptomatic shedding at the time of labor probably occurs much more frequently than has been appreciated in the past based upon standard viral isolation techniques. It also implies that although many infants are exposed during birth, neonatal herpes is rare. HSV is more likely to be present in the genital tract at the onset of labor as a result of asymptomatic rather than symptomatic disease and is responsible for almost all neonatal infections (Brown et al., 1991; Sullivan-Bolyai et al., 1983; Prober et al., 1988; Whitley et al., 1988; Arvin et al., 1982). In addition, unpublished data from the University of Washington suggest that the viral load of HSV in the genital tract at the time of labor in women with asymptomatic shedding may be comparable to or in some cases greater than in women with symptomatic recurrences (Brown et al., 1998).

EPIDEMIOLOGY OF CURRENT OBSTETRIC PRACTICE

Genital herpes is the most common ulcerative sexually transmitted disease in North America (Fleming et al., 1997; Quinn and Cates, 1992). Current obstetric practice is guided by the unsubstantiated belief that symptomatic recurrence of HSV infection at the onset of labor is the primary risk factor for neonatal transmission. This belief, coupled with anxiety among both patients and health care providers, has resulted in an increase in the rate of cesarean sections in an attempt to prevent transmission. In spite of this, the incidence of neonatal herpes has appeared to increase in some populations, probably as a result of parallel increases in the frequency of the infection in the adult population (Nahmias et al., 1990; Stone et al., 1989). In Seattle, King County, Wash., between 1966 and 1985, the incidence of neonatal herpes rose from 3.2 to approximately 15 cases per 100,000 live births (Sullivan-Bolyai et al., 1983). This occurred in spite of a cesarean section rate over the same period approaching 70% for women entering pregnancy with symptomatic recurrent genital HSV (Wolfe, 1990). Since 1985, the rates of neonatal herpes have decreased to about 11 cases per 100,000 live births and have remained at that level to the present. Rates of neonatal herpes, however, vary widely throughout the United States and Europe. For example, the current rate of neonatal HSV at the University of Washington is approximately 1 in 1,800 live births, which is higher than that found in most other areas of the country, where reported rates vary from 1 case per 2,000 to 1 case per 10,000 live births (Brown et al., 1991; Stone et al., 1989; Garland, 1992; Chuang, 1988). Although the mortality and morbidity of neonatal herpes have decreased with the advent of antiviral chemotherapy, more than 40% of neonates with the infection still die or are impaired (Whitley et al., 1991b).

A conservative estimate of the cost of this excess cesarean section rate nationally can be made by making several assumptions. If we assume a delivery rate in the United States of approximately 4 million births per year and an incidence of symptomatic genital herpes of 10% in the reproductive-age population, 400,000 women with a history of symptomatic recurrent genital herpes will deliver annually. If we further assume a baseline cesarean section rate of 20%, the excess cesarean section rate of 20% attributable to genital herpes will result in about 80,000 cesarean sections for the indication of genital herpes. If we assume that a cesarean section costs approximately $3,000 more than a vaginal delivery, the national costs for these excess cesarean sections due to recurrent genital herpes may approximate $225,000,000 annually. To this must be added the indirect costs such as the increased recovery time and increased time lost from work, the cost of repeat cesarean sections, and the myriad social consequences to the immediate family and the community. Thus, current obstetrical practice not only has failed to reduce the incidence of neonatal herpes, but also has significantly increased the rate of cesarean section and postpartum complications such as endometritis among women entering pregnancy with a history of recurrent genital herpes (Randolph et al., 1993).

Until recently, strategies to prevent maternal-fetal transmission centered on pregnant women with recurrent HSV-2, with the assumption that it was this population of women who, by reactivating their genital herpes near parturition, were at greatest risk of transmitting the infection to their infants. It was thought that women whose disease reactivated in the last several weeks prior to the onset of labor were at risk of having infectious virus persist in their genital tracts at the onset of labor and therefore underwent cesarean section. This thinking led to the practice of weekly HSV antepartum cultures from 34 weeks to term and was in large part responsible for the high rates of cesarean sections in women with a history of symptomatic recurrent genital herpes. A recent study has demonstrated that antepartum asymptomatic shedding of HSV as determined by weekly HSV cultures does not predict whether HSV will be present in the genital tract at the onset of labor (Arvin et al., 1991). In addition, the duration of asymptomatic shedding during pregnancy is brief, seldom more than 3 days (Brown et al., 1985).

Recent studies have demonstrated that most of the morbidity and the majority of cases of neonatal herpes in pregnancy are due not to women whose genital herpes reactivated at the onset of labor but to women acquiring genital herpes, frequently asymptomatically, in late pregnancy (Brown et al., 1987, 1997). In a recent study performed at the University of Washington, subclinical shedding at the time of labor was detected in 116 women. Of these, 20 patients had asymptomatic shedding secondary to first-episode disease and 96 had asymptomatic shedding secondary to recurrent disease. The rates of neonatal transmission were significantly higher in the mothers with asymptomatic shedding secondary to first-episode than those with recurrent disease (40 and 1%, respectively; $P = 0.001$). Among the 96 women with subclinical shedding secondary to recurrent disease, 7 were shedding HSV-1 and 89 were shedding HSV-2 (Brown et al., 1998). Of the seven shedding HSV-1, one (14%) transmitted the infection to her newborn. Of 89 women shedding HSV-2, none (0%) transmitted the infection. Even though asymptomatic shedding of HSV-1 was much less common than of HSV-2, HSV-1 appeared to be transmitted significantly more readily to the fetus irrespective of the stage of maternal disease. However, when neonatal infection with HSV-1 occurred, the neurodevelopmental consequences were significantly less severe than in neonatal infections due to HSV-2 (Whitley et al., 1991b). The use of fetal scalp electrodes in mothers in labor with a history of recurrent genital herpes was demonstrated to be a risk factor for neonatal herpes (Brown et al., 1991).

In a companion study at the University of Washington of 7,046 patients who were susceptible to acquiring an HSV infection, sera for HSV antibody tests were obtained at the first prenatal visit and again at the time of labor (Brown et al., 1997). Of these, 94 (1.3%) seroconverted, 64 (68%) acquired HSV-2, and 30 (32%) acquired HSV-1 antibodies. The median interval between serologic tests was 202 days (range, 26 to 257 days). The overall chance of seroconversion during pregnancy, adjusted for a 40-week gestation, was 2.1% (Table 1). Rates of seroconversion to HSV-2 among HSV-seronegative and HSV-1-seropositive women were similar, suggesting that prior HSV-1 infection does not protect against the acquisition of HSV-2. However, the rate of seroconversion to HSV-1 among HSV-seronegative women was significantly higher than that of HSV-2-seropositive women, suggesting that prior HSV-2 infection protects against the acquisition of HSV-1 (2.3 and 0%, respectively; $P = 0.002$).

Among the 94 women who seroconverted by the time of labor, 60 (64%) had subclinical infections and 34 (36%) had clinical infections (32 had gen-

Table 1 Antenatal HSV seroconversion among 7,046 HSV serologically susceptible women

Type of seroconversion	% who seroconverted $(n)^a$	Adjusted % seroconversion (SE)[b]
Any	1.3% (94/7,046)	2.1% (0.2)
HSV negative → any positive	2.4% (49/2,033)	3.7% (0.5)
HSV negative → HSV-1 positive	1.4% (30/2,033)	2.3% (0.4)
HSV negative → HSV-2 positive	1.0% (19/2,033)	1.4% (0.3)
HSV-1 positive → HSV-1 and HSV-2 positive	1.1% (45/4,074)	2.3% (0.3)
HSV-2 positive → HSV-1 and HSV-2 positive	0.0% (0/939)	0.0%

[a]Number who seroconverted/number at risk for seroconversion over 201.5 days (median) of observation.

[b]Estimated chance of seroconversion adjusted for a 280-day gestation. Assumes uniform seroconvertion over the entire length of pregnancy. SE was estimated by "bootstrap" resampling.

ital infections) (Table 2). The rate of seroconversion appeared to be uniform over the course of pregnancy. Among these 94 women, there were no cases of neonatal HSV or any increase in the frequency of pregnancy complications compared to 6,009 women who did not seroconvert. In contrast,

Table 2 Frequency of symptoms and trimester of acquisition among women seroconverting to HSV during pregnancy

Seroconversion	No. who seroconverted		Total (n = 94)
	Symptomatic (n = 34 [36%])	Subclinical (n = 60 [64%])	
By type			
HSV negative → HSV-1 positive	8[a]	22	30 (32%)
HSV negative → HSV-2 positive	8	11	19 (20%)
HSV-1 positive → HSV-1 and HSV-2 positive	18	27	45 (48%)
By trimester			
First	7	11	18 (19%)
Second	15	3	18 (20%)
Third	12	12	24 (25%)
First or second	n/a[b]	3	3 (3%)
Second or third	n/a	22	22 (23%)
Unable to define	n/a	9	9 (10%)

[a]Two oral only; one oral and genital; five genital only.

[b]n/a, not applicable.

among nine mothers who had their first episode of genital HSV at or near the time of labor, neonatal HSV developed in four. Neonatal herpes was significantly more frequent among those with first-episode HSV at the time of labor (4 of 9) than those whose seroconversion was complete by the time of labor (0 of 94) ($P < 0.001$). Among 2,182 of these women for whom sera were also obtained from their partners, the rate of seroconversion for HSV-seronegative women with an HSV-2-seropositive partner was 13% and that for HSV-1-seropositive women with an HSV-2-seropositive partner was 7.2% (Brown et al., 1997).

It is important to emphasize that even with best care, many cases of neonatal herpes cannot be prevented (Prober et al., 1992). Even if every patient entering pregnancy with symptomatic recurrent genital herpes underwent a cesarean section, only a minority of cases of neonatal herpes would be prevented. Cesarean section may even decrease the transplacental transmission of protective anti-HSV antibodies (Bujko et al., 1989). In addition, about 5% of infants with neonatal HSV are born with the disease, suggesting that the infection was acquired in utero (Nahmias et al., 1983).

STRATEGIES TO REDUCE THE FREQUENCY OF NEONATAL HERPES AND CESAREAN SECTIONS FOR RECURRENT GENITAL HERPES

Type-Specific Serologic Testing

HSV type-specific serologic testing should be performed at the first prenatal visit and will have three identifiable purposes.

First, women who are serologically at risk for acquiring genital herpes in late pregnancy will be identified (i.e., women who are HSV seronegative or HSV-1 seropositive). This will permit serologic testing of their partners and the identification of serologically discordant couples. Since women who acquire genital herpes and are seroconverting at the time of labor are at significant risk for neonatal HSV transmission, HSV serologically discordant couples should be counseled about methods of preventing the woman from acquiring genital herpes. Depending on the type of serologic discordancy (for example, an HSV-seronegative patient and an HSV-1- and HSV-2-seropositive partner), counseling should include recommending abstinence, avoidance of oral-genital sex, use of condoms, and/or suppressive antiviral chemotherapy for the male partner for the duration of pregnancy.

Second, it will identify women who are already HSV-2 seropositive at the time of their initial prenatal visit. Knowledge of their HSV-2 seropositivity, with its attendant risk of subclinical shedding at the time of labor, would suggest that invasive obstetrical procedures such as electronic fetal-monitoring scalp electrodes, early artificial rupture of the fetal membranes, or use of forceps and vacuum extractors should be used only for strict obstetrical indications. A patient who is HSV-2 seropositive and presents in labor with a lesion could be considered for vaginal delivery if she is appropriately informed regarding the very small but measurable risks to the newborn. However, it is important to emphasize that the determination of HSV-2 seropositivity should be precise and based upon a type-specific and sensitive HSV serologic test. Women who have genital recurrent HSV-1 or who are seroconverting to either HSV-1 or HSV-2 at the time of labor and present in labor with an active lesion are not candidates for vaginal delivery.

Lastly, routine serologic testing of sexually active, reproductive-age women would identify a large number of HSV-2-seropositive, asymptomatic women who are unaware of their disease. This would permit appropriate education about their infection, the recognition of recurrences, and the methods of avoiding transmission to sexual partners.

Acyclovir Treatment

Studies in progress suggest that acyclovir may suppress symptomatic reactivation of genital herpes at term and therefore obviate the need for cesarean section.

Acyclovir is a nucleoside analog which has a selective activity that enables it to inhibit the replication of HSV when present at concentrations up to 3,000-fold lower than those that inhibit mammalian cellular functions. Because of its remarkable specificity for cells already infected with HSV, it has proven remarkably safe in mammalian fetal test systems (Gnann et al., 1983). Several large studies have been unable to demonstrate any evidence of fetal teratogenicity or toxicity (Kingsley, 1986; Andrews et al., 1992). Even though acyclovir is cleared by the kidneys, recent pharmacokinetic studies in pregnancy have demonstrated that steady-state acyclovir levels for doses of 200 mg or 400 mg every 8 h are comparable to those expected in nonpregnant women (Frenkel et al., 1991). Surprisingly, the increased volume of distribution of pregnant women and the increased renal blood flow in late pregnancy do not alter the steady-state pharmacokinetics. Acyclovir is highly concentrated in the amniotic fluid and milk but does not accumulate in the fetus (Frenkel et al., 1991; Lau et al., 1987). The mean maternal/infant plasma ratio at delivery is 1.3:1.

Acyclovir is extremely effective in suppressing both symptomatic recurrences and asymptomatic shedding in nonimmunosuppressed, nonpregnant adults (Kaplowitz et al., 1991; Wald et al., 1996, 1997). Of the three small studies of acyclovir suppression in late pregnancy, two (only one was controlled and prospective) were able to demonstrate that treatment reduced symptomatic recurrences at the time of labor (Stray-Pedersen, 1990; Scott et al., 1996). The third study, which was stopped because of difficulty in recruiting patients (Brocklehurst et al., 1998), was unable to demonstrate effectiveness. Until the prospective studies of prophylactic acyclovir in late pregnancy which are in progress have been completed and evaluated for safety and efficacy, the prophylactic use of acyclovir in late pregnancy must be approached with caution and certainly only after complete informed consent is given by the patient.

REFERENCES

Andrews, E. B., B. C. Yankaskas, J. F. Cordero, K. Schoeffler, S. Hampp, and the Acyclovir in Pregnancy Registry Advisory Committee. 1992. Acyclovir in pregnancy registry: six years experience. *Obstet. Gynecol.* **79:**7–13.

Arvin, A. M., A. S. Yeager, F. W. Bruhn, and M. Grossman. 1982. Neonatal herpes simplex infection in the absence of mucocutaneous lesions. *J. Pediatr.* **100:**715–721.

Arvin, A. M., P. A. Hensleigh, C. G. Prober, D. S. Au, L. L. Yasukawa, A. E. Wittek, P. E. Palumbo, S. G. Paryani, and A. S. Yeager. 1991. Failure of antepartum maternal cultures to predict the infant's risk of exposure to herpes simplex virus at delivery. *N. Engl. J. Med.* **324:**1237–1252.

Ashley, R. L. 1993. Laboratory techniques in the diagnosis of herpes simplex infection. *Genitourin. Med.* **69:**174–183.

Boucher, F. D., L. L. Yasukawa, R. N. Bronzan, P. A. Hensleigh, A. M. Arvin, and C. G. Prober. 1990. A prospective evaluation of primary genital herpes simplex virus type 2 infections acquired during pregnancy. *Pediatr. Infect. Dis. J.* **9:**499–504.

Brocklehurst, P., G. Kinghorn, O. Carney, K. Helsen, E. Ross, E. Ellis, R. Shen, F. Cowan, and A. Mindel. 1998. A randomized placebo controlled trial of suppressive acyclovir in late pregnancy in women with recurrent genital herpes infection. *Br. J. Obstet. Gynecol.* **105:**275–280.

Brown, Z. A., L. A. Vontver, J. Benedetti, C. W. Critchlow, D. E. Hickok, C. J. Sells, S. Berry, and L. Corey. 1985. Genital herpes in pregnancy: risk factors associated with recurrences and asymptomatic viral shedding. *Am. J. Obstet. Gynecol.* **153:**24–30.

Brown, Z. A., L. A. Vontver, J. Benedetti, C. W. Critchlow, C. J. Sells, S. Berry, and L. Corey. 1987. Effects on infants of a first episode of genital herpes during pregnancy. *N. Engl. J. Med.* **317:**1246–1251.

Brown, Z. A., J. Beneditti, R. Ashley, S. Burchett, S. Selke, S. Berry, L. A. Vontver, and L. Corey. 1991. Neonatal herpes simplex virus infection in relation to asymptomatic maternal infection at the time of labor. *N. Engl. J. Med.* **324:**1247–1252.

Brown, Z. A., A. Anholm, R. Ashley, S. Berry, S. Selke, J. Zeh, and L. Corey. 1993. HSV serological discordancy among sexual partners and rates of seroconversion during pregnancy, p. 36. *Program and Abstracts of the Infectious Disease Society for Obstetrics and Gynecology,* Stowe, Vt., August 4–7, 1993.

Brown, Z. A., J. K. Benedetti, D. H. Watts, S. Selke, S. Berry, R. L. Ashley, and L. Corey. 1995. A comparison between detailed and simple histories in the diagnosis of genital herpes complicating pregnancy. *Am. J. Obstet. Gynecol.* **172:**1299–1303.

Brown, Z., S. Selke, J. Zeh, R. Ashley, K. Brady, J. Kopelman, S. Berry, K. Mohan, M. Herd, and L. Corey. 1997. The acquisition of herpes simplex virus during pregnancy. *N. Engl. J. Med.* **337:**509–515.

Brown Z., R. F. Hume, S. Selke, J. Zeh, R. Ashley, D. H. Watts, S. Berry, M. Herd, and L. Corey. 1998. Subclinical shedding of herpes simplex virus (HSV) at the time of labor. 18th Annual Meeting of the Society of Perinatal Obstetricians, February 2–7, 1998, Miami Beach, Fla. *Am. J. Obstet. Gynecol.* **178:**S3.

Bujko, M., V. Sulovic, G. Sbutetga-Milosevic, and V. Zwanovic. 1989. Mode of delivery and level of passive immunity against herpes simplex virus. *Clin. Exp. Obstet. Gynecol.* **16:**6–8.

Centers for Disease Control and Prevention. 1986. Genital herpes infection—United States, 1966–1984. *Morbid. Mortal. Weekly Rep.* **35:**402–403.

Chuang, T. 1988. Neonatal herpes incidence, prevention and consequences. *Am. J. Prev. Med.* **4:**47–53.

Cone, R. W., A. C. Hobson, Z. A. Brown, R. Ashley, S. Berry, C. Winter, and L. Corey. 1994. Frequent detection of genital herpes simplex virus DNA by polymerase chain reaction among pregnant women. *JAMA* **272:**792–796.

Corey, L., H. G. Adams, Z. A. Brown, and K. K. Holmes. 1983. Genital herpes simplex virus infections: clinical manifestations, course, and complications. *Ann. Intern. Med.* **98:**958–972.

Fleming, D. T., G. D. McQuillan, R. F. Johnson, A. J. Nahmias, S. O. Aral, F. K. Lee, and M. E. St. Louis. 1997. Herpes simplex virus type 2 in the United States, 1976 to 1994. *N. Engl. J. Med.* **337:**1105–1111.

Frenkel, L. M., Z. A. Brown, Y. J. Bryson, L. Corey, J. D. Unadkat, P. A. Hensleigh, A. M. Arvin, C. G. Prober, and J. D. Connor. 1991. Pharmacokinetics of acyclovir in the term human pregnancy and neonate. *Am. J. Obstet. Gynecol.* **164:**569–576.

Garland, S. M. 1992. Neonatal herpes simplex: Royal Women's Hospital 10 year experience with management guidelines for herpes in pregnancy. *Aust. N.Z.J. Obstet. Gynecol.* **32:**331–334.

Gnann, J. W., N. H. Barton, and R. J. Whitley. 1983. Acyclovir: mechanism of action, pharmacokinetics, safety and clinical applications. *Pharmacotherapy* **3:**275–283.

Hensleigh, P., W. Andrews, Z. Brown, J. Greenspoon, L. Yasukawa, and C. G. Prober. 1997. Genital herpes during pregnancy: inability to distinguish primary and recurrent infections clinically. *Obstet. Gynecol.* **89:**891–895.

Kaplowitz, L. G., D. Baker, L. Gelb, J. Blythe, R. Hale, P. Frost, C. Crumpacker, S. Rabinovich, J. E. Peacock, Jr., J. Herndon, et al. 1991. Prolonged continuous acyclovir treatment of normal adults with frequently recurring genital herpes simplex virus infection. *JAMA* **265:**747–751.

Kingsley, S. 1986. Fetal and neonatal exposure to acyclovir. Unpublished data.

Koutsky, L. A., C. E. Stevens, K. K. Holmes, R. L. Ashley, N. B. Kiviat, C. W. Critchlow, and L. Corey. 1992. Underdiagnosis of genital herpes by current clinical and viral-isolation procedures. *N. Engl. J. Med.* **326:**1533–1539.

Kulhanjian, J. A., V. Soroush, D. S. Au, R. N. Bronzan, L. L. Yasukawa, L. E. Weylman, A. M. Arvin, and C. G. Prober. 1992. Identification of women at unsuspected risk of primary infection with herpes simplex virus type 2 during pregnancy. *N. Engl. J. Med.* **326:**916–920.

Langenberg, A., J. Benedetti, J. Jenkins, R. Ashley, C. Winter, and L. Corey. 1989. Development of clinically recognizable genital lesions among women previously identified as having "asymptomatic" herpes simplex virus type 2 infection. *Ann. Intern. Med.* **110:**882–887.

Lau, R. J., M. G. Emery, and R. E. Galinsky. 1987. Unexpected accumulation of acyclovir in breast milk. *Obstet. Gynecol.* **69:**468–471.

Mertz, G. J., O. Schmidt, J. L. Jourden, M. E. Guinana, M. L. Remington, A. Fahnlander, C. Winter, K. K. Holmes, and L. Corey. 1985. Frequency of acquisition of first-episode genital infection with herpes simplex virus from symptomatic and asymptomatic source contacts. *Sex. Transm. Dis.* **12:**33–39.

Nahmias, A. J., H. H. Keyserling, and G. M. Kerrick. 1983. Herpes simplex, p. 636–678. *In* J. S. Remington and J. O. Klein (ed.), *Infectious Diseases of the Fetus and Newborn Infant*, 2nd ed. W. B. Saunders Co., Philadelphia, Pa.

Nahmias, A. J., F. K. Lee, and S. Beckman-Nahmias. 1990. Sero-epidemiological and sociological patterns of herpes simplex virus infection in the world. *Scand. J. Infect. Dis. Suppl.* **69:**19–36.

Prober, C. G., P. A. Hensleigh, F. D. Boucher, L. L. Yasukawa, D. S. Au, and A. M. Arvin. 1988. Use of routine viral cultures at delivery to identify neonates exposed to herpes simplex virus. *N. Engl. J. Med.* **318:**887–891.

Prober, C. G., L. Corey, Z. A. Brown, P. A. Hensleigh, L. M. Frenkel, Y. J. Bryson, R. J. Whitley, and A. M. Arvin. 1992. The management of pregnancies complicated by genital infections with herpes simplex virus. *Clin. Infect. Dis.* **15:**1031–1038.

Quinn, T. C., and W. Cates. 1992. Epidemiology of sexually transmitted diseases in the 1990s, p. 1–37. *In* T. C. Quinn (ed.), *Sexually Transmitted Diseases.* Raven Press, New York, N.Y.

Randolph, A. G., A. E. Washington, and C. G. Prober. 1993. Cesarean delivery for women presenting with genital herpes lesions. *JAMA* **270:**77–82.

Scott, L. L., P. J. Sanchez, G. L. Jackson, F. Zeray, and G. Wendel. 1996. Acyclovir suppression to prevent cesarean delivery after first-episode genital herpes. *Obstet. Gynecol.* **87:**69–73.

Stone, K. M., C. A. Brooks, M. E. Guinan, and E. R. Alexander. 1989. National surveillance for neonatal herpes simplex virus infections. *Sex. Transm. Dis.* **16:**152–156.

Stray-Pedersen, B. 1990. Acyclovir in late pregnancy to prevent neonatal herpes simplex. *Lancet* **336:**756.

Sullivan-Bolyai, J., H. F. Hull, C. Wilson, and L. Corey. 1983. Neonatal herpes simplex virus infection in King County, Washington: increasing incidence and epidemiologic correlates. *JAMA* **250:**3059–3062.

Wald, A., J. Zeh, G. Barnum, G. Davis, and L. Corey. 1996. Suppression of subclinical shedding of herpes simplex virus type 2 with acyclovir. *Ann. Intern. Med.* **125:** 776–779.

Wald, A., L. Corey, R. Cone, A. Hobson, G. Davis, and J. Zeh. 1997. Frequent genital herpes simplex virus 2 shedding in immunocompetent women effect of acyclovir treatment. *J. Clin. Invest.* **99:**1092–1097.

Whitley, R. J., L. Corey, A. Arvin, F. D. Lakeman, C. V. Sumaya, P. F. Wright, L. M. Dunkle, R. W. Steele, S. J. Soong, A. J. Nahamias, C. A. Alford, D. A. Powell, V. San Joaquin, and the NIAID Collaborative Antiviral Study Group. 1988. Changing presentation of herpes simplex virus infection in neonates. *J. Infect. Dis.* **158:**109–116.

Whitley, R., A. Arvin, C. Prober, S. Burchett, L. Corey, D. Powell, S. Plotkin, S. Starr, C. Alford, J. Connor, R. Jacobs, A. Nahmias, and S.-J. Soong. 1991a. A controlled trial comparing vidarabine with acyclovir in neonatal herpes simplex virus infection. *N. Engl. J. Med.* **324:**444–449.

Whitley, R., A. Arvin, C. Prober, L. Corey, S. Burchett, S. Plotkin, S. Starr, R. Jacobs, D. Powell, A. Nahmias, C. Sumaya, K. Edwards, C. Alford, G. Caddell, S. J. Soong, and the NIAID Collaborative Antiviral Study Group. 1991b. Predictors of morbidity and mortality in neonates with herpes simplex virus infections. *N. Engl. J. Med.* **324:**450–454.

Wolfe, M. 1990. Obstetrical course and complications of women with symptomatic genital herpes: a population based analysis. Ph.D. thesis. University of Washington, Seattle.

15
Genital Herpesvirus Infections: Rationale for a Vaccine Strategy

Ann M. Arvin

One of the most serious consequences of genital herpes as a sexually transmitted disease is the infection of infants who are exposed to the virus at the time of delivery (Nahmias et al., 1971; Whitley et al., 1991a, 1991b; Prober and Arvin, 1989; Brown et al., 1997; Arvin and Prober, 1997). Studies of genital herpes in pregnancy have been a major source of new knowledge about the herpes simplex virus (HSV) infections of the genital tract and the epidemiology of HSV-1 and HSV-2 transmission by sexual contact (Prober and Arvin, 1989; Brown et al., 1987, 1991, 1997; Arvin and Prober, 1997; Arvin et al., 1986; Prober et al., 1987, 1988; Kulhanjian et al., 1992; Wald et al., 1995; Boggess et al., 1997). Data from these studies require a change in basic concepts about the prevalence of genital herpes, which has turned out to be much higher than was previously perceived. Furthermore, most infections are acquired from asymptomatic partners. Finally, primary and recurrent infections are usually asymptomatic.

HSV INFECTIONS IN PREGNANCY AND THE NEWBORN

The transmission of HSV to infants usually results from exposure, during delivery, to maternal genital secretions that contain infectious virus. Since both HSV-1 and HSV-2 can cause genital herpes, neonatal infection can be due to either virus type, but most cases in the United States are due to HSV-2. Neonatal herpes is classified as localized mucocutaneous infection, disseminated infection, or herpes encephalitis. Although intrauterine infections and transmissions from nonmaternal contacts occur occasionally, most

Ann M. Arvin, Department of Pediatrics, Stanford University School of Medicine, Stanford, CA 94305.

Sexually Transmitted Diseases and Adverse Outcomes of Pregnancy
Edited by P. J. Hitchcock, H. T. MacKay, J. N. Wasserheit, and R. Binder
©1999 American Society for Microbiology, Washington, D.C.

herpetic disease in the newborn is a consequence of peripartum infection of the maternal genital tract.

In the past, concern about exposure of the infant to HSV focused on mothers who were known to have genital herpes (Prober et al., 1992). However, the clinical experience of pediatricians with cases of neonatal herpes demonstrates that most infants who acquire neonatal herpes are born to women who have no history of genital herpes and no signs of infection during pregnancy or at the time of delivery. These infections have now been shown to be due to asymptomatic infection of the mother in most instances. Only about 5% of adults in the United States have a clinical history of genital herpes, but seroepidemiologic studies show prevalence rates of HSV-2 infection, which is the usual cause of genital herpes, that range from a minimum of 15% to as high as 60% in women of childbearing age and in men of comparable ages (Arvin and Prober, 1994; Fleming et al., 1997; Sullender et al., 1988; Ashley et al., 1988; Bernstein et al., 1985). In contrast to the perception that primary genital herpes causes severe, progressive localized lesions, studies performed by serologic methods that detect HSV-2-specific antibodies document that most individuals acquire genital HSV-2 infection silently or that initial symptoms are nonspecific (Brown et al., 1995). Unfortunately, these clinically silent or unrecognized infections, whether primary or recurrent, are associated with the shedding of infectious virus at genital sites, thereby facilitating viral transmission to other susceptible individuals by sexual contact or to the newborn at the time of delivery.

In current clinical practice, only those few pregnant women who have a history of genital herpes can be identified as being at risk for transmitting the virus to their infants at the time of delivery (Prober et al., 1992). The vast majority of pregnant women who are at risk of HSV-2 reactivation from asymptomatic genital HSV infections or who have acquired asymptomatic primary HSV-2 infection during pregnancy cannot be identified by history or by laboratory evaluation. In part, this problem arises because most adults have been infected with HSV-1 in childhood and commercially available serologic screening tests do not differentiate HSV-1 from HSV-2 infection. Clinicians are often misled, since diagnostic laboratories often report serologic results as " HSV-1 titer" and "HSV-2 titer," despite the known cross-reactivity of antibodies to the two virus types (Ashley et al., 1991). Many physicians therefore believe, incorrectly, that it is possible to make a reliable serologic diagnosis of HSV-2 infection. Lack of access to accurate serologic testing remains a persistent, unresolved problem in the clinical management of HSV-2 infections in pregnancy, even though accurate methods for differentiating these infections have been available in the research setting for more than 10 years.

When the medical community recognized the risk of HSV transmission from mothers with silent infection to their newborns, cultures of antepartum samples from herpetic women were recommended as an approach to the management of pregnancies, especially for women with a history of pregnancy complications due to genital herpes. The purpose of these weekly or twice-weekly cultures was to detect episodes of asymptomatic shedding late in pregnancy, providing an indication for elective cesarean delivery of the infant if maternal cultures were positive during the last week of gestation. However, antepartum cultures failed to predict the risk of infection and disease of the infant because the period of viral reactivation proved to be very short and the interval required to culture the virus was too long to provide timely information about the mother's status (Arvin, 1986). In theory, a more rapid viral detection method could be used to screen women for the presence of virus at delivery. However, none of the direct HSV antigen assays, based upon enzyme immunoassay or immunofluorescence techniques, are sensitive or reliable enough to detect asymptomatic genital HSV infection or viral infection not associated with identifiable lesions. While PCR methods have the required sensitivity, they have not yet been adapted for widespread clinical use (Boggess et al., 1997; Hardy et al., 1990; Cone et al., 1994).

FACTORS INFLUENCING THE RISK OF NEONATAL INFECTION FOLLOWING EXPOSURE TO MATERNAL HSV INFECTION

Exposure to HSV at delivery does not lead inevitably to neonatal herpes. In fact, as is true for many other pathogens, most exposed infants escape infection (Prober and Arvin, 1989; Brown et al., 1987; Prober et al., 1987). Assuming that about 25% of pregnant women are infected with HSV-2 and that there is a 1 to 2% risk of viral reactivation on the day of delivery, a high attack rate would result in many more infected infants than the observed incidence of approximately 1 per 5,000 births. This discrepancy occurs because the transmission rate for neonatal infection is less than 2% when the infant is born to a mother who has known recurrent HSV-2 infection or who is experiencing a first symptomatic episode of HSV-2 infection due to infection acquired at some time in the past.

In contrast, while the odds that a woman will have a newly acquired genital HSV infection late in pregnancy are very low, the risk of viral transmission to the infant is much higher. Based upon combined data from four studies, 41% of infants (15 of 34) born to mothers with first-episode genital HSV infections at delivery developed neonatal herpes (Prober and Arvin, 1989). In a recent study, four of seven infants who were born before maternal seroconversion and who were exposed at delivery became infected (Brown et al., 1997). The high transmission rate among infants exposed to first-episode maternal HSV infection can be attributed to several factors. The titers of infectious virus present in the genital tract are usually very high, so that the infant is likely to be exposed to a larger viral inoculum.

Cervical infection is also much more likely in first-episode genital herpes as opposed to recurrent disease, permitting prolonged exposure during the birth process. Infants born to mothers with primary HSV infection late in pregnancy often have not acquired any transplacental antibodies with the capacity to neutralize HSV or to mediate antibody-dependent cellular cytotoxicity at the time of inoculation. Analysis by serologic assays for type-specific antibodies also suggests that transplacentally acquired HSV-1 antibodies have a limited effect in cross-protecting infants exposed to primary HSV-2 infection in the mother (Prober and Arvin, 1989; Brown et al., 1997; Sullender et al., 1988).

ACQUISITION OF PRIMARY HSV-2 INFECTION IN PREGNANCY

Since primary HSV-2 infection acquired during pregnancy is a significant cause of neonatal and possibly fetal morbidity, we have examined the sero-epidemiologic patterns of infection in pregnant women. Of 1,580 pregnant women who were susceptible at the onset of pregnancy, 0.2% acquired HSV-2 infection prior to delivery, for an annualized rate of acquisition of 0.58% (Boucher et al., 1990). The rate of acquisition of HSV-2 during pregnancy is not significantly different from seroconversion rates among nonpregnant adults (Brown et al., 1997).

HSV-2 antibodies were also measured to assess the frequency with which pregnant women remain susceptible to HSV-2 despite having a long-term sexual partner who is infected (Kulhanjian et al., 1992). In a prospective study of 190 couples, the absence of antibodies to HSV-2 was observed in 18 women (9.5%) whose partners were seropositive. Ten of the infected partners (56%) had no history of symptomatic genital herpes. Based on this study, approximately 1 in 20 women can be expected to be at unsuspected risk of exposure to HSV-2 by an asymptomatic, HSV-2-infected partner despite several years of sexual contact. Of the 18 seronegative women with a seropositive partner, 1 acquired HSV-2 infection during pregnancy. The prospective evaluation of pregnant women by the HSV-2 immunoglobulin G (IgG) antibody assay also confirmed the seroprevalence rate of 32% in this upper-middle-class population. Despite careful questioning, two-thirds of the women with HSV-2 IgG antibodies had no history of genital herpes, which was consistent with previous observations (Sullender, 1988; Brown, 1991) that most infected women who are at risk of HSV-2 reactivation during pregnancy have clinically silent infections.

CURRENT APPROACHES TO THE MANAGEMENT OF INFANTS WITH NEONATAL HERPES OR EXPOSURE TO MATERNAL INFECTION AT DELIVERY

Since most neonatal exposures to HSV remain undetected despite optimal obstetrical care, recognition of the signs of neonatal herpes in infants usually provides the only opportunity to intervene with appropriate antiviral therapy (Whitley et al., 1991a, 1991b). Pediatricians must identify mucocutaneous, disseminated, or central nervous system infections based upon clinical and laboratory evaluations to determine whether an infant should be treated with acyclovir. Neonates infected with HSV have a very poor induction of active immunity to the virus (Sullender et al., 1987, 1988; Kohl et al., 1989; Arvin, 1992). As in other immunocompromised patients with herpesvirus infections, antiviral therapy can compensate to some extent for these deficiencies in host response. Antiviral therapy has been most effective in infants whose initial clinical signs are limited to mucocutaneous lesions (Whitley et al., 1991a, 1991b). Some benefit in decreasing the morbidity and mortality caused by disseminated herpes and herpes encephalitis has been demonstrated in clinical trials of acyclovir and vidarabine therapy, but persistent high mortality rates and a high incidence of severe sequelae indicate the need for more effective approaches to this infection in the newborn.

Cesarean delivery is recommended if lesions of genital herpes are present at the onset of labor. However, clinical circumstances arise, such as precipitous delivery or the presence of atypical lesions that are recognized as herpetic only after delivery, which result in a known exposure of the infant. Cultures of samples obtained at delivery because of a maternal history of primary genital herpes in pregnancy may also demonstrate that the mother had active asymptomatic infection when the infant was born.

If a history of recurrent maternal disease is elicited, the parents can be advised that the risk of infection is low despite exposure. However, the parents and other caregivers should be instructed to report any signs of lethargy, poor feeding, fever, or skin lesions immediately so that antiviral therapy can be initiated if necessary. Obtaining surface samples for culture from the infant at the time the exposure is identified and performing weekly surveillance cultures of samples from the eyes, nose, mouth, and skin for 4 to 6 weeks after delivery has been recommended (Prober et al., 1992). However, whether these cultures will lead to the earlier identification of infected infants than will simply observing them for clinical signs of infection is not known. Some limitation in their sensitivity can be anticipated, since infants with localized herpes encephalitis often have negative cultures from these sites at the time of diagnosis. Any cutaneous lesions that are suspected to be herpetic should be evaluated by direct immunofluorescence methods for rapid diagnosis (Arvin and Prober, 1995). Serologic evaluation of the infant for IgG antibodies to HSV is not helpful because it will reflect the presence of transplacentally acquired antibodies. Since infected infants are known to have no HSV IgM response or a response that is delayed for several weeks, this serologic test cannot be used to guide the timely initiation of antiviral therapy. From a technical standpoint, HSV IgM assays also have a high false-positive rate. Giving acyclovir to the infant as prophylaxis is not justified when the mother has recurrent infection, because (i) there are no criteria to identify the (estimated) 3 of 100 exposed infants who will become infected, (ii) intravenous administration is required to provide adequate central nervous system penetration, and (iii) administration for the duration of disease would entail at least 3 weeks of treatment.

When a neonate is exposed to a first episode of maternal genital herpes, viral cultures of the eyes, throat, urine, stool, and cerebrospinal fluid (CSF) are recommended at 48 h or when the exposure is identified (Prober et al., 1992). Infants whose CSF is abnormal or who have positive cultures from specimens obtained at more than 48 h of age should be treated with intravenous acyclovir. Infants born to mothers with primary HSV infections appear to be at higher risk of the disseminated form of neonatal herpes, which presents with signs similar to those of bacterial sepsis; these infants are more likely to have positive cultures from superficial sites than are those with localized central nervous system infection. Standard serologic methods can be used to determine whether the mother's first episode of symptoms is true primary genital herpes, which is defined as a new herpesvirus infection in a mother who has never been infected with either HSV-1 or HSV-2. These methods can also be used to document whether the infant has any detectable HSV antibodies, regardless of their type specificity. However, there are no current recommendations directed specifically to the management of the infant whose mother has true primary genital herpes during pregnancy or the infant who lacks HSV antibodies. Passive antibody prophylaxis may be an approach to the management of these infants in the future, but high-titer HSV immune globulin preparations are not available currently (Whitley, 1994).

It is very important to note that some apparently first episodes of genital herpes represent the first symptomatic manifestation of a preexisting HSV-2 infection when analyzed by research methods to measure levels of type-specific antibodies to HSV-2. In this circumstance, the risk to the infant is likely to be equivalent to an exposure due to recurrent maternal disease, but current clinical diagnostic methods do not permit the identification of this subgroup.

As with infants exposed to recurrent maternal genital herpes, no data exist to establish the efficacy of empirical antiviral therapy in asymptomatic infants born to mothers with new HSV-2 infections, and there are no criteria to determine the duration of administration. Prophylaxis could have adverse effects by acting only to prolong the incubation period, with disease appearing when the prophylaxis was discontinued, or by interfering with the immune response. Observation with immediate initiation of acyclovir therapy when symptoms occur or when surveillance cultures become positive is a reasonable approach to the management of these infants.

RATIONALE FOR DEVELOPING HSV VACCINES TO REDUCE THE MORBIDITY AND MORTALITY OF NEONATAL HERPES

A comprehensive assessment of the problems encountered in preventing the exposure of newborns to HSV due to maternal asymptomatic genital herpes and the limitations of antiviral therapy in reducing the severe consequences of neonatal herpes indicates that the development of effective vaccines may be an important strategy to prevent neonatal herpes.

The potential impact of immunization against HSV-2 on the incidence of neonatal herpes is suggested by the observation that primary maternal HSV-2 infections acquired during late gestation account for approximately 45% of the cases of neonatal herpes each year. A targeted-vaccine approach is feasible because susceptible women can be identified by screening for HSV-2 IgG antibodies. One might anticipate that an effective vaccine would prevent systemic infection in the mother or that it might shorten the duration of virus shedding at genital sites. The potential beneficial effects of immunization include a reduction in the risk of maternal acquisition of HSV-2 infection despite exposures during pregnancy, as well as a reduction in the risk of exposure of the infant even if the mother becomes infected with HSV-2.

It is more difficult to predict the potential benefit of maternal immunization to reduce the risk of neonatal herpes caused by recurrent HSV-2 infections in the mother. However, maternal immunization could result in less frequent episodes of viral reactivation, a decrease in the amount of virus shed, or a shorter duration of virus shedding with episodes of reactivation, thereby reducing the chance of infection of the infant at delivery. Even if reactivation is not blocked, a lower rate of transmission of the virus to the infant might occur as a result of higher titers of transplacentally acquired antibodies. Higher antibody titers may also diminish morbidity even if the infant becomes infected, by enhancing the likelihood that the infection will be localized rather than systemic.

REFERENCES

Arvin, A. M. 1992. Relationships between maternal immunity to herpes simplex virus and the risk of neonatal herpes virus infection. *Rev. Infect. Dis.* **13:**S953–S956.

Arvin, A. M., and C. G. Prober. 1994. Analysis of the epidemiology and pathogenesis of herpes simplex virus infections in pregnant women and infants using the 2 glycoprotein G antibody assay. *Infect. Agents Dis.* **2:**375–382.

Arvin, A. M., and C. G. Prober. 1995. Herpes simplex viruses, p. 876–883. *In* P. R. Murray, E. J. Baron, M. A. P. Faller, F. C. Tenover, and R. H. Yolken (ed.), *Manual of Clinical Microbiology*, 6th ed. American Society for Microbiology, Washington, D.C.

Arvin, A. M., and C. G. Prober. 1997. Herpes simplex virus type 2: a persistent problem. Editorial. *N. Engl. J. Med.* **337:**1158–1159.

Arvin, A. M., P. A. Hensleigh, C. G. Prober, D. S. Au, L. L. Yasukawa, A. E. Wittek, P. E. Palumbo, S. G. Paryani, and A. S. Yeager. 1986. Failure of antepartum maternal cultures to predict the infant's risk of exposure to herpes simplex virus at delivery. *N. Engl. J. Med.* **315:**796–800.

Ashley, R. L., J. Militoni, F. Lee, A. Nahmias, and L. Corey. 1988. Comparison of Western blot (immunoblot) and glycoprotein G-specific immunodot enzyme assay for detecting antibodies to herpes simplex virus types 1 and 2 in human sera. *J. Clin. Microbiol.* **26:**662–667.

Ashley, R., A. Cent, V. Maggs, A. Nahmias, and L. Corey. 1991. Inability of enzyme immunoassays to discriminate between infections with herpes simplex virus types 1 and 2. *Ann. Intern. Med.* **115:**520–526.

Bernstein, D. I., Y. J. Bryson, and M. A. Lovett. 1985. Antibody response to type common and type-unique epitopes of herpes simplex virus polypeptides. *J. Med. Virol.* **515:**251–263.

Bogges, K. A., D. H. Watts, A. C. Hobson, R. L. Ashley, Z. A. Brown, and L. Corey. 1997. Herpes simplex virus type 2 detection by culture and polymerase chain reaction and relationship to genital symptoms and cervical antibody status during the third trimester of pregnancy. *Am. J. Obstet. Gynecol.* **176:**443–451.

Boucher, F. D., L. L. Yasukawa, R. N. Bronzan, P. A. Hensleigh, A. M. Arvin, and C. G. Prober. 1990. A prospective evaluation of primary genital herpes simplex virus type 2 infections acquired during pregnancy. *Pediatr. Infect. Dis. J.* **9:**499–504.

Brown, Z. A., L. A. Vontver, J. Benedetti, C. W. Critchlow, C. J. Sells, S. Berry, and L. Corey. 1987. Effects of infants of a first episode of genital herpes during pregnancy. *N. Engl. J. Med.* **317:**1246–1251.

Brown, Z. A., J. Benedetti, R. Ashley, S. Burchett, S. Selke, S. Berry, L. A. Vontver, and L. Corey. 1991. Neonatal herpes simplex virus infection in relation to asymptomatic maternal infection at the time of labor. *N. Engl. J. Med.* **324:**1247–1252.

Brown, Z. A., J. K., Benedetti, D. H. Watts, S. Selke, S. Berry, R. L. Ashley, and L. Corey. 1995. A comparison between detailed and simple histories in the diagnosis of genital herpes complicating pregnancy. *Am. J. Obstet. Gynecol.* **172:**1299–1303.

Brown, Z. A., S. Selke, J. Zeh, J. Kipelman, A. Maslow, R. L. Ashley, D. H. Watts, S. Berry, M. Herd, and L. Corey. 1997. The acquisition of herpes simplex virus during pregnancy. *N. Engl. J. Med.* **337:**509–515.

Cone, R. W., A. C. Hobson, Z. Brown, R. Ashley, S. Berry, C. Winter, and L. Corey. 1994. Frequent detection of genital herpes simplex virus DNA by polymerase chain reaction among pregnant women. *JAMA* **272:**792–796.

Fleming, D. T., G. M. McQuillan, R. E. Johnson, A. J. Nahmias, S. O. Aral, F. K. Lee, and M. E. St. Louis. 1997. Herpes simplex virus type 2 in the United States, 1976 to 1994. *N. Engl. J. Med.* **337:**1105–1111.

Hardy, D. A., A. M. Arvin, L. L. Yasukawa, D. M. Lewinsohn, P. A. Hensleigh, and C. G. Prober. 1990. The successful identification of asymptomatic genital simplex infection at delivery using the polymerase chain reaction. *J. Infect. Dis.* **162:** 1031–1035.

Kohl, S., M. S. West, C. G. Prober, W. M. Sullender, L. S. Loo, and A. M. Arvin. 1989. Neonatal antibody-dependent cellular cytotoxic antibody levels are associated with the clinical presentation of neonatal herpes simplex virus infection. *J. Infect. Dis.* **160:**770–776.

Kulhanjian, J. A., V. Soroush, D. S. Au, R. N. Bronzan, L. L. Yasukawa, L. E. Weylman, A. M. Arvin, and C. G. Prober. 1992. Identification of women at unsuspected risk of contracting primary herpes simplex virus type 2 infections during pregnancy. *N. Engl. J. Med.* **326:**916–920.

Nahmias, A. J., W. E. Josey, Z. M. Naib, M. G. Freeman, R. J. Fernandez, and J. H. Wheeler. 1971. Perinatal risk associated with maternal genital herpes simplex infection. *Am. J. Obstet. Gynecol.* **110:**825–837.

Prober, C. G., W. M. Sullender, L. L. Yasukawa, D. S. Au, A. S. Yeager, and A. M. Arvin. 1987. Low risk of herpes simplex virus infections in neonates exposed to the virus at the time of vaginal delivery to mothers with recurrent herpes simplex virus infections. *N. Engl. J. Med.* **316:**240–244.

Prober, C. G., P. A. Hensleigh, F. D. Boucher, L. L. Yasukawa, D. S. Au, and A. M. Arvin. 1988. Use of routine viral cultures at delivery to identify neonates exposed to herpes simplex virus. *N. Engl. J. Med.* **318:**887–891.

Prober, C. G., and A. M. Arvin. 1989. Genital herpes and the pregnant woman. *In* M. Swartz, and J. S. Remington (ed.), *Current Clinical Topics in Infectious Diseases*, vol. 10. Blackwell Scientific Publications Ltd., Oxford, United Kingdom.

Prober, C. G., L. Corey, Z. A. Brown, P. A. Hensleigh, L. M. Frenkel, Y. J. Bryson, R. J. Whitley, and A. M. Arvin. 1992. The management of pregnancies complicated by genital infections with herpes. IDSA position paper. *Clin. Infect. Dis.* **15:** 1031–1038.

Sullender, W. M., J. L. Miller, L. L. Yasukawa, J. S. Bradley, S. B. Black, A. S. Yeager, and A. M. Arvin. 1987. Humoral and cellular immunity in neonates with herpes simplex virus infection. *J. Infect. Dis.* **155:**28–37.

Sullender, W. M., L. L. Yasukawa, M. Schwartz, L. Pereira, P. A. Hensleigh, C. G. Prober, and A. M. Arvin. 1988. Type-specific antibodies to herpes simplex virus type 2 (HSV-2) glycoprotein G in pregnant women, infants exposed to maternal HSV-2 infections at delivery, and infants with neonatal herpes. *J. Infect. Dis.* **157:** 164–171.

Wald, A., J. Zeh, S. Selke, R. L. Ashley, and L. Corey. 1995. Virologic characteristics of subclinical and symptomatic genital herpes infections. *N. Engl. J. Med.* **333:**770–775.

Whitley, R. J. 1994. Neonatal herpes simplex virus infections: is there a role for immunoglobulin in disease prevention and therapy? *Pediatr. Infect. Dis. J.* **13:**432–438.

Whitley, R., A. M. Arvin, C. G. Prober, L. Corey, S. Burchett, S. Plotkin, S. Starr, R. Jocobs, D. Powell, A. Nahmias, and members of the Collaborative Antiviral Study Group. 1991a. Predictors of morbidity and mortality in neonates with herpes simplex virus infections. *N. Engl. J. Med.* **324:**450–454.

Whitley, R., A. M. Arvin, C. G. Prober, L. Corey, S. Burchett, S. Plotkin, S. Starr, C. Alford, J. Connor, and members of the Collaborative Antiviral Study Group. 1991b. A controlled trial comparing vidarabine with acyclovir in neonatal herpes simplex virus infection. *N. Engl. J. Med.* **324:**444–449.

16
Congenital Cytomegalovirus Infection

William J. Britt

Human cytomegalovirus (HCMV) is a well-known cause of opportunistic infection in immunocompromised hosts. In the posttransplantation period, allograft recipients are at risk for serious HCMV infections (Britt and Alford, 1996). HCMV infections are an important cause of death in certain transplant populations, such as recipients of bone marrow allografts from major histocompatibility complex (MHC)-matched but unrelated donors (Winston et al., 1990). In the initial description of patients with AIDS, HCMV was identified as an important opportunistic pathogen (Gottlieb et al., 1981). As more effective antiretroviral antiviral agents extended the survival of AIDS patients, HCMV became a common cause of debilitating infections in this population. Prior to the introduction of highly active antiretroviral therapy, HCMV was the most frequent cause of opportunistic infections in patients in the late stages of AIDS (Gallant et al., 1992; Munoz et al., 1993). Common disease syndromes associated with HCMV in this population included encephalitis, colitis/enteritis, and retinitis. HCMV retinitis was observed in as many as 25% of long-lived patients with AIDS (Gross et al., 1990; Skolnik, 1992). Current antiviral therapy for invasive HCMV infections is often toxic and only marginally effective in many patients (Palestine et al., 1991; Skolnik, 1992; Spector et al., 1993).

Although this is less well appreciated, HCMV is a major cause of disease in congenitally infected infants (Fowler et al., 1992b). Natural-history studies have estimated rates of congenital HCMV infection ranging between 2 and 40 in 1,000 live births in the United States, making it the most common congenital viral infection in humans (Table 1) (Fowler et al., 1992b;

William J. Britt, Departments of Pediatrics and Microbiology, University of Alabama at Birmingham, 1600 7th Ave. South, Suite 752, Birmingham, AL 35233.

Sexually Transmitted Diseases and Adverse Outcomes of Pregnancy
Edited by P. J. Hitchcock, H. T. MacKay, J. N. Wasserheit, and R. Binder
©1999 American Society for Microbiology, Washington, D.C.

Table 1 HCMV as a cause of congenital infection in the United States[a]

Parameter	Value
Estimated rate of live births	4,000,000
Rate of congenital HCMV infection	1%
No. of infected infants	40,000
No. with symptoms[b]	2,800 (7%)
No. without symptoms[c]	37,200 (93%)
No. of infected infants with permanent sequelae[d]	6,000

[a] Modified from Fowler et al., 1992b.

[b] Infants with symptomatic infection in the newborn period secondary to congenital infection. The estimated rate is given in parentheses.

[c] Infants without clinically apparent infection in the newborn period. The estimated rate is given in parentheses.

[d] The number of infants with permanent sequelae following intrauterine HCMV infection includes approximately 90% of those with symptomatic infection as newborns and 15% of those without symptoms of congenital infection.

Stagno et al., 1982a, 1986). Approximately 10% of infected infants will exhibit permanent neurodevelopmental sequelae as a result of this intrauterine infection (Stagno et al., 1986). Based on current birth rates in the United States, it has been estimated that each year approximately 4,000 to 7,000 infants will suffer neurologic damage secondary to congenital HCMV infection (Table 1) (Fowler et al., 1992b). This rate appears to be similar to the incidence of central nervous system (CNS) damage secondary to congenital rubella syndrome during the rubella pandemics which occurred in the United States before the initiation of widespread rubella immunization. Because an effective vaccine for congenital HCMV is not currently available, infection with HCMV during pregnancy represents a significant risk for the developing fetus and thus is an important cause of adverse outcomes of pregnancy. This chapter describes some of the key epidemiologic characteristics of this maternal-fetal infection, including sources of maternal infection and maternal populations with increased rates of infection and fetal transmission, and provides a limited description of maternal immune responses associated with protection from fetal transmission and disease.

NATURAL HISTORY OF CONGENITAL HCMV INFECTIONS: IMPORTANCE OF THE TYPE AND SOURCES OF MATERNAL INFECTION

The seemingly complex natural history of congenital HCMV infection can be greatly simplified by an understanding of the maternal component of this maternal-fetal infection. Because the maternally derived immune response to HCMV determines both the frequency of transmission of the virus to the fetus and the virulence of the ensuing infection, maternal immunity represents a key element in the natural history of this intrauterine infection. In women infected with HCMV prior to pregnancy, maternal immunity prior to conception (preconceptional immunity) has been consistently associated with a reduced rate of fetal transmission (Stagno et al., 1982a, 1986). The rate of fetal transmission has been reported to range between 25 and 75% (mean, 40%) in women undergoing primary infection during pregnancy (defined as seroconversion during pregnancy or the presence of HCMV-specific immunoglobulin [IgM] antibodies in maternal serum obtained in the first trimester), on the basis of seven independent studies, whereas women with recurrent infection and/or reinfection (infection in the presence of preexisting immunity, defined as the presence of HCMV-specific IgG antibodies prior to pregnancy) during pregnancy have rates of fetal infection ranging from 0.2 to 2%, depending on socioeconomic status (SES) (see below) (Stagno et al., 1982a, 1986). The finding that preconceptional serologic immunity can dramatically lower the rate of fetal infection but not completely prevent intrauterine transmission is unique to HCMV and represents one of the least understood characteristics of this perinatal infection. It also indicates that active immunization might be an effective strategy to prevent fetal infection.

Primary infection during pregnancy can develop as a result of exposure to infectious virus from several sources. Epidemiologic studies have documented that exposure to infected children and sexual exposure represent the two most common modes of community acquisition of HCMV (Adler, 1989; Chandler et al., 1985; Drew et al., 1981; Handsfield et al., 1985; Pass et al., 1987; Sohn et al., 1991). Additional risk factors associated with an increased rate of maternal infection during pregnancy include multiple sexual partners and young maternal age (Fowler and Pass, 1991; Sohn et al., 1991). Exposure to secretions from young children excreting HCMV represents an obvious source of infection for susceptible women of childbearing age. In contrast, the risk of virus acquisition following sexual activity appears dependent on both exposure and age.

Over 20 years ago, differences in SES between groups of pregnant women were shown to influence the rate of congenital infection. Approximately 2% of infants born to women of lower SES were reported to be infected with HCMV, compared to a rate of 0.2% in women of upper-middle and high SES (Stagno et al., 1982a). Further analysis of these groups revealed that the women from the lower SES group were younger and had an increased number of sexual partners and a higher incidence of other sexually transmitted diseases (Fowler and Pass, 1991). Because sexual transmission of HCMV has been documented in sexually active women, homosexual men, and adolescent females, a likely explanation for differences in the rate of congenital HCMV infection between populations of low and high SES was increased sexual exposure. However, this explanation may be too simplistic, since other aspects of the biology of this virus could contribute to the increased rate of maternal infection during pregnancy in women from the lower SES group. When viewed simply by age, young age is itself a significant risk factor for congenital HCMV infection even in a population with increased rates of sexually transmitted disease in all age groups (Table 2). Perhaps the immune response to HCMV of young, pregnant females is markedly different from that of older women. Pathogenic mechanisms which could account for such differences remain unknown, but in laboratory studies, HCMV is able to replicate in hormonally sensitive tissue, suggesting several endocrine explanations for maternal age-related effects on transmission.

Maternal immunity can limit fetal transmission by 50-fold. Recent results from a case-control study indicated that maternal seroimmunity to HCMV was associated with a 91% reduction in the incidence of congenital HCMV infection compared to that in women without preconception seroimmunity (Fowler et al., 1997b). The molecular and cellular basis of protective maternal immunity is unknown, but several studies have suggested that virus-neutralizing antibodies correlate with prevention of both maternal and fetal infection (Adler et al., 1995; Boppana and Britt, 1995). Moreover, it appears that the quantity of virus-neutralizing antibodies in maternal serum can be correlated with a protective effect (Boppana and Britt, 1995). Two studies have suggested that virus-neutralizing antibodies may modulate the course of retinitis in AIDS patients, providing additional support for a protective role for this specific class of neutralizing antibodies (Boppana et al., 1995). The contribution of cellular immune responses, specifically virus-specific MHC-restricted $CD8^+$ cytotoxic T lymphocytes, to the natural history of congenital HCMV infections remains to be defined.

Recent findings from this laboratory have provided evidence for the importance of both the quantity and quality of antiviral antibodies induced by primary maternal infection during pregnancy in prevention of fetal infection. Comparison of serum antibody responses in a group of women undergoing primary HCMV infection during pregnancy revealed that women who transmitted virus to their offspring had lower levels of both

Table 2 Influence of maternal age on prevalence of congenital HCMV infection[a]

Maternal age (yr)	No. positive/no. tested	Prevalence (%)
<20	97/4,125	23.5
Total population	215/17,163	12.5
Total population ≤20	118/13,038	9.1

[a] Modified from Fowler et al., 1993.

neutralizing antibodies and high-avidity antibodies (specific for HCMV and its major envelope glycoprotein) than did women who did not transmit virus (Boppana and Britt, 1995). Because affinity maturation of an antibody response has been reported to require T-lymphocyte help, it could be postulated that failure to produce high-avidity antibodies reactive with HCMV represents a subtle, virus-specific immune dysfunction in this group of women. In women of childbearing age, HCMV is rarely associated with a clinically significant maternal infection, so that such a deficiency in antibody responses could be expected to be of minimal consequence. In contrast, the inability to mount an immune response capable of limiting viral dissemination and transmission to the fetus is quite significant.

Maternal acquisition of HCMV and subsequent transmission to the developing fetus involve a complex interplay between maternal immunity and undefined effects of young maternal age. As detailed in the previous section, several important sources of virus exposure have been associated with an increased incidence of maternal infection and subsequent fetal transmission (Adler, 1989; Fowler and Pass, 1991; Fowler et al., 1993; Pass et al., 1987; Stagno et al., 1984). Because adolescent females have one of the highest rates of HCMV infection during pregnancy, more effective approaches to reduction of maternal exposure are required. Together, these data would suggest that vaccination of women of childbearing of age to induce specific immunity similar to that observed following natural infection would offer the greatest likelihood of success (Adler et al., 1995; Fowler et al., 1992b).

ADVERSE OUTCOME OF PREGNANCY FOLLOWING MATERNAL HCMV INFECTION: IMPORTANCE OF MATERNAL IMMUNITY

The consequences of intrauterine HCMV infection can range from mild, clinically inapparent infection to severe, life-threatening multiorgan disease (Boppana et al., 1992; Stagno et al., 1983). Organ involvement can be divided into CNS disease and non-CNS disease. The long-term sequelae of HCMV infection are almost entirely related to CNS damage. Severe, clinically apparent congenital HCMV infection presents in the newborn period with multiple-organ involvement (Boppana et al., 1992). The most commonly observed non-CNS abnormalities include hepatobiliary disease, splenomegaly, and thrombocytopenia (Table 3) (Boppana et al., 1992). Fortunately, almost all of these manifestations of congenital HCMV infections are self-limited and usually resolve during the first several months of life. Although mortality rates in newborn infants with severe infections have been reported to be as high as 20%, the most recent studies have reported mortality rates on the order of 11%, usually as the result of multiorgan failure, including pneumonitis (Boppana et al., 1992; McCracken et al., 1969). Other, less common manifestations of congenital HCMV infection

Table 3 Clinical and laboratory abnormalities of neonates associated with symptomatic congenital HCMV infection[a]

Abnormality	No. positive/total no. (%)
Clinical	
Prematurity	36/106 (34)
Small for gestational age	53/106 (50)
Petechiae/rash	80/106 (76)
Hepatosplenomegaly	63/106 (60)
Jaundice	69/103 (67)
Microcephaly	54/102 (53)
Laboratory	
Abnormal liver function tests	46/58 (83)
Decreased platelet counts	62/81 (77)
Conjugated hyperbilirubinemia	55/68 (81)
Hemolysis	37/72 (51)

[a]Modified from Boppana et al., 1992.

include dental enamel dysplasia and an increased frequency of inguinal hernias (Britt and Alford, 1996; Stagno et al., 1982b).

Intrauterine infection of the CNS invariably leads to permanent sequelae, probably because of the limited self-renewal capacity of the CNS. CNS damage can be readily apparent, such as when it manifests as microcephaly, or may be detected following imaging studies or during assessment of perceptual-organ function (Boppana et al., 1997; Conboy et al., 1987). Non-sight-threatening retinitis is detected in approximately 10 to 15% of infants with clinically apparent congenital HCMV infection (Boppana et al., 1994). The presence of retinitis has been associated with more severe CNS involvement (Conboy et al., 1987). Hearing loss is by the far the most common symptom associated with CNS involvement. This sequela can be documented in 60 to 80% of infants with clinically apparent infection and up to 15% of infants without symptoms of congenital HCMV infection at birth (Fowler et al., 1992b). A more recent study of a screened population has documented hearing loss in approximately 7.2% of infants with asymptomatic congenital infection (Fowler et al., 1997b). The hearing loss is often bilateral, sensorineural (damage to inner ear and/or eighth cranial nerve), and progressive (see below). Because of the frequency of hearing loss associated with congenital HCMV infection and the prevalence of congenital HCMV, hearing loss following congenital HCMV infection is the most common cause of nonfamilial hearing loss in the United States (Hicks et al., 1993).

The severity of HCMV infection in the newborn period has been related directly to the qualitative and quantitative nature of maternal immunity

(Table 2). Symptomatic newborn infection following recurrent infection or reinfection in women with preconceptional seroimmunity has been described very infrequently. In infected infants born to women with immunity, the incidence of long-term sequelae is reduced (Fowler et al., 1992b; Stagno et al., 1986). Together, these findings suggest that the maternal immune response can limit the severity of fetal infection. Although the nature of protective maternal responses is unknown, it must be assumed that antiviral antibodies, possibly virus-neutralizing antibodies, play a significant role in limiting fetal disease because of their capacity to cross the placenta and enter the fetal circulation. Studies have documented that neutralizing antibodies directed against the major envelope glycoprotein of HCMV are of the immunoglobulin G_1 (IgG) subclass (Urban et al., 1994). This IgG subclass represents the vast majority of maternal IgG antibodies in the fetal circulation, because of its abundance in maternal serum and because of an active placental transport system specific for IgG_1 antibodies. Because placental transport mechanisms for antibodies are not fully developed until early in the third trimester, it could be postulated that fetuses infected early in gestation would have decreased quantities of transplacentally derived maternal antiviral antibodies. Epidemiological studies have shown that fetuses exposed to virus in the first or early second trimester are more likely to have significant sequelae than are those born to women infected in the third trimester (Stagno et al., 1986). Lastly, recently described findings from a rhesus monkey model of congenital HCMV infection are consistent with the concept that the quantity of antiviral antibodies in the fetal circulation could determine the outcome of in utero infections (Tarantal et al., 1998).

Several additional observations must be included in any description of the pathogenesis of intrauterine HCMV infection. Because the timing of transmission cannot be ascertained precisely, the correlation between first- or early-second-trimester maternal infection and severe fetal infection must be considered only an association and not evidence for a specific pathogenic mechanism of this intrauterine infection. Studies in experimental-animal models have suggested that there is a lengthy interval between maternal viremia and fetal transmission (Griffith et al., 1990). Thus, the apparent relationship between maternal seroconversion early in pregnancy and severe fetal infection may not be chronologically related. Another characteristic unique to this intrauterine disease is the differential susceptibility of various organ systems to HCMV replication during fetal development. The stage of cellular differentiation influences viral replication and may contribute to the extent of organ involvement in the infected fetus. However, recent information has indicated that even fetuses infected in the last trimester of pregnancy are at risk for disease (Pass et al., 1994). This result is in contrast to data from previous studies and provides further evidence that the pathogenesis of congenital HCMV is complex and probably involves additional, as yet undefined mechanisms.

LONG-TERM SEQUELAE OF CONGENITAL HCMV INFECTION: PROGRESSION OF CENTRAL NERVOUS SYSTEM DAMAGE DURING INFANCY AND EARLY CHILDHOOD

Although CNS damage following congenital HCMV infection has been recognized since the disease was first described, only recently have clinicians appreciated the progression of CNS dysfunction during infancy and early childhood. Sensorineural hearing loss which follows intrauterine HCMV infection can progress during the first 5 years of life (Fowler et al., 1997a). Similar progression of retinal lesions has been documented in up to 23% of infants with retinitis following congenital HCMV infection (Boppana et al., 1995). Because of the lack of precision in cognitive testing during infancy and early childhood, it has been difficult to demonstrate the progression of intellectual deficits in infants with HCMV-induced CNS damage.

Progressive hearing loss is limited almost exclusively to infants with congenital infections which follow primary maternal infection (Fowler et al. 1992b). It has been documented in up to 64% of infants with clinically apparent congenital infection (Boppana et al., 1992). Hearing loss progresses in about 50% of infants with subclinical congenital infection (Fowler et al., 1992a, 1997a; Williamson et al., 1992). Studies have also identified characteristics of the primary maternal infection associated with hearing loss. These have included maternal infection early in pregnancy, sustained serologic responses following infection, and elevated IgG anti-HCMV antibodies in maternal serum at the time of delivery (Boppana et al., 1993). The persistent elevation of the antiviral antibody response in this group of women may represent indirect evidence of sustained viral replication (Boppana et al., 1993). In contrast to these findings, progression of hearing deficits has not been associated with specific serologic responses in infected infants (Boppana et al., 1996; Britt and Vugler, 1989). Higher (transient) levels of perinatal HCMV-specific antibodies are observed in infants with hearing loss than in infants without hearing loss (Boppana et al., 1996; Britt and Vugler, 1989). This observation is consistent with transplacental transfer of maternal antibodies and thus probably does not reflect the antibody response of the newborn infant.

The pathogenesis of hearing loss following congenital HCMV infection is unknown. Two mechanisms have been proposed. The first involves direct virus-induced cytopathologic changes with loss of cellular components of the cochlea and possibly the eighth cranial nerve. Consistent with this proposed mechanism has been the demonstration of hair cell loss and histopathologic changes in the eighth cranial nerve and cochlea of rhesus monkeys inoculated in utero with rhesus CMV (Barry, personal communication; Tarantal et al., 1998). The second proposed mechanism invokes pathogenic antiviral immune responses as the major component of cellular destruction. Evidence for both has been found in experimental-animal models (Griffith and Aquino-de Jesus, 1991; Woolf et al., 1989). In addition, either mechanism can easily be reconciled with the observed progression of hearing loss in infancy and early childhood. However, appropriate therapeutic interventions are markedly different depending on the pathogenic mechanism. Future efforts aimed at defining this process will require more clinical studies of affected children as well as extensive use of animal models of virus-induced hearing loss (Tarantal et al., 1998; Griffith and Aquino-de Jesus, 1991).

PREVENTION OF DAMAGING CONGENITAL HCMV INFECTIONS

Approaches that attempt to limit exposure risks by altering specific behavior could offer a cost-effective solution for prevention of significant congenital HCMV infection. Findings from studies of hospital personnel have shown that attention to routine hygienic practices, such as hand washing, can limit HCMV acquisition even with repeated nonsexual exposure to HCMV (Dworsky et al., 1983). Likewise, studies from group day care centers have identified sources of HCMV exposure that can be minimized by simple hygienic measures such as routine hand washing after changing of diapers, designated areas for changing and disposal of soiled diapers, and education of child care workers and parents of young children about the sources and routes of transmission of HCMV (Hutto et al., 1985).

The most obvious method of limiting disease caused by intrauterine HCMV infection is to develop and use an effective vaccine. This may be accomplished by active vaccination, as has been demonstrated by universal rubella immunization. Live, replicating HCMV vaccines have been proposed as a means of doing this, but to date no direct evidence has been provided to suggest that current live virus vaccine formulations can provide such immunity (Adler et al., 1995). A recent investigation with the guinea pig model of congenital HCMV infection has provided very encouraging data supporting the concept that vaccine immunity induced by a single viral protein can prevent congenital infection (Harrison and Britt, 1994). This animal model uses intrauterine infection of fetal guinea pigs with guinea pig CMV (gpCMV). Additional studies with this model have suggested that passive transfer of antibodies against the gpCMV homologue of envelope glycoprotein B prevented severe fetal infection following maternal challenge with gpCMV (Harrison and Britt, 1997). A human trial with a recombinant HCMV envelope protein as a candidate vaccine has been partially completed, and the early results have indicated that the vaccine is safe and highly immunogenic. Other vaccine candidates which will soon enter clinical trials include genetically attenuated, replicating virus vaccines (Laughlin, personal communication).

Acknowledgments
This work was supported in part by National Institutes of Health grants from NICHD (P01 HD10699) and NIAID (R01 AI30105). I thank Karen Fowler, Robert Pass, and Suresh Boppana for critical discussions and access to unpublished data.

REFERENCES

Adler, S. P. 1989. Cytomegalovirus and child day care. Evidence for an increased infection rate among day-care workers. *N. Engl. J. Med.* **321:**1290–1296.

Adler, S. P., S. E. Starr, S. A. Plotkin, S. H. Hempfling, J. Buis, M. L. M. Manning, and A. M. Best. 1995. Immunity induced by primary human cytomegalovirus infection protects against secondary infection among women of childbearing age. *J. Infect. Dis.* **171:**26–32.

Barry, P. A. Personal communication.

Boppana, S. B., and W. J. Britt. 1995. Antiviral antibody responses and intrauterine transmission following primary maternal cytomegalovirus infection. *J. Infect. Dis.* **171:**1115–1121.

Boppana, S. B., R. F. Pass, W. J. Britt, S. Stagno, and C. A. Alford. 1992. Symptomatic congenital cytomegalovirus infection: neonatal morbidity and mortality. *Pediatr. Infect. Dis. J.* **11:**93–99.

Boppana, S. B., R. F. Pass, and W. J. Britt. 1993. Virus-specific antibody responses in mothers and their newborn infants with asymptomatic congenital cytomegalovirus infections. *J. Infect. Dis.* **167:**72–77.

Boppana, S., C. Amos, W. Britt, S. Stagno, C. Alford, and R. Pass. 1994. Late onset and reactivation of chorioretinitis in children with congenital cytomegalovirus infection. *Pediatr. Infect. Dis. J.* **13:**1139–1142.

Boppana, S. B., M. A. Polis, A. A. Kramer, W. J. Britt, and S. Koenig. 1995. Virus specific antibody responses to human cytomegalovirus (HCMV) in human immunodeficiency virus type 1-infected individuals with HCMV retinitis. *J. Infect. Dis.* **171:**182–185.

Boppana, S. B., J. Miller, and W. J. Britt. 1996. Transplacentally acquired antiviral antibodies and outcome in congenital human cytomegalovirus infection. *Viral Immunol.* **9:**211–218.

Britt, W. J., and C. A. Alford. 1996. Cytomegalovirus, p. 2493–2523. *In* B. N. Fields, D. M. Knipe, and P. M. Howley (ed.), *Virology*, 3rd ed. Raven Press, New York, N.Y.

Britt, W. J., and L. Vugler. 1989. Antiviral antibody responses in mothers and their newborn infants with clinical and subclinical congenital cytomegalovirus infections. *J. Infect. Dis.* **161:**214–219.

Chandler, S. H., K. K. Holmes, B. B. Wentworth, L. T. Gutman, P. J. Wiesner, E. R. Alexander, and H. H. Handsfield. 1985. The epidemiology of cytomegaloviral infection in women attending a sexually transmitted disease clinic. *J. Infect. Dis.* **152:**597–605.

Conboy, T. J., R. F. Pass, S. Stagno, C. A. Alford, G. J. Myers, W. J. Britt, F. P. McCollister, M. N. Summers, C. E. McFarland, and T. J. Boll. 1987. Early clinical manifestations and intellectual outcome in children with symptomatic congenital cytomegalovirus infection. *J. Pediatr.* **111:**343–348.

Drew, W. L., L. Mintz, R. C. Miner, M. Sands, and B. Ketterer. 1981. Prevalence of cytomegalovirus infection in homosexual men. *J. Infect. Dis.* **143:**188–192.

Dworsky, M., K. Welch, G. Cassady, and S. Stagno. 1983. Occupational risk for primary cytomegalovirus infection among pediatric health care workers. *N. Engl. J. Med.* **309:**950–953.

Fowler, K. B., and R. F. Pass. 1991. Sexually transmitted diseases in mothers of neonates with congenital cytomegalovirus infection. *J. Infect. Dis.* **164:**259–264.

Fowler, K., F. McCollister, R. Pass, A. Dahle, S. Stagno, and W. Britt. 1992a. Childhood deafness: the importance of congenital cytomegalovirus screening. *Am. J. Epidemiol.* **136:**954.

Fowler, K. B., S. Stagno, R. F. Pass, W. J. Britt, T. J. Boll, and C. A. Alford. 1992b. The outcome of congenital cytomegalovirus infection in relation to maternal antibody status. *N. Engl. J. Med.* **326:**663–667.

Fowler, K. B., S. Stagno, and R. F. Pass. 1993. Maternal age and congenital cytomegalovirus infection: screening of two diverse newborn populations, 1980–1990. *J. Infect. Dis.* **168:**552–556.

Fowler, K. B., F. P. McCollister, A. J. Dahle, S. Boppana, W. J. Britt, and R. F. Pass. 1997a. Progressive and fluctuating sensorineural hearing loss in children with asymptomatic congenital cytomegalovirus infection. *J. Pediatr.* **130:**624–630.

Fowler, K. B., R. F. Pass, and S. Stagno. 1997b. Congenital cytomegalovirus infection risk in future pregnancies and maternal CMV infection, abstr. 191. *In 6th International Cytomegalovirus Workshop.*

Gallant, J. E., R. D. Moore, D. D. Richman, J. Keruly, and R. E. Chaisson. 1992. Incidence and natural history of cytomegalovirus disease in patients with advanced human immunodeficiency virus disease treated with zidovudine. *J. Infect. Dis.* **166:**1223–1227.

Gottlieb, M. S., R. Schroff, and H. M. Schanker. 1981. Pneumocystis carinii pneumonia and mucosal candidiasis in previously healthy homosexual men. Evidence of a new acquired cellular immunodeficiency. *N. Engl. J. Med.* **305:**1425–1431.

Griffith, B. P., and M. J. Aquino-de Jesus. 1991. Guinea pig model of congenital cytomegalovirus infection. *Transplant. Proc.* **23:**29–31.

Griffith, B. P., M. Chen, and H. C. Isom. 1990. Role of primary and secondary maternal viremia in transplacental guinea pig cytomegalovirus transfer. *J. Virol.* **64:**1991–1997.

Gross, J. G., S. A. Bozzette, W. C. Mathews, S. A. Spector, I. S. Abramson, J. A. McCutchan, T. Mendex, D. Munguia, and W. R. Freeman. 1990. Longitudinal study of cytomegalovirus retinitis in acquired immune deficiency syndrome. *Ophthalmology* **97:**681–686.

Handsfield, H. H., S. H. Chandler, V. A. Caine, J. D. Meyers, L. Corey, E. Medeiros, and J. K. McDougall. 1985. Cytomegalovirus infection in sex partners: evidence for sexual transmission. *J. Infect. Dis.* **151:**344–348.

Harrison, C. J., and W. J. Britt. 1994. Pre-pregnancy immunization with the major envelope glycoprotein of guinea pig cytomegalovirus: immune responses and pregnancy outcome after first trimester primary gpCMV infection. *Pediatr. Res.* **35:** 181A.

Harrison, C. J., and W. Britt. 1997. Modified disease in mothers and pups after passive guinea pig CMV glycoprotein B antibody administration during primary maternal gestational guinea pig CMV infection, abstr. 153. *In 6th International Cytomegalovirus Workshop*, Orange Beach, Alabama.

Hicks, T., K. Fowler, M. Richardson, A. Dahle, L. Adams, and R. Pass. 1993. Congenital cytomegalovirus infection and neonatal auditory screening. *J. Pediatr.* **123:** 779–782.

Hutto, S. C., R. E. Ricks, M. Garvie, and R. F. Pass. 1985. Epidemiology of cytomegalovirus infections in young children: day care vs home care. *Pediatr. Infect. Dis. J.* **4:**149–152.

Laughlin, C. Personal communication.

McCracken, G. J., H. R. Shinefield, K. Cobb, A. R. Rausen, M. R. Dische, and H. F. Eichenwald. 1969. Congenital cytomegalic inclusion disease. A longitudinal study of 20 patients. *Am. J. Dis. Child.* **117:**522–539.

Munoz, A., L. K. Schrager, H. Bacellar, I. Speizer, S. H. Vermund, R. Detels, A. J. Saah, L. A. Kingsley, D. Seminara, and J. P. Phair. 1993. Trends in the incidence of outcomes defining acquired immunodeficiency syndrome (AIDS) in the Multicenter AIDS Cohort Study: 1985–1991. *Am. J. Epidemiol.* **137:**423–438.

Palestine, A. G., M. A. Polis, M. D. De Smet, B. F. Baird, J. Falloon, J. A. Kovacs, R. T. Davey, J. J. Zurlo, K. M. Zunich, and M. Davis. 1991. A randomized, controlled trial of foscarnet in the treatment of cytomegalovirus retinitis in patients with AIDS. *Ann. Intern. Med.* **115:**665–673.

Pass, R. F., E. A. Little, S. Stagno, W. J. Britt, and C. A. Alford. 1987. Young children as a probable source of maternal and congenital cytomegalovirus infection. *N. Engl. J. Med.* **316:**1366–1370.

Pass, R. F., K. B. Fowler, S. Stagno, W. J. Britt, S. B. Boppana, and C. A. Alford. 1994. Gestational age at time of maternal infection and outcome of congenital cytomegalovirus infection. *Pediatr. Res.* **35:**191A.

Skolnik, P. R. 1992. Treatment of CMV retinitis. *N. Engl. J. Med.* **326:**1701.

Sohn, Y. M., M. K. Oh, K. B. Balcarek, G. A. Cloud, and R. F. Pass. 1991. Cytomegalovirus infection in sexually active adolescents. *J. Infect. Dis.* **163:**460–463.

Spector, S. A., T. Weingeist, R. B. Pollard, D. T. Dieterich, T. Samo, C. A. Benson, D. F. Busch, W. R. Freeman, P. Montague, and H. J. Kaplan. 1993. A randomized, controlled study of intravenous ganciclovir therapy for cytomegalovirus peripheral retinitis in patients with AIDS. AIDS Clinical Trials Group and Cytomegalovirus Cooperative Study Group. *J. Infect. Dis.* **168:**557–563.

Stagno, S., R. F. Pass, M. E. Dworsky, R. E. Henderson, E. G. Moore, P. D. Walton, and C. A. Alford. 1982a. Congenital cytomegalovirus infection: the relative importance of primary and recurrent maternal infection. *N. Engl. J. Med.* **306:**945–949.

Stagno, S., R. F. Pass, J. P. Thomas, J. M. Navia, and M. E. Dworsky. 1982b. Defects of tooth structure in congenital cytomegalovirus infection. *Pediatrics.* **69:**646–648.

Stagno, S., R. F. Pass, M. E. Dworsky, and C. A. Alford. 1983. Congenital and perinatal cytomegaloviral infections. *Semin. Perinatol.* **7:**31–42.

Stagno, S., G. Cloud, R. F. Pass, W. J. Britt, and C. A. Alford. 1984. Factors associated with primary cytomegalovirus infection during pregnancy. *J. Med. Virol.* **13:** 347–353.

Stagno, S., R. F. Pass, G. Cloud, W. J. Britt, R. E. Henderson, P. D. Walton, D. A. Veren, F. Page, and C. A. Alford. 1986. Primary cytomegalovirus infection in pregnancy. Incidence, transmission to fetus, and clinical outcome. *JAMA* **256:**1904–1908.

Tarantal, A. F., M. S. Salamar, W. J. Britt, P. A. Luciw, A. G. Hendrickx, and P. A. Barry. 1998. Neuropathogenesis induced by rhesus cytomegalovirus in fetal rhesus monkeys (*Macaca mulatta*). *J. Infect. Dis.* **177:**446–450.

Urban, M., T. Winkler, M. P. Landini, W. Britt, and M. Mach. 1994. Epitope-specific distribution of IgG subclasses against antigenic domains on glycoproteins of human cytomegalovirus. *J. Infect. Dis.* **169:**83–90.

Williamson, W. D., G. J. Demmler, A. K. Percy, and F. I. Catlin. 1992. Progressive hearing loss in infants with asymptomatic congenital cytomegalovirus infection. *Pediatrics* **90:**862–866.

Winston, D. J., W. G. Ho, and R. E. Champlin. 1990. Cytomegalovirus infections after bone marrow transplantation. *Rev. Infect. Dis.* **12:**S776–S792.

Woolf, N. K., F. J. Koehrn, J. P. Harris, and D. D. Richman. 1989. Congenital cytomegalovirus labyrinthitis and sensorineural hearing loss in guinea pigs. *J. Infect. Dis.* **160:**929–937.

17
Laryngeal Papillomatosis

Thomas M. Becker

Despite the remarkably high prevalence of genital human papillomavirus (HPV) infections among women worldwide (Munoz and Bosch, 1992), the complications of HPV associated with mother-child transmission are extremely rare. Nonetheless, when maternally acquired HPV-associated disorders become manifest, the complications may be severe and represent major challenges to clinical management. This chapter briefly summarizes maternally transmitted HPV infections in children and problems associated with HPV-related diseases among pregnant women near parturition. Most of the discussion focuses on juvenile-onset laryngeal papillomatosis (recurrent respiratory papillomatosis [RRP]), the most challenging and costly of the diseases associated with mother-child HPV transmission.

CLINICAL MANIFESTATIONS

Laryngeal papillomatosis is the most common benign neoplasm of the larynx. The lesions are characterized by recurrent tumors, which cause hoarseness and upper airway obstruction. The common sites of tumor growth are the true vocal cords, subglottis, laryngeal surface of the epiglottis, nasal vestibule, soft palate, carina, bronchi, bronchioles, and peripheral lung fields. Commonly used adjectives to describe these lesions include "relentless, proliferative, invasive, and vexing" (McCabe and Clark, 1983). Although benign, the growths are life-threatening and often require surgical removal at frequent intervals to achieve control. Treatment for cure is possible in some proportion of patients; however, recurrence of growths is com-

Thomas M. Becker, Department of Public Health and Preventive Medicine, Oregon Health Sciences Center, 3181 S.W. Sam Jackson Park Road, Portland, OR 97201-3098.

Sexually Transmitted Diseases and Adverse Outcomes of Pregnancy
Edited by P. J. Hitchcock, H. T. MacKay, J. N. Wasserheit, and R. Binder
©1999 American Society for Microbiology, Washington, D.C.

mon, particularly among children. Long periods of remission—up to many years—may be followed by recrudescence of clinically apparent lesions.

Two major forms of RRP have been identified on the basis of age at occurrence. Juvenile-onset RRP cases can become clinically manifest shortly after birth, during infancy, or during the preschool years. The juvenile-onset "cutoff point" has been variably defined as age 12 years or age 16 years, depending on the series reported. Adult-onset cases usually occur after age 20 years and have been found in patients in their 70s. Approximately half of all cases are juvenile-onset cases. Histologically, the juvenile- and adult-onset cases are identical; HPV-6 and HPV-11, common causes of genital warts, are the most common causes of both forms of RRP (Steinberg and Abramson, 1985; Mounts et al., 1982; Corbitt et al., 1988). Rare cases in which there is DNA evidence of HPV-16, a high-risk type causing cervical cancer, in RRP lesions have been reported (Bauman and Smith, 1996; Pou et al., 1995). Because these HPV types are associated with genital HPV infections, maternal genital transmission and sexual transmission have been accepted by many researchers as the likely modes of transmission for juvenile- and adult-onset RRP, respectively.

EPIDEMIOLOGY

Although laryngeal warts, papillomata, have been recognized as a clinical entity since the 1600s, little progress has been made in defining the extent of these lesions in various populations. The incidence of both juvenile-onset and adult-onset papillomatosis is unknown, and the prevalence of disease has not been accurately assessed. Kashima et al. (1990) suggested that the proportion of infants who later develop RRP could range as widely as 1 in 80 to 1 in 1,500 live births, with offspring of mothers with condylomata acuminata at high risk (1 in 400 births). If maternal genital transmission is the true mechanism of infection leading to juvenile-onset laryngeal papillomatosis (the most widely accepted theory), it is clear that, given the high prevalence of genital HPV-6 and HPV-11 infections in women, only a very small proportion of exposed infants exposed to maternal genital HPV develop juvenile-onset RRP. Data collected in New Mexico (Becker et al., 1994) indicate that approximately 4% of women of childbearing age have asymptomatic cervical HPV-6 or HPV-11 infection as detected by PCR techniques on a single sample. For this example, let us consider that an additional 0.5% of women have clinically apparent genital warts at delivery. If 3.5 million live births occur in the country each year and 20% of the infants are delivered by cesarean section, then 126,000 newborns would potentially be exposed each year to HPV from a cervical or external vulvar source. If 1,500 new cases of RRP occur per year (based on conservative estimate from Kashima et al. [1990 report]), only a very small proportion (1.2%) of potentially exposed children will develop clinically manifest disease. This proportion would be even lower if subclinical vaginal and vulvar infections represent sources of HPV exposure during delivery.

The strongest support for maternal genital transmission of HPV to children who later develop juvenile-onset RRP stems primarily from two lines of evidence, i.e., observations that most RRP lesions contain DNA from HPV-6 and HPV-11 on immunohistochemical, immunohistologic, and hyridization studies (Steinberg et al., 1987; Mounts et al., 1982) and that high proportions of affected offspring have mothers who report genital warts (20 to 60% of mothers from different case series) (Quick et al., 1980; Kashima et al., 1990; Holinger et al., 1950; Bauman and Smith, 1996). Of interest to future viral transmission studies are reports of infants with RRP who were delivered to HPV-infected mothers via cesarean section (Kashima et al., 1990; Steinberg and Abramson, 1985; Bauman and Smith, 1996). Adult-onset RRP has also been associated with HPV-6 and HPV-11, presumably acquired from orogenital contact with infected partners. Cofactors associated with RRP have not been extremely well characterized, although Kashima et al. (1992) carried out a small study of juvenile- and adult-onset cases and controls without RRP, selected from ear, nose, and throat clinics. That study showed that juvenile-onset cases, compared to controls, were more likely to be firstborn, via vaginal delivery, to young mothers (Kashima et al., 1992). Patients with adult-onset cases were more likely than controls to report a large number of sex partners and frequent orogenital sex (Kashima et al., 1992). This study supports the theory that the modes of transmission for these two forms of RRP vary substantially (Mounts et al., 1982). Unfortunately, the study failed to collect data on maternal genital warts and possible exposures through contact with condylomata at delivery. The development of RRP in at least five children delivered by cesarean section suggests that ascending infection with HPV is a possible mode of transmission (Bauman and Smith, 1996).

Although abundant published data have described the often severe clinical manifestations of RRP in different case series (Steinberg and Abramson, 1985; Holinger et al., 1950; Steinberg et al., 1987), few data have addressed host immunity and host factors relevant to the development of disease. Kashima et al. (1990) observed that siblings of affected children never develop RRP and that family members who provide tracheostomy care of affected individuals and thus have substantial exposure to secretions of affected patients never develop RRP. In the research field of cervical neoplasia and HPV, we and others have suggested that the genetics of the HLA system may be relevant to disease development and that certain HLA types are associated with development of cervical dysplasia (Apple et al., 1994; Wank and Thomssen, 1991). This area has not yet been adequately explored. The influence of hormones, suggested by improvement in juvenile-onset RRP patients as they approach puberty, also warrants further evaluation.

TREATMENT

From a historic viewpoint, the many and various treatments for laryngeal papillomatosis indicate the inadequacy of any single strategy in ability to eradicate disease. The various forms of therapy have included different ablative and surgical techniques, topical and oral medical therapies, interferon, and laser therapy. Most of these treatment strategies have been evaluated by means of uncontrolled trials (Abramson et al., 1988, 1992; Steinberg et al., 1988; McCabe and Clark, 1983; Dedo and Jackler, 1982; Smith et al., 1980), although a few well-designed controlled clinical trials have evaluated the effects of intramuscular interferon as an adjunct therapy for control of RRP (Healy et al., 1988; Leventhal et al., 1988). Endoscopic excision has remained the standard of care, and the benefits of interferon appear to be controversial (Healy et al., 1988; Leventhal et al., 1991). Additional recent adjuvant therapy trials have included indole-3-carbinol, acyclovir, ribavirin, retinoic acid, and photodynamic therapy. To date, none of the therapeutic combinations has been shown to be highly efficacious in achieving complete remission of RRP (Bauman and Smith, 1996; Avidano and Singleton, 1995).

RESEARCH NEEDS

A few research groups in the United States and in Europe have directed substantial efforts to understanding the etiologic factors associated with development of RRP, and measurable progress has been documented, especially in laboratory investigations. Recent national collaborative clinical trials of interferon treatment of RRP have surpassed the small uncontrolled trials, demonstrating further progress in the field. Nonetheless, substantial groundwork in defining the epidemiology of these infections and the resultant diseases remains to be done. The data needed to define the incidence and prevalence of RRP are inadequate. The literature in this field indicates that most of the epidemiologic information results from case series by particular physicians or hospitals, and there are no population-based perspectives to characterize the extent of these infections and the associated diseases. Population-based registries could certainly help to define the extent of clinically manifest RRP. Although some effort has gone into the development of an RRP registry at the Federal level, additional resources to assist in this effort must be made available. The possibility of adding this disease to existing SEER Registries and their surveillance system should be explored. To date, no population-based case-control or cohort studies to characterize the risks associated with development of RRP have been undertaken. Cohort studies of infants born to mothers with overt condylomata may be feasible in large hospitals where women seek treatment for condylomata during pregnancy. Such specialty clinics exist in several medical communities. Treatment trials will have to be expanded to include different treatment regimens and combination therapies. The specific clinical lesions associated with transmission of HPV and the cofactors associated with development of RRP must be identified in multicenter studies. Specific HPV types associated with aggressive behavior of juvenile RRP lesions also must be further examined with a population-based perspective. Researchers have disagreed about the relevance of specific HPV types to the clinical behavior of RRP lesions (Mounts and Kashima, 1984; Steinberg and Abramson, 1985). In a case series of 16 patients, Bonagura et al. (1994) suggested that enhanced expression of certain HLA class II haplotypes, coupled with decreased expression of specific class I antigens, resulted in a poor host response to HPV infections that cause RRP. The genetics of the host-virus interaction among RRP patients clearly warrants examination through appropriately designed studies. Screening of high-risk infants has so far not been possible—this area also deserves further consideration to determine the feasibility of screening in certain groups, such as infants born to young mothers with genital warts. Another area that warrants more thorough investigation is the role of other viral infections as potential cofactors in the prognosis of RRP. Pou et al. (1995), in a case series, suggested that coinfection with members of the herpesvirus family may lead to the development of aggressive forms of RRP.

CONGENITAL CONDYLOMATA ACUMINATA

Congenital condylomata acuminata is a rarely reported disease of newborns and infants. Several case reports, however, clearly indicate the occurrence of maternal-fetal transmission even in the absence of fetal exposure to the maternal genital tract through cesarean delivery (Tang et al., 1978; Rogo and Nyansera, 1989; Weiss et al., 1986). The presence of condylomata in infants may suggest sexual abuse; nonetheless, the reports of condylomata in newborns document that congenital acquisition is possible although infrequent. Although the rarity of this event does not argue strongly for new public health measures to prevent the occurrence of congenital condylomata, investigation of the biological factors that affect the development of congenital warts may be relevant to other HPV-related diseases.

Other obstetric challenges associated with HPV infection near term include the accelerated growth of maternal condylomata with advancing pregnancy and the management of sometime rapidly advancing cervical neoplastic lesions that are caused by cervical HPV infection. Although these conditions may be relevant to the health of offspring, they are not the primary pediatric problem of viral transmission and are not discussed further in this chapter.

CONCLUSION

Research in the field of maternal transmission of HPV to infants has been hampered by the same limitations that have slowed progress in studies of genital HPV and cervical neoplasia—inability to culture or propagate the virus and uncertain test characteristics (sensitivity and specificity) in identification of HPV infection. However, recent progress with PCR-based tests to identify HPV genes has helped move the field forward. In addition, studies of RRP and of congenital transmission of condylomata have been hampered by the small numbers of cases, by lack of a screening test for RRP, and by the difficulties in designing population-based research in the absence of incidence data. Multicenter clinical trials can and should continue, however, even in the absence of baseline epidemiologic data—especially since no form of therapy has yet been shown to be adequate. With appropriate resources devoted to the collection of basic epidemiologic information in studies of RRP, substantial strides can be taken to improve the understanding and treatment of these disorders during the coming decade.

The RRP Task Force

In collaboration with the Centers for Disease Control and Prevention, the RRP Task Force was developed by interested laypersons, researchers, and clinicians to determine the most effective management of pregnant women with HPV infections of the genital tract. Another goal of the task force is to establish a national registry of RRP patients and a national tissue bank to aid studies of this disease. This type of collaborative government-private interaction is a promising alliance that should further the field in the next decade.

The RRP Foundation

The RRP Foundation was developed by laypersons and medical personnel to create a broader public awareness of RRP, provide a support system for families with affected members, and advance the research in disease treatment, prevention, and eradication. Information can be obtained by writing the RRP Foundation, 50 Wesley Drive, Hamilton Square, NJ 08690.

Acknowledgments

I acknowledge the following people for their assistance with this manuscript: Stephanie D. Kaplan, Catherine D. Pedersen, and the staff of Children's Hospital, Seattle, Wash.

REFERENCES

Abramson, A. L., V. Mullooly, M. S. Horowitz, and B. M. Steinberg. 1988. Clinical effects of alpha interferon dose variation on laryngeal papillomas. *Laryngoscope* **98:**1324–1329.

Abramson, A. L., M. J. Shikowitz, V. M. Mullooly, B. M. Steinberg, C. A. Amella, and H. R. Rothstein. 1992. Clinical effects of photodynamic therapy on recurrent laryngeal papillomas. *Arch. Otolaryngol. Head Neck Surg.* **118:**25–29.

Apple, R. J., H. A. Erlich, W. Klitz, M. M. Manos, T. M. Becker, and C. M. Wheeler. 1994. HLA DR-DQ disease associations in Hispanic cervical carcinoma are HPV type-specific. *Nat. Genet.* **6**(2)**:**157–162.

Avidano, M. A., and G. T. Singleton. 1995. Adjuvant drug strategies in the treatment of recurrent respiratory papillomatosis. *Otolaryngol. Head Neck Surg.* **112:**197–202.

Bauman, N., and R. Smith. 1996. Recurrent respiratory papillomatosis. *Pediatr. Otol.* **43:**1385–1401.

Becker, T. M., C. M. Wheeler, N. S. McGough, C. A. Parmenter, C. A. Stidley, M. H. Dorin, and S. W. Jordan. 1994. Sexually transmitted diseases and other risk factors for cervical dysplasia in southwestern Hispanic and non-Hispanic white women. *JAMA* **271:**1181–1188.

Bonagura, V. R., F. P. Siegal, A. L. Abramson, F. Santiago-Schwartz, M. E. O'Reilly, K. Shah, D. Drake, and B. M. Steinberg. 1994. Enriched HLA-DQ3 phenotype and decreased class I major histocompatibility complex antigen expression in recurrent respiratory papillomatosis. *Clin. Diagn. Lab. Immunol.* **1:**357–360.

Corbitt, G., A. P. Zarod, J. R. Arrand, M. Longson, and W. T. Farrington. 1988. Human papillomavirus genotypes associated with laryngeal papilloma. *J. Clin. Pathol.* **41:**284–288.

Dedo, H. H., and R. K. Jackler. 1982. Laryngeal papilloma: results of treatment with the CO_2 laser and podophyllin. *Am. Otol. Rhinol. Laryngol.* **91:**425–430.

Healy, G. B., R. D. Gelber, A. L. Trowbridge, K. M. Grundfast, R. J. Ruben, and K. N. Price. 1988. Treatment of recurrent respiratory papillomatosis with human leukocyte interferon. *N. Engl. J. Med.* **319:**401–407.

Holinger, P. H., K. C. Johnston, and G. C. Anison. 1950. Papilloma of the larynx: a review of 109 cases with a preliminary report of aureomycin therapy. *Ann. Otol. Rhinol. Laryngol.* **59:**547–559.

Kashima, H. K., K. Shah, and M. Goodstein. 1990. Recurrent respiratory papillomatosis, p. 889–893. *In* K. K. Holmes, P.-A. Mardh, F. Sparling, and P. Weisner (ed.), *Sexually Transmitted Diseases.* McGraw-Hill Book Co., New York, N.Y.

Kashima, H., F. Shah, A. Lyles, R. Glackin, N. Muhammad, L. Turner, S. Van Zandt, W. Whitt, and K. Shah. 1992. A comparison of risk factors in juvenile onset and adult onset recurrent respiratory papillomatosis. *Laryngoscope* **102:**9–13.

Leventhal, B. G., H. K. Kashima, P. W. Weck, P. Mounts, J. K. Whisnant, K. L. Clark, S. Cohen, H. H. Dedo, D. J. Donovan, B. W. Fearon, L. J. Gardiner, R. P. Lusk, H. R. Muntz, M. A. Richardson, G. T. Singleton, A. S. Yonkers, and D. Wold. 1988. Randomized surgical adjuvant trial of interferon alpha-n1 in recurrent papillomatosis. *Arch. Otolaryngol. Head Neck Surg.* **114:**1163–1169.

Leventhal, B. G., H. K. Kashima, P. Mounts, L. Thurmond, S. Chapman, S. Buckley, and D. Wold. 1991. Long-term response of recurrent respiratory papillomatosis to treatment with lymphoblastoid interferon alfa-n1. *N. Engl. J. Med.* **325:** 613–617.

McCabe, B. F., and K. F. Clark. 1983. Interferon and laryngeal papillomatosis: the Iowa experience. *Ann. Otol. Laryngol.* **92:**2–7.

Mounts, P., and H. Kashima. 1984. Association of human papillomavirus subtype and clinical course in respiratory papillomatosis. *Laryngoscope* **94:**28–32.

Mounts, P., K. Shah, and H. Kashima. 1982. Viral etiology of juvenile and adult onset squamous papilloma of the larynx. *Proc. Natl. Acad. Sci. USA* **79:**5425–5429.

Munoz, N., and F. X. Bosch. 1992. Review of case-control and cohort studies, p. 251–260. *In* N. Munoz, F. X. Bosch, K. Shah, and A. Meheus (ed.), *The Epidemiology of Cervical Cancer and Human Papillomavirus.* IARC, Lyon, France.

Pou, A. M., F. L. Rimell, J. A. Jordan, P. Barua, D. L. Shoemaker, J. C. Post, J. T. Johnson, and G. D. Ehrlich. 1995. Adult respiratory papillomatosis: human papillomavirus type and viral coinfections as predictors of prognosis. *Ann. Otol. Rhinol. Laryngol.* **104:**758–762.

Quick, C. A., S. L. Watts, R. A. Krzyzek, and A. J. Faras. 1980. Relationship between condylomata and laryngeal papillomata. *Ann. Otol.* **89:**467–471.

Rogo, K. O., and P. N. Nyansera. 1989. Congenital condylomata acuminata with meconium staining of amniotic fluid and fetal hydrocephalus: case report. *East Afr. Med. J.* **66:**411–413.

Smith, H. G., C. W. Vaughan, G. B. Healy, and M. S. Strong. 1980. Topical chemotherapy of recurrent respiratory papillomatosis. *Ann. Otol.* **89:**473–478.

Steinberg, B. M., and A. L. Abramson. 1985. Laryngeal papillomas. *Clin. Dermatol.* **3:**130–138.

Steinberg, B. M., A. L. Abramson, and B. Winkler. 1987. Laryngeal papillomatosis: clinical, histopathologic, and molecular studies. *Laryngoscope* **97:**678–685.

Steinberg, B. M., T. Gallagher, M. Stotler, and A. L. Abramson. 1998. Persistence and expression of human papillomavirus during interferon therapy. *Arch. Otolaryngol. Head Neck Surg.* **114:**27–32.

Tang, C., D. W. Shermeta, and C. Wood. 1978. Congenital condylomata acuminata. *Am. J. Obstet. Gynecol.* **131:**912–913.

Wank, R., and C. Thomssen. 1991. High risk of squamous cell carcinoma of the cervix for women with HLA-DQw3. *Nature* **352:**723–725.

Weiss, J. P., S. November, and C. T. Curtin. 1986. Recurrent penile condylomata in a 17-month old boy. *J. Urol.* **136:**468–469.

ANIMAL MODELS

18
Chlamydial Diseases of the Reproductive Tract of Domestic Ruminants

Gareth E. Jones

Clinicians and microbiologists interested in human genital tract diseases involving chlamydial infection should be aware that there are two analogous conditions that occur naturally in domestic ruminants and that might offer valuable comparative insights. The first is chlamydial abortion in sheep, goats, and cattle as a result of *Chlamydia psittaci* infection; humans are also very occasionally affected by the same agent and with similar outcomes. This disease is relatively well documented. The other, much more recently recognized, condition is chlamydial endometritis, salpingitis (inflammation of the uterine lining and fallopian tubes, respectively), and infertility of cattle as a result of *Chlamydia pecorum* infection. This review is intended to highlight aspects of these two diseases which are likely to be of interest to workers in the field of human chlamydiosis.

CHLAMYDIAL ABORTION OF SHEEP AND OTHER RUMINANTS

Chlamydial abortion of sheep was first described by Greig (1936) as a disease entity called enzootic abortion of ewes (EAE). The cause was subsequently identified by Stamp et al. (1950). Since then, chlamydial abortion has become recognized as an important reproductive disease in sheep and goats in several European, North American, and African countries, although it has not been found in Australasia. Cattle (Storz and McKercher, 1962; Kwapien et al., 1970; Nabeya et al., 1991; Holliman et al., 1994) and pigs (Woollen et al., 1990; Papadopoulos, personal communication) also may be affected by the same agent, but the disease in these species is much less commonly diagnosed. In Canada and the United Kingdom, EAE is

Gareth E. Jones, Moredun Research Institute; present address, YAbA Ltd., Pentlands Science Park, Bush Loan, Penicuik EH26 0PZ, United Kingdom.

Sexually Transmitted Diseases and Adverse Outcomes of Pregnancy
Edited by P. J. Hitchcock, H. T. MacKay, J. N. Wasserheit, and R. Binder
©1999 American Society for Microbiology, Washington, D.C.

responsible for approximately 45% of all diagnosed ovine abortions (Dohoo et al., 1985; VIDA, 1992). In the United Kingdom, the prevalence has been estimated at 8.6% of flocks, involving some 1.5 million sheep (Leonard et al., 1993). The incidence of outbreaks appeared to increase sharply in the United Kingdom from the late 1970s (VIDA, 1992), probably because of increased trade in, and movement of, sheep at that time, resulting in wide-scale mixing of sheep from different flocks.

Etiology

The causal agent of EAE is the ovine abortifacient form of *C. psittaci*, previously designated biotype 1 (Spears and Storz, 1979) and immunotype 1 (Perez-Martinez and Storz, 1985). Most studies have reported a remarkable degree of homogeneity of strains of *C. psittaci* in molecular terms (McClenaghan et al., 1984, 1991; Denamur et al., 1991; Griffiths et al., 1992). However, one recent study found 2 of 28 strains to differ from the others in polypeptide profiles, inclusion morphology, and reactivity with monoclonal antibodies (Vretou et al., 1996). Furthermore, biological differences were found when experimental sheep and mouse systems were used. Apparent antigenic differences detected in sheep by homologous/heterologous vaccination/challenge experiments (Aitken et al., 1981, 1986) have been corroborated by using a similar approach with mice (Johnson and Hobson, 1986; Johnson and Clarkson, 1986; Siarkou, 1992); four subgroups of abortifacient *C. psittaci* were identified by these means. Differences in the virulence of the invasive abortifacient strains also have been detected by using mice (Buzoni-Gatel and Rodolakis, 1983) and sheep (Rodolakis and Souriau, 1989).

Ruminants also can be infected by *C. pecorum* (Fukushi and Hirai, 1992), a chlamydial species which is heterogeneous in all respects, most notably molecular composition (Fukushi and Hirai, 1993; Herring, 1993; Anderson et al., 1996), antigenicity (Fukushi and Hirai, 1993), and pathogenicity. Infections have been linked to polyarthritis, conjunctivitis, encephalitis, and enteritis, but are also often inapparent. Infection with an "enteric" subtype of *C. pecorum* appears to be ubiquitous in sheep (Clarkson and Philips, 1997). *C. pecorum* strains share several antigens and epitopes with abortifacient *C. psittaci* strains (Baghian et al., 1996).

Clinical Expression

Infection of ewes may result in abortion or in the production of stillborn lambs in the last 5 weeks of gestation (normally ~146 days). These events may be preceded for up to 5 days by signs of malaise. Placentas from infected ewes usually have necrotic areas (which may cover the entire surface); a purulent vaginal discharge is also evident (Aitken, 1991). Postpartum uterine infection may occur as an associated complication, but this may be due to secondary bacterial invasion. Inapparent fetal loss before 105 days of gestation also has been reported (Papp et al., 1993).

In primary outbreaks, the usual pattern is one of a small number of abortions in year 1, often overlooked or ignored; an abortion "storm" in year 2, often involving 30% or more of all ewes; and a final enzootic phase from year 3 onward, in which only flock newcomers abort (generally in their second lambing, having become infected in the first pregnancy). In year 3, the abortion rate stabilizes at 5 to 15% per annum (Aitken, 1991). A deviation from this pattern is seen when the lambing season in a flock is extended; then a biphasic incidence rate is observed. In the first wave, infected ewes excrete chlamydiae. Other ewes, due to lamb later, will subsequently abort (Blewett et al., 1982).

When EAE is experimentally reproduced in naive ewes by subcutaneous injection or by dosing via the oropharyngeal route, abortions usually occur in 40 to 50% of animals, with 75 to 90% excreting chlamydiae at lambing or at abortion (Jones et al., 1995).

Epidemiology

Infection is introduced into flocks by acquisition of infected ewes. Sources of infectious material are conceptuses, particularly the placenta; vaginal discharges at parturition; and feces for several weeks after lambing or abortion (Aitken, 1991). Infection is thought to be primarily by the oropharyngeal route, with evidence indicating that tonsillar tissue or gastric epithelium may be the systemic portal of entry (Jones and Anderson, 1988; Amin and Wilsmore, 1995). The occurrence and importance of infection via the respiratory route by inhalation of aerosols are unknown. Ewes and ewe lambs can become infected at any age and season, although lambing time represents the period of highest risk.

It now appears that *C. psittaci* can also be transmitted venereally, although field evidence for this is confined to one report at present (Bernstein and Yaakobowitz, 1990). Experimental attempts to mimic infection by this route have yielded conflicting results. A small experiment by Wilsmore et al. (1984) failed to establish infection in ewe lambs inseminated with semen infected with chlamydia. A similar study by Appleyard et al. (1985) induced detectable infection but no abortions. However, the work of Papp and Shewen (1996a) demonstrated that intravaginal infection both before mating and during pregnancy could induce detectable infection at parturition, with production of weak lambs or aborted or stillborn fetuses. Infection of the genital tract of rams has been reported on several occasions (Storz et al., 1976; Rodolakis and Bernard, 1977; Schutte and Pienaar, 1977; Lozano, 1986).

The minimum infective dose of *C. psittaci* has not been established. Early workers discovered that a very high challenge dose led to fewer abortions than did a lower challenge dose of the same infective material, which suggested to them that the high-dose inoculum may be stimulating the development of partial immunity (McEwen et al., 1951).

Pathogenesis

Sheep

Infection. Following experimental infection of nonpregnant animals by subcutaneous injection or instillation via the tonsillar crypts, the organism enters an eclipse phase and cannot be cultured, even in animals treated with immunosuppressants such as prednisolone, azathioprine, or cyclosporin A (Huang et al., 1990; Jones and Anderson, unpublished). Other than fever following injection, no clinical or serologic signs of infection are detectable until pregnancy.

Latency. Suppression of chlamydial growth (both *C. trachomatis* and *C. psittaci*) has been shown in a variety of in vitro and in vivo systems to involve multiple mechanisms, which include gamma interferon (IFN-γ), tumor necrosis factor alpha (TNF-α), and nitric oxide (Shemer-Avni et al., 1989; Williams et al., 1990; Rank et al., 1992; Lacy et al., 1992; Beatty et al., 1993; Mayer et al., 1993). One chlamydiastatic mechanism mediated by IFN-γ is the induction of indoleamine-2,3-dioxygenase, which degrades tryptophan and therefore makes it unavailable to the chlamydia (Carlin et al., 1989; Thomas et al., 1993). A study of sheep cells has shown that recombinant ovine IFN-γ inhibits growth of the EAE agent, an effect which was largely reversible by addition of exogenous L-tryptophan (Graham et al., 1995).

Quiescent infection in nonpregnant sheep is reactivated during pregnancy by mechanisms which remain unknown. Two studies of the kinetics of placental infection in pregnant ewes both showed that chlamydiae could not be cultured from the placenta until 90 to 95 days of gestation regardless of when the animals were infected (Buxton et al., 1990; Papp et al., 1993). However, in one of these studies, chlamydial antigen (lipopolysaccharide) was detected in placental tissue by enzyme-linked immunosorbent assay (ELISA) as early as 65 days of gestation (Papp et al., 1993). These findings suggest that the metabolic form of *C. psittaci*, i.e., reticulate bodies, may be present in the placenta at least 25 to 30 days before maturation into infective elementary bodies can occur. The stimulus for development and reorganization into infectious elementary bodies at 90 days of gestation is unknown, but it is at this stage in pregnancy that the fetal lamb begins to grow rapidly, with accompanying increases in circulating levels of progesterone, estrone sulfate, and prostaglandin E_2 (PGE_2) in the dam (Thorburn, 1991).

Tropism. The site of colonization is a layer in the placenta, the trophectoderm (Buxton et al., 1990). In vitro studies have shown that uninucleate trophoblast cells are highly susceptible to infection with *C. psittaci* and that they respond to infection by producing large quantities of PGE_2 (Livingstone et al., unpublished). In view of the accompanying observation that systemic PGE_2 levels rise at the same time that chlamydiae can be isolated from the infected sheep placenta, it is tempting to speculate that this hormone could constitute a growth stimulus or maturation factor for *C. psittaci*. Another possible growth factor is erythritol, which induces the localization of *Brucella abortus* in the bovine placenta (Smith et al., 1962). Erythritol is also detected in the ovine placenta, where it exerts a similar effect on *Brucella melitensis* (Keppie et al., 1965). However, the absence of erythritol in human placental tissue (Keppie et al., 1965), which is susceptible to infection with the abortifacient strain of *C. psittaci*, suggests that erythritol may not be an essential growth factor for *C. psittaci*.

Cause(s) of abortion. Another aspect of *C. psittaci* infection that remains uncertain is the pathogenesis of abortion or premature parturition. The pathologic changes which occur must undoubtedly decrease placental function by interfering with the fetal-maternal exchange of nutrients, waste materials, and gases. However, the extent of macroscopic placental lesions does not always correlate with survival of the lambs or with the time of parturition, suggesting that additional factors are involved in these events. Leaver et al. (1989) observed, in ewes experimentally infected with the abortifacient strain of *C. psittaci*, decreased peripheral levels of progesterone in plasma, increased levels of 17β-estradiol in amniotic fluid and peripheral plasma, and perhaps increased PGE_2 levels. The changes in both progesterone and PGE_2 levels were noted to be "temporally related to the morphological and histochemical changes characteristic of trophoblast infection." Our in vitro studies at Moredun Research Institute (Livingstone et al., unpublished) suggest that trophoblast cells were probably responsible for the raised PGE_2 levels seen by Leaver et al. (1989). Elevated PGE_2 levels stimulate cortisol production by the ovine fetus, leading to a series of hormone-mediated changes, both fetal and maternal. The end stage consists of uterine contractions, leading to premature birth.

Chlamydial induction of PGE_2 production by trophoblast cells is likely to occur through the action of TNF-α, in turn stimulated by chlamydial lipopolysaccharide (Dayer et al., 1985; Brade et al., 1986; Holtmann et al., 1990). The lipopolysaccharide of *C. psittaci* lacks typical endotoxin properties such as lethal toxicity, pyrogenicity, and local Shwartzman reactivity (Brade et al., 1986). However, since some of the symptoms of human abortion due to *C. psittaci* have been ascribed to lipopolysaccharide (Buxton, 1986) (see below), it is possible that the lipopolysaccharide contributes to lowered fetal survivability in sheep. In summary, at least three factors may contribute to premature parturition and fetal survival: (i) mechanical interference with placental function as a result of pathologic changes in the placenta; (ii) the production of high levels of PGE_2, possibly by the trophectoderm; and (iii) endotoxic shock to the fetus.

Susceptibility. Biparous ewes are significantly more likely to abort than are uniparous ewes (Jones, unpublished), but in abortions involving twins, one lamb and its placenta may show little or no evidence of disease compared with its dead sibling. This suggests that whether *C. psittaci* induces disease in the naive ewe is determined by the fetus, specifically by the susceptibility of the individual placenta to infection and subsequent multiplication of the organism. Alternatively, it may be that the infectious agent colonizes the placenta(s) from the site(s) of latency irregularly and that the placental infection is inefficient; i.e., both placentas do not always become infected.

Humans

C. psittaci also causes abortion in women, but there are several important differences in the diseases of sheep and humans (Wong et al., 1985; Buxton, 1986). Latency does not appear to develop in humans, and abortion has been recorded only in women pregnant at the time of exposure to the organism. As in the sheep, the preferred site of infection is the placental trophoblast. However, unlike the sheep, pregnancy loss can happen at any time. Although the majority of recorded cases were in pregnancies of 24 weeks or later, at least one abortion occurred at 8 weeks. The premature infant invariably dies, and the mother can experience severe disease and can die. Symptoms include disseminated intravascular coagulation, thrombocytopenia, and hepatic and renal failure. It has been suggested that some of these symptoms may be due to the release of chlamydial lipopolysaccharide into the maternal circulation (Buxton, 1986).

Immunity

Ewes which have aborted once as a result of *C. psittaci* infection will not abort from this cause again, but this immunity is not sterilizing in all animals; consequently, shedding can occur during the estrus cycle (Papp et al., 1994; Papp and Shewen, 1996b) and at subsequent lambings (Jones and Livingstone, unpublished). Papp and Shewen (1996b) detected *C. psittaci* in vaginal, uterine, and oviduct samples from ewes that had been infected the previous year and that had subsequently aborted or produced weak lambs. No obvious pathologic findings were associated with these persistent infections, although an increase in the presence of plasma cells and lymphocytes in the uterus was noted. The exact mechanisms of protective immunity against *C. psittaci* are largely unknown, but both humoral and cell-mediated immune mechanisms appear to be involved (McCafferty, 1990). With respect to humoral immunity, the serologic correlates of protection are unknown and in vitro attempts to demonstrate neutralizing antibodies in the sera of immune animals have given variable, often contradictory results.

In a study by Tan et al. (1990), a preparation of the major outer membrane protein of *C. psittaci*, which comprised over 90% of the total immunogen administered, provided a high degree of protection against experimental infection with *C. psittaci*. This observation, which suggested that this protein might be an important protective immunogen, has been supported by studies of a pregnant mouse model. In this model, monoclonal antibodies to the major outer membrane protein can prevent fetal infection although not placental infection (Buzoni-Gatel et al., 1990). The monoclonal antibodies used in that study have been shown subsequently to be specific for the major outer membrane protein (McCafferty and Anderson, personal communication).

A monoclonal antibody against another surface-expressed antigen of *C. psittaci*, an 89-kDa protein, reduced infection by 60% in a tissue culture model (Cevenini et al., 1991), suggesting that antibodies against this protein may also be involved in acquired immunity.

Cell-mediated immunity probably contributes to resistance against *C. psittaci* infection. Most of the evidence for this is derived from mouse models (Buzoni-Gatel et al., 1987, 1992). However, sheep which have aborted because of *C. psittaci* infection and are therefore very unlikely to abort from this cause again develop a delayed hypersensitivity response. Furthermore, sheep that had a poor delayed hypersensitivity response following vaccination were found to be more likely to abort following experimental challenge than were sheep showing good hypersensitivity responses (Dawson et al., 1986), suggesting that cell-mediated immunity is important in resistance.

Vaccination

Three principal antigenic preparations have been used in vaccines: (i) inactivated forms of the cultured organism; (ii) a temperature-sensitive, attenuated mutant; and (iii) protein extracted from genetically engineered bacteria expressing the major outer membrane protein.

Inactivated Forms of the Cultured Organisms

A *C. psittaci* vaccine made from egg-grown formalin-fixed organisms was commercially available in the United Kingdom from the 1950s (McEwen et al., 1955) until 1992, when it was taken off the market because of production difficulties. The duration of immunity engendered by the original inactivated egg-grown vaccine was considered to be at least 3 years (Foggie, 1959). Two inactivated vaccines have been described in the United States. One, produced from tissue culture-grown organisms, was found to reduce experimentally induced abortion in sheep (Waldhalm et al., 1982). The other, a combination vaccine containing inactivated *Campylobacter* species, *Salmonella* species, and *Escherichia coli* antigens in addition to those of *C. psittaci*, was tested in a small field trial and found to provide significant protection against *Chlamydia*- and *Campylobacter*-associated abortions but not against those involving *Salmonella* (Hansen et al., 1990). More recently, trials with an inactivated, tissue culture-grown, semipurified preparation demonstrated that protection occurred in a dose-dependent manner and was also influenced by the adjuvant used (Jones et al., 1995). The best of four adjuvants (including Marcol 52/Arlacel A, Novasomes, and Alhydrogel) was immune-stimulating complex (ISCOM) matrix. The marginal antibody response to ISCOM matrix vaccination suggested that humoral immunity may be a minor component of the observed protection. The vaccine-related protection persisted for over 1 year; administration of a booster injection in the second year enhanced the resistance to experimental challenge.

Temperature-Sensitive Attenuated Vaccine

A temperature-sensitive strain of *C. psittaci* was produced in Nouzilly, France, in the early 1980s by mutagenesis (Rodolakis and Souriau, 1983). This strain, which grows only below 39.5°C, was highly efficacious in experimental challenge studies (Rodolakis, 1983; Rodolakis and Bernard, 1984; Chalmers et al., 1997). The most recent experimental study with a commercial form of this vaccine (now available in the United Kingdom) showed an abortion rate of 7.1% in the vaccinated group compared with 80% in the unvaccinated group; the vaccine also reduced the number of infected animals (Chalmers et al., 1997). However, preliminary reports of field trials suggest that the vaccine is less efficacious under field conditions, for reasons which are unclear.

Recombinant Protein Vaccines

The demonstration that the major outer membrane protein constituted an essential immunogen of *C. psittaci* (Tan et al., 1990) led to experiments with various forms of recombinant major outer membrane protein expressed in bacteria. Although partial protection was observed, the results were variable and the recombinant antigen was not as good as were proteins prepared from chlamydiae (Jones et al., 1992; Jones et al., unpublished). At least two explanations are possible: (i) the proper tertiary structure was not achieved in the recombinant protein and therefore antibodies against this did not bind (well) to infectious elementary bodies, or (ii) other chlamydial antigens (Tan et al., 1990) are also required for good protective immunity.

Model Systems for Screening Candidate Vaccines

Candidate vaccines have generally been tested by using oropharyngeal or subcutaneous challenge with infectious organisms (McEwen et al., 1955;

Wilsmore et al., 1990; Jones et al., 1995). Such experiments take approximately 8 months to complete, and only one experiment per year is possible because of the breeding cycle of the sheep. Accordingly, mouse models have been developed as a more efficient system for screening vaccine candidates. Three different mouse models have been described by workers in Nouzilly, France (Buzoni-Gatel and Rodolakis, 1983; Rodolakis et al., 1989). In a variant of one of these models developed by Jones et al. (unpublished), mice treated with the test vaccines are subsequently challenged by intraperitoneal injection of 2×10^6 inclusion-forming units of *C. psittaci*. A comparison of 11 different strains of mice, based on the *H2* locus of the major histocompatibility complex, showed large variations in the susceptibility to *C. psittaci* and in the protective response following vaccination; only one strain (a CBA subline) was found to be satisfactory in both respects (Jones et al., unpublished). A second model has been developed in which sheep immune serum is incubated with chlamydiae before intraperitoneal inoculation of mice (Hughes, 1997). This model appears to be superior to the active-immunization model, since it correlates with findings in experimentally vaccinated sheep (Hughes, 1997).

Treatment

Long-acting oxytetracycline can be effectively used to prevent chlamydial abortion, provided that the treatment is administered between 95 and 110 days of gestation. A second injection 2 weeks later improves protection. Treatment later in gestation provides only marginal benefit (Greig and Linklater, 1985).

BOVINE CHLAMYDIAL INFERTILITY, METRITIS, AND SALPINGITIS

Etiology

The agent involved is a subtype of *C. pecorum* (Fukushi and Hirai, 1992, 1993; Anderson, personal communication). PCR-based analysis of the major outer membrane protein gene has shown variations within this subtype (Anderson, personal communication), but the full extent of variation is unknown. Neither is it known whether there is a distinct subtype of *C. pecorum* which causes metritis in cattle or whether most subtypes of this species are pathogenic when inoculated into the uterus of cows in estrus.

Clinical Expression and Pathologic, Microbiological, and Serologic Findings

Due to the relatively recent recognition of bovine chlamydial infertility, metritis, and salpingitis, the most reliable descriptions of its clinical expression are provided by experimental infection studies (Bowen et al., 1978; Wittenbrink et al., 1993). A detailed description of the more recent work of Wittenbrink et al. (1993) follows, because of its relevance to human chlamydial infection.

Experimental Infections

The infective inoculum for this set of experiments was a chlamydia strain isolated from the uterus of a cow at a slaughterhouse (BovEnd 11/88). This isolate was thought to be *C. psittaci*, but subsequent molecular fingerprinting has shown it to be a subtype of *C. pecorum* (Anderson, personal communication). Two experiments were performed in previously unmated (virgin) cows. Experiment 1 used two infected cows; experiment 2 used six infected and two uninfected animals. The intrauterine inoculations, performed at estrus, delivered either 1.07×10^9 (first experiment) or 2.14×10^8 (second experiment) 50% chicken embryo lethal doses.

In the first experiment, animals developed fever within 24 h of inoculation and were depressed and anorexic for 36 h. A vaginal discharge, initially grey and later thick and yellowish, developed 2 or 3 days after inoculation and lasted until the animals were killed on day 7. At necropsy, the uterus of each animal was filled with a thick, yellow exudate. Histopathologically, widespread necrosis and ulceration of the uterine epithelium were evident; the mucosa was infiltrated with neutrophils, lymphocytes, plasma cells, and macrophages.

In the second experiment, two of the six infected cows became febrile and anorexic. All developed a purulent vaginal discharge that continued for 10 to 18 days and then became intermittent, lasting, in one animal, until week 19. Examination of these discharges revealed chlamydial elementary bodies for up to 12 weeks postinoculation in five animals and 20 weeks postinoculation in one animal. Fecal shedding of chlamydiae for up to 12 months also was noted in all infected cows and in one control cow. However, these organisms were not characterized, and they may have been an enteric, rather than the experimental (genital), form of *C. pecorum*. Insemination of all six infected animals was attempted on five occasions. Four failed to conceive, and two did so only after the fifth insemination. The two control animals conceived after the first or second insemination. Two infected animals were killed at 19 weeks and two at 26 weeks postinoculation. Lesions in these were confined to the uterus; there was moderate, chronic endometritis. Chlamydiae were isolated from the vaginal and uterine mucosa and from the small and large intestines of one cow killed at 19 weeks postinoculation and of one killed at 26 weeks postinoculation. Serologic examinations revealed that five animals seroconverted at 4 weeks postinoculation, and all six showed increased ELISA titers.

In another study, an isolate obtained from a cow with metritis was compared with an isolate obtained from a cow which had aborted; these isolates were typed (by molecular fingerprinting) as *C. pecorum* and abortifacient *C. psittaci*, respectively (Jones et al., in preparation). Each strain was inoculated, at estrus, into the uterus and cervix of three previously unmated (virgin) cattle. The total dose administered was 2×10^7 inclusion-forming units. Two animals inoculated with the "metritis" (*C. pecorum*) strain developed histopathologic lesions of metritis and salpingitis; one (killed at 21 days postinoculation) also had endometritis, with copious quantities of thick, yellow, purulent material in the uterus. Of those challenged with the abortifacient strain of *C. psittaci*, one (killed at 21 days post-inoculation) had subacute metritis with cellular infiltration of the uterine mucosa. No other abnormalities were detected in any animal, including the two controls, nor were any other clinical signs observed. Chlamydiae were detected by PCR in three animals. The single animal inoculated with the "metritis" strain and killed at 21 days postinoculation was positive in one uterine horn and one associated lymph node; and two animals inoculated with the abortifacient *C. psittaci* strain and killed at 42 and 63 days postinoculation were positive in medial iliac lymph nodes. Despite the absence of disease, two of the "metritis" strain group seroconverted at 2 weeks postinoculation and two from the "abortion" strain group seroconverted at 3 weeks postinoculation.

Both studies clearly demonstrate that certain forms of *C. pecorum* can cause endometritis when inoculated directly into the uteri of cattle. In contrast, only minor pathologic changes were observed following inoculation of an abortifacient form of *C. psittaci*. The two studies used different strains of *C. pecorum*, which differed in the restriction fragment fingerprint of the gene of the major outer membrane protein (Appino and Anderson, unpublished). It therefore appears that variations in virulence can occur between "metritis" strains of *C. pecorum*. Curiously, one strain also induced salpingitis, a feature not described in the other study (Jones et al., in preparation; Wittenbrink et al., 1993). It is also of note that despite the absence of outward clinical signs, the pathologic changes observed at necropsy were severe enough to cause infertility. Infection was detected serologically, but as yet there are no means by which to distinguish antibodies raised by "metritis" forms of *C. pecorum* from those raised by other subtypes of this species or by *C. psittaci*.

CONCLUSIONS

Both forms of chlamydial infection of ruminants offer useful comparative features for human reproductive tract disease. Enzootic abortion of ewes is an acute disease that does not have an obvious parallel in humans. However, the causal organism persists in the reproductive tract (and possibly other sites) in 20% of animals that have suffered a disease episode and that (because of that episode) are immune from further clinical disease. The factor(s) that permits this carrier state is unknown, as are the precise mechanisms of excretion of the organism at estrus and during lambing. Bovine chlamydial infertility, due to metritis and salpingitis, in contrast has direct parallels with human chlamydial genital disease, in particular the development of salpingitis following infection. The bovine disease is still in the very early stages of characterization, and so the full extent of its usefulness as a model for human disease remains to be determined.

Acknowledgments

The unpublished studies referred to in this chapter and performed at MRI were funded by the Scottish Office, Agriculture, Environment and Forestry Department and by the EU (project CT93-957).

REFERENCES

Aitken, I. D. 1991. Enzootic (chlamydial) abortion, p. 43–49. *In* W. B. Martin and I. D. Aitken (ed.), *Disease of Sheep.* Blackwell Scientific Publications Ltd., Oxford, United Kingdom.

Aitken, I. D., G. W. Robinson, and I. E. Anderson. 1981. Recent experimental studies on chlamydial abortion in ewes. *Sheep Vet. Soc. Proc.* **5:**553–560.

Aitken, I. D., I. E. Anderson, and G. W. Robinson. 1986. Ovine chlamydial abortion: limitations of inactivated vaccine, p. 55–65. *In* I. D. Aitken (ed.), *Chlamydial Disease of Ruminants.* CEC publication EUR 10056 EN. Office for Official Publications of the European Communities, Luxembourg.

Amin, J. D., and A. J. Wilsmore. 1995. Studies on the early phase of the pathogenesis of ovine enzootic abortion in the non-pregnant ewe. *Br. Vet. J.* **151:**141–155.

Anderson, I. E. Personal communication.

Anderson, I. E., S. I. F. Baxter, S. Dunbar, A. G. Rae, H. L. Philips, M. J. Clarkson, and A. J. Herring. 1996. Analyses of the genomes of chlamydial isolates from ruminants and pigs support the adoption of the new species *Chlamydia pecorum. Int. J. Syst. Bacteriol.* **46:**245–251.

Appino, S., and I. E. Anderson. Unpublished data.

Appleyard, W. T., I. D. Aitken, and I. E. Anderson. 1985. Attempted venereal transmission of *Chlamydia psittaci* in sheep. *Vet. Rec.* **116:**535–538.

Baghian, A., K. Kousoulas, R. Truax, and J. Storz. 1996. Specific antigens of *Chlamydia pecorum* and their homologues in *C. psittaci* and *C. trachomatis. Am. J. Vet. Res.* **57:**1720–1725.

Beatty, W. L., G. L. Byrne, and R. P. Morrison. 1993. Morphologic and antigenic characterization of interferon γ-mediated persistent *Chlamydia trachomatis* infection *in vitro. Proc. Natl. Acad. Sci. USA* **90:**3998–4002.

Bernstein, M., and J. Yaakobowitz. 1990. The identification and prevention of venereal transmission of *C. psittaci* in sheep. *Isr. J. Vet. Med.* **45:**192.

Blewett, D. A., F. Gisemba, J. K. Miller, F. W. A. Johnson, and M. J. Clarkson. 1982. Ovine enzootic abortion: the acquisition of infection and consequent abortion within a single lambing season. *Vet. Rec.* **111:**499–501.

Bowen, R. A., P. Spears, J. Storz, and G. E. Seidel. 1978. Mechanisms of infertility in genital tract infections due to *C. psittaci* transmitted through contaminated semen. *J. Infect. Dis.* **138:**95–98.

Brade, L., S. Schramek, U. Schade, and H. Brade. 1986. Chemical, biological and immunochemical properties of the *Chlamydia psittaci* lipopolysaccharide. *Infect. Immun.* **54:**568–574.

Buxton, D. 1986. Potential danger to pregnant women of *Chlamydia psittaci* from sheep. *Vet. Rec.* **118:**510–511.

Buxton, D., R. M. Barlow, J. Finlayson, I. E. Anderson, and A. Mackellar. 1990. Observations on the pathogenesis of *Chlamydia psittaci* infection of pregnant sheep. *J. Comp. Pathol.* **102:**221–237.

Buzoni-Gatel, D., and A. Rodolakis. 1983. A mouse model to compare virulence of abortive and intestinal ovine strains of *Chlamydia psittaci*: influence of the route of inoculation. *Ann. Microbiol. (Inst. Pasteur)* **134A:**91–99.

Buzoni-Gatel, D., A. Rodolakis, and M. Plommet. 1987. T cell mediated and humoral immunity in a mouse *Chlamydia psittaci* systemic infection. *Res. Vet. Sci.* **43:** 59–63.

Buzoni-Gatel, D., F. Bernard, A. Andersen, and A. Rodolakis. 1990. Protective effect of polyclonal and monoclonal antibodies against abortion in mice infected by *Chlamydia psittaci. Vaccine* **8:**342–346.

Buzoni-Gatel, D., L. Guilloteau, F. Bernard, S. Bernard, T. Chardes, and A. Rocca. 1992. Protection against *Chlamydia psittaci* in mice conferred by Lyt-2^+ T cells. *Immunology* **77:**284–288.

Carlin, J. M., E. C. Borden, and G. I. Byrne. 1989. Interferon-induced indoleamine 2,3-dioxygenase activity inhibits *Chlamydia psittaci* replication in human macrophages. *J. Interferon Res.* **9:**329–337.

Cevenini, R., M. Donati, E. Brocchi, F. de Simone, and M. la Placa. 1991. Partial characterization of an 89-kDa highly immunoreactive protein from *Chlamydia psittaci* A/22 causing abortion. *FEMS Microbiol. Lett.* **81:**111–116.

Chalmers, W. S. K., J. Simpson, S. J. Lee, and W. Baxendale. 1997. Use of a live chlamydial vaccine to prevent ovine enzootic abortion. *Vet. Rec.* **141:**63–67.

Clarkson, M. J., and H. L. Philips. 1997. Isolation of faecal chlamydia from sheep in Britain and their characterization by cultural properties. *Vet. J.* **153:**307–311.

Dawson, M., A. Zaghloul, and A. J. Wilsmore. 1986. Ovine enzootic abortion: experimental studies of immune responses. *Res. Vet. Sci.* **40:**59–64.

Dayer, J. M., B. Beutler, and A. Cerami. 1985. Cachectin/tumor necrosis factor stimulates collagenase and prostaglandin E_2 production by human synovial cells and dermal fibroblasts. *J. Exp. Med.* **162:**2163–2168.

Denamur, E., C. Sayada, A. Souriau, J. Orfila, A. Rodolakis, and J. Elion. 1991. Restriction pattern of the major outer-membrane protein gene provides evidence for a homogeneous invasive group among ruminant isolates of *Chlamydia psittaci. J. Gen. Microbiol.* **137:**2525–2530.

Dohoo, I. R., R. A. Curtis, and G. G. Finlay. 1985. A survey of sheep disease in Canada. *Can. J. Comp. Med.* **49:**239–247.

Foggie, A. 1959. The duration of immunity in ewes following vaccination against ovine enzootic abortion virus. *Vet. Rec.* **71:**741–742.

Fukushi, H., and K. Hirai. 1992. Proposal of *Chlamydia pecorum* sp. nov. for *Chlamydia* strains derived from ruminants. *Int. J. Syst. Bacteriol.* **42:**306–308.

Fukushi, H., and K. Hirai. 1993. *Chlamydia pecorum*—the fourth species of genus *Chlamydia. Microbiol. Immunol.* **37:**515–522.

Graham, S. P., G. E. Jones, M. Livingstone, and G. Entrican. 1995. Recombinant ovine interferon gamma inhibits the multiplication of *Chlamydia psittaci* in ovine cells. *J. Comp. Pathol.* **112:**185–195.

Greig, J. R. 1936. Enzootic abortion in ewes. *Vet. Rec.* **48:**1225–1227.

Greig, A., and K. A. Linklater. 1985. Field studies on the efficacy of a long acting preparation of oxytetracycline in controlling outbreaks of enzootic abortion of sheep. *Vet. Rec.* **117:**627–628.

Griffiths, P. C., H. L. Philips, M. Dawson, and M. J. Clarkson. 1992. Antigenic and morphological differentiation of placental and intestinal isolates of *Chlamydia psittaci* of ovine origin. *Vet. Microbiol.* **30:**165–177.

Hansen, D. E., O. R. Hedstrom, R. J. Sonn, and S. P. Snyder. 1990. Efficacy of a vaccine to prevent *Chlamydia*- or *Campylobacter*-induced abortions in ewes. *J. Am. Vet. Med. Assoc.* **196:**731–734.

Herring, A. J. 1993. Typing *Chlamydia psittaci*—a review of methods and recent findings. *Br. Vet. J.* **149:**455–475.

Holliman, A., R. G. Daniel, J. G. Parr, P. C. Griffiths, B. J. Bevan, T. C. Martin, R. G. Hewinson, M. Dawson, and R. Munro. 1994. Chlamydiosis and abortion in a dairy herd. *Vet. Rec.* **134:**500–502.

Holtmann, H., Y. Shemer-Avni, K. Wessel, I. Sarov, and D. Wallach. 1990. Inhibition of growth of *Chlamydia trachomatis* by tumor necrosis factor is accompanied by increased prostaglandin synthesis. *Infect. Immun.* **58:**3168–3172.

Huang, H.-S., D. Buxton, and I. E. Anderson. 1990. The ovine immune response to *Chlamydia psittaci*: histopathology of the lymph node. *J. Comp. Pathol.* **102:**89–97.

Hughes, S. 1997. Ph.D. thesis, University of Edinburgh, Edinburgh, Scotland.

Johnson, F. W. A., and M. J. Clarkson. 1986. Ovine abortion isolates: antigenic variations detected by mouse infection, p. 129–132. *In* I. D. Aitken (ed.), *Chlamydial Diseases of Ruminants.* CEC publication EUR 10056 EN. Office for Official Publications of the European Communities, Luxembourg.

Johnson, F. W. A., and D. Hobson. 1986. Intracerebral infection of mice with ovine strains of *Chlamydia psittaci*: an animal screening test for the assay of vaccines. *J. Comp. Pathol.* **96:**497–505.

Jones, G. E. Manuscript in preparation.

Jones, G. E. Unpublished data.

Jones, G. E., and I. E. Anderson. 1988. *Chlamydia psittaci*: is tonsillar tissue the portal of entry in ovine enzootic abortion? *Res. Vet. Sci.* **44:**260–261.

Jones, G. E., and I. E. Anderson. Unpublished data.

Jones, G. E., and M. Livingstone. Unpublished data.

Jones, G. E., A. J. Herring, J. Machell, T. W. Tan, I. E. Anderson, and S. Dunbar. 1992. Preliminary studies with a recombinant major outer membrane protein vaccine: clinical efficacy of several vaccine formulations against experimental enzootic abortion of ewes, p. 63. *In* P.-A. Mardh, M. la Placa, and M. Ward (ed.), *Proceedings of the European Society of Chlamydial Research*, vol. 2. Uppsala University Centre for STD Research, Uppsala, Sweden.

Jones, G. E., K. A. Jones, J. Machell, J. Brebner, I. E. Anderson, and S. How. 1995. Efficacy trials with tissue-culture grown, inactivated vaccines against chlamydial abortion in sheep. *Vaccine* **13:**715–723.

Jones, G. E., A. Donn, J. Machell, and B. Biolatti. Manuscript in preparation.

Jones, G. E., J. Machell, S. Hughes, and M. Livingstone. Unpublished data.

Keppie, J., A. E. Williams, K. Witt, and H. Smith. 1965. The role of erythritol in the tissue localization of the *Brucellae*. *Br. J. Exp. Pathol.* **46:**104–108.

Kwapien, R. P., S. D. Lincoln, D. E. Reed, C. E. Whiteman, and T. L. Chow. 1970. Pathologic changes of placentas from heifers with experimentally induced epizootic bovine abortion. *Am. J. Vet. Res.* **31:**999–1015.

Lacy, D., G. I. Byrne, and D. Paulnock. 1992. Chlamydia-induced immunosuppression in mice is the result of multiple mechanisms, p. 86. *In* P.-A. Mardh, M. la Placa, and M. Ward (ed.), *Proceedings of the European Society of Chlamydial Research*, vol. 2. Uppsala University Centre for STD Research, Uppsala, Sweden.

Leaver, H. A., A. Howie, I. D. Aitken, B. W. Appleyard, I. E. Anderson, G. Jones, L. A. Hay, G. E. Williams, and D. Buxton. 1989. Changes in progesterone, oestradiol 17β, and intrauterine prostaglandin E_2 during late gestation in sheep experimentally infected with an ovine abortion strain of *Chlamydia psittaci*. *J. Gen. Microbiol.* **135:**565–573.

Leonard, C., G. L. Caldow, and G. J. Gunn. 1993. An estimate of the prevalence of enzootic abortion of ewes in Scotland. *Vet. Rec.* **133:**180–183.

Livingstone, M., G. Jones, and N. Poyser. Unpublished data.

Lozano, E. A. 1986. Etiologic significance of bacterial isolates from rams with palpable epidydimitis. *Am. J. Vet. Res.* **47:**1153–1156.

Mayer, J., M. L. Woods, Z. Vavrin, and J. B. Hibbs, Jr. 1993. Gamma interferon-induced nitric oxide production reduces *Chlamydia trachomatis* infectivity in McCoy cells. *Infect. Immun.* **61:**491–497.

McCafferty, M. C. 1990. Immunity to *Chlamydia psittaci* with particular reference to sheep. *Vet. Microbiol.* **25:**87–99.

McCafferty, M. C., and I. E. Anderson. Personal communication.

McClenaghan, M., A. J. Herring, and I. D. Aitken. 1984. Comparison of *Chlamydia psittaci* isolates by DNA restriction endonuclease analysis. *Infect. Immun.* **45:**384–389.

McClenaghan, M., N. F. Inglis, and A. J. Herring. 1991. Comparison of isolates of *Chlamydia psittaci* of ovine, avian and feline origin by analysis of polypeptide profiles from purified elementary bodies. *Vet. Microbiol.* **26:**269–278.

McEwen, A. D., A. I. Littlejohn, and A. Foggie. 1951. Enzootic abortion in ewes. Some aspects of infection and resistance. *Vet. Rec.* **63:**489–492.

McEwen, A. D., J. B Dow, and R. D. Anderson. 1955. Enzootic abortion in ewes. An adjuvant vaccine prepared from eggs. *Vet. Rec.* **67:**393–394.

Nabeya, M., K. Kaneko, H. Ogino., D. Nakabayashi, T. Watanabe, J. Murayama, K. Hayashi, H. Fukushi, T. Yamagushi, K. Hirai, Y. Inaba, and M. Matumoto. 1991. Abortion in Japanese cows caused by *Chlamydia psittaci*. *Vet. Microbiol.* **29:**261–265.

Papadopoulos, O. Personal communication.

Papp, J. R., and P. E. Shewen. 1996a. Pregnancy failure following vaginal infection of sheep with *Chlamydia psittaci* prior to breeding. *Infect. Immun.* **64:**1116–1125.

Papp, J. R., and P. E. Shewen. 1996b. Localization of chronic *C. psittaci* infection in the reproductive tract of sheep. *J. Infect. Dis.* **174:**1296–1302.

Papp, J. R., P. E. Shewen, and C. J. Gartley. 1993. *Chlamydia psittaci* infection and associated infertility in sheep. *Can. J. Vet. Res.* **57:**185–189.

Papp, J. R., P. E. Shewen, and C. J. Gartley. 1994. Abortion and subsequent excretion of chlamydiae from the reproductive tract of sheep during estrus. *Infect. Immun.* **62:**3786–3792.

Perez-Martinez, J. A., and J. Storz. 1985. Antigenic diversity of *Chlamydia psittaci* of mammalian origin determined by microimmunofluorescence. *Infect. Immun.* **50:** 905–910.

Rank, R. G., K. H. Ramsey, E. A. Pack, and D. M. Williams. 1992. Effect of gamma interferon on resolution of murine chlamydial genital infection. *Infect. Immun.* **60:** 4427–4429.

Rodolakis. A. 1983. In vitro and in vivo properties of chemically induced temperature-sensitive mutants of *Chlamydia psittaci* var. *ovis*: screening in a murine model. *Infect. Immun.* **42:**525–530.

Rodolakis, A., and K. Bernard. 1977. Isolation of *Chlamydia ovis* from genital organs of rams with epidydimitis. *Bull. Acad. Vet. France* **50:**65–69.

Rodolakis, A., and F. Bernard. 1984. Vaccination with temperature-sensitive mutant of *Chlamydia psittaci* against enzootic abortion of ewes. *Vet. Rec.* **114:**193–194.

Rodolakis, A., and A. Souriau. 1983. Response of ewes to temperature-sensitive mutants of *Chlamydia psittaci* (var *ovis*) obtained by NTG mutagenesis. *Ann. Rech. Vet.* **14:**155–161.

Rodolakis, A., and A. Souriau. 1989. Variations in the virulence of strains of *Chlamydia psittaci* for pregnant ewes. *Vet. Rec.* **125:**87–190.

Rodolakis, A., F. Bernard, and F. Lantier. 1989. Mouse models for evaluation of virulence of *Chlamydia psittaci* isolated from ruminants. *Res. Vet. Sci.* **46:**34–39.

Schutte, A. P., and J. G. Pienaar. 1977. Chlamydiosis in sheep and cattle in South Africa. *J. S. Afr. Vet. Assoc.* **48:**261–265.

Shemer-Avni, Y., D. Wallach, and I. Sarov. 1989. Reversion of the antichlamydial effect of tumor necrosis factor by tryptophan and antibodies to beta interferon. *Infect. Immun.* **57:**3484–3490.

Siarkou, V. 1992. Ph.D. thesis. Aristotle University, Thessaloniki, Greece.

Smith, H., A. E. Williams, J. H. Pearce, J. Keppie, P. W. Harris-Smith, R. B. Fitzgeorge, and K. Witt. 1962. Fetal erythritol: a cause of the localization of *Brucella abortus* in bovine contagious abortion. *Nature* **193:**47–49.

Spears, P., and J. Storz. 1979. Biotyping of *Chlamydia psittaci* based on inclusion morphology and response to diethylaminoethyl-dextran and cycloheximide. *Infect. Immun.* **24:**224–232.

Stamp, J. T., A. D. McEwen, J. A. A. Watt, and D. I. Nisbet. 1950. Enzootic abortion in ewes. 1. Transmission of the disease. *Vet. Rec.* **62:**251–254.

Steven, D. H., K. A. Mallon, and P. W. Nathanielsz. 1980. Sheep trophoblast in monolayer cell culture. *Placenta* **1:**209–221.

Storz, J., and D. G. McKercher. 1962. Etiological studies on epizootic bovine abortion. *Zen. Veterinaer-med.* **9:**411–427.

Storz, J., E. J. Carroll, E. H. Stephenson, L. Bull, and A. K. Eugster. 1976. Urogenital infection and seminal excretion after inoculation of bulls and rams with chlamydiae. *Am. J. Vet. Res.* **37:**517–5200.

Tan, T. W., A. J. Herring, I. E. Anderson, and G. E. Jones. 1990. Protection of sheep against *Chlamydia psittaci* infection with a subcellular vaccine containing the major outer membrane protein. *Infect. Immun.* **58:**3101–3108.

Thomas, S. M., L. F. Garrity, C. R. Brandt, C. S. Schobert, G.-S. Feng, M. W. Taylor, J. M. Carlin, and G. I. Byrne. 1993. IFN-γ-mediated antimicrobial response. Indoleamine 2,3-dioxygenase-deficient mutant host cells no longer inhibit intracellular *Chlamydia* spp. or *Toxoplasma* growth. *J. Immunol.* **150:**5529–5534.

Thorburn, G. D. 1991. The placenta, prostaglandins and parturition: a review. *Reprod. Fertil. Dev.* **3:**277–294.

VIDA. 1992. *Veterinary Investigation Diagnosis Analysis II (VIDA), 1992 and 1985–92.* MAFF, CVL, Weybridge, England.

Vretou, E., H. Loutrari, L. Mariani, K. Costelidou, P. Eliades, G. Conidou, S. Karamanou, O. Mangana, V. Siarkou, and O. Papadopoulos. 1996. Diversity among abortion strains of *C. psittaci* demonstrated by inclusion morphology, polypeptide profiles and monoclonal antibodies. *Vet. Microbiol.* **51:**275–289.

Waldhalm, D. G., W. J. DeLong, and R. F. Hall. 1982. Efficacy of a bacterin prepared from *Chlamydia psittaci* grown in cell culture for experimental immunization of ewes. *Vet. Microbiol.* **7:**493–498.

Williams, D. M., D. M. Magee, L. F. Bonewald, J. G. Smith, C. A. Bleicker, G. I. Byrne, and J. Schachter. 1990. A role in vivo for tumor necrosis factor alpha in host defense against *Chlamydia trachomatis. Infect. Immun.* **58:**1572–1576.

Wilsmore, A. J., V. Parsons, and M. Dawson. 1984. Experiments to demonstrate routes of transmission of ovine enzootic abortion. *Br. Vet. J.* **140:**380–391.

Wilsmore, A. J., B. C. Wilsmore, G. J. R. Dagnall, K. A. Izzard, R. M. Woodland, M. Dawson, and C. Venables. 1990. Clinical and immunological responses of ewes following vaccination with an experimental formalin-inactivated *Chlamydia psittaci (ovis)* vaccine and subsequent challenge with the live organism during pregnancy. *Br. Vet. J.* **146:**341–348.

Wittenbrink, M. M., H. A. Schoon, D. Schoon, R. Mansfeld, and W. Bisping. 1993. Endometritis in cattle experimentally induced by *Chlamydia psittaci. J. Vet. Med. Ser. B.* **40:**437–450.

Wong, S. Y., E. S. Gray, D. Buxton, J. Finlayson, and F. W. A. Johnson. 1985. Acute placentitis and spontaneous abortion caused by *Chlamydia psittaci* of sheep origin: a histological and ultrastructural study. *J. Clin. Pathol.* **38:**707–711.

Woollen, N., E. K. Daniels, T. Yeary, H. W. Leipold, and R. M. Phillips. 1990. Chlamydial infection and perinatal mortality in a swine herd. *J. Am. Vet. Med. Assoc.* **197:**600–601.

19
Bovine Trichomoniasis

Lynette B. Corbeil and Robert H. BonDurant

Bovine trichomoniasis has many similarities to human trichomoniasis. Both protozoan infections are sexually transmitted and are characterized by clinical signs that vary from asymptomatic to purulent discharge after weeks to months of infection. Bovine trichomoniasis, caused by *Tritrichomonas foetus* (Fig. 1), has been associated with infertility due to spontaneous abortion in the first trimester or later (Abbitt and Meyerholz, 1979; BonDurant, 1985; Parsonson et al., 1976; Rhyan et al., 1988; Skirrow and BonDurant, 1988). More recently, human trichomoniasis, caused by *Trichomonas vaginalis*, has been associated with premature rupture of the membranes and preterm delivery and/or low-birth-weight infants in the last trimester of pregnancy (Hillier et al., 1995; Cotch et al., 1997; Read et al., 1993; Grice, 1974; Gibbs et al., 1992; Minkoff et al., 1984). The reduction of preterm birth rates achieved by treatment with metronidazole during mid-pregnancy supports this conclusion (Morales et al., 1994; Hauth et al., 1995; Fleury et al., 1977; Saurina and McCormack, 1997). Trichomoniasis is also associated with an increased rate of human immunodeficiency virus infection in female prostitutes (Laga et al., 1993).

Animal models of human trichomoniasis have been problematic. Early studies of small laboratory animals involved systemic inoculation that did not mimic sexual transmission. More recently, murine models of vaginal infection in estrogenized mice have been developed for both *T. vaginalis* (McGroy and Garber, 1992) and *T. foetus* (Hook et al., 1995). In these models, the route of infection mimics sexual transmission and relatively persistent

---

Lynette B. Corbeil, Department of Pathology, University of California, San Diego, San Diego, CA 92103-8416. **Robert H. BonDurant,** Department of Population Health and Reproduction, University of California, Davis, Davis, CA 95616.

Sexually Transmitted Diseases and Adverse Outcomes of Pregnancy
Edited by P. J. Hitchcock, H. T. MacKay, J. N. Wasserheit, and R. Binder
©1999 American Society for Microbiology, Washington, D.C.

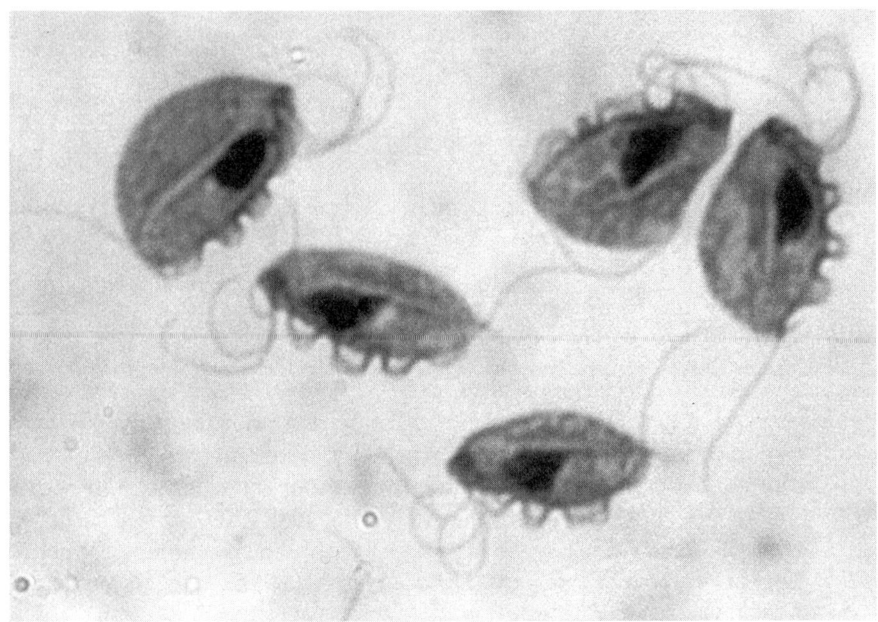

Figure 1 Giemsa stain of *T. foetus.* The tear-shaped motile protozoa have a single nucleus, three anterior flagella, and an undulating membrane with a protruding single posterior flagellum. Courtesy of John Thomford, University of California, San Diego.

vaginal infection results. However, pretreatment with estrogen affects immune system responses (Wira and Sandoe, 1987, 1989), thus altering host-parasite relationships. Also, it is not yet clear whether the pathogenesis of *T. vaginalis* infection is the same for mice as for humans. For example, attachment to cells, hemolysis, and cytotoxicity might be specific to a host. This could explain the species specificity of these infections. The host specificity of *T. vaginalis* confounds the interpretation of studies of mice. However, since bovine trichomoniasis is a naturally occurring sexually transmitted infection, it can better serve as a model for human trichomoniasis (Corbeil, 1995). Both *T. vaginalis* and *T. foetus* are anaerobic motile protozoa with one-stage life cycles. Both survive only in the male and female reproductive tracts in nature, although they may be readily cultured in vitro with complex media. Both pathogens adhere to vaginal epithelial cells, bind to host cell surface proteins, digest immunoglobulins with extracellular proteinases, and produce hemolysins and cytotoxins (Corbeil, 1995; Graves and Gardner, 1993). The bovine infection causes significant economic loss due to reproductive failure and consequently has been well studied. The use of this model to help understand human infection may be quite productive for two reasons: (i) the similarities in host-pathogen relationships may imply similarities in immune mechanisms of protection; and (ii) the early loss of pregnancy in bovine trichomoniasis should stimulate research on adverse outcomes in the first and second trimester of pregnancy in women with trichomoniasis.

NATURAL HISTORY

Trichomoniasis is a common disease in cattle where natural breeding is used (Table 1). A total of 40% of Australian herds (19 of 47) were reported to be infected (Dennett et al., 1974). In the United States, prevalences have varied from 16% of herds in California (BonDurant et al., 1990) to 44% in Nevada (Kvasnicka et al., 1989). Prevalence rates in individual bulls range from 25% in Australia (Dennett et al., 1974) to 71% in Nigeria (Akinboade, 1980) to 5% in California (BonDurant et al., 1990). Prevalence rates in cows were lower: 42 and 6.4% in the Nigerian and Australian studies, respectively (Akinboade, 1980; Dennett et al., 1974). The difference in prevalence in cows and bulls reflects the difference in the duration of infection (it is shorter in females than in males). The infection is self-limiting in females, although the duration is variable (ranging from 12 to 22 weeks or longer [Skirrow and BonDurant, 1988]). The duration of experimental infections in females ranges between 8 weeks (BonDurant et al., 1993) and 19.5 weeks (Skirrow and BonDurant, 1990a). The duration may depend on the number of parasites in the ejaculate, since a higher experimental innoculum (7×10^6 parasites) takes longer to cure spontaneously than do doses of 1×10^6, and animals given 10^4 or 10^2 parasites resolved infection even more quickly

Table 1 Prevalence of bovine trichomoniasis

Percent infection of:		Herds	Location	Reference
Bulls	Cows			
3–14		27–44	Nevada	Kvasnicka et al., 1989
5		16	California	BonDurant et al., 1990
8			Oklahoma	Wilson et al., 1979
7			Florida	Abbitt and Meyerholz, 1979
25	6	40	Australia	Dennett et al., 1974
71	42		Nigeria[a]	Akinboade, 1980
4–6		7–16	Costa Rica	Perez et al., 1992
56			Argentina[a]	Campero et al., 1987

[a]These two studies were done on single large herds rather than being surveys of geographic areas.

(BonDurant et al., 1993; Skirrow and BonDurant, 1990a). Bulls older than 4 years usually remain infected for long periods (or for life), whereas 2- to 4-year-old bulls are more resistant to infection and are infected for a shorter duration (Clark et al., 1974; Skirrow and BonDurant, 1988). The experimental dose to achieve infection in females is low; a dose of 10^2 parasites was enough to infect 4 of 8 females inoculated intravaginally whereas all 15 females given 10^6 parasites became infected (BonDurant et al., 1993).

Trichomoniasis in cattle is generally associated with a lack of overt clinical signs. The bull is an asymptomatic carrier, although the female usually develops mild to moderate vaginitis, cervicitis, endometritis, and sometimes salpingitis. The initial infection period in the female is silent. In the only published study of the time course of lesion development, no inflammatory infiltrate was detected in the vagina, cervix, or uterus of cows killed prior to 50 days of infection (Parsonson et al., 1976), suggesting that the parasite suppressed host responses for some time. Inflammation was apparent after 60 days, and fetal loss occurred between 60 and 90 days (Parsonson et al., 1976). Others have reported the range of fetal loss from immediately after implantation (at day 16 to 17) through 5 to 7 months of gestation (in a 9-month gestation period), although early losses are more common than mid- to late-gestation losses (BonDurant, 1985; Rhyan et al., 1988; Skirrow and BonDurant, 1988). Fetal lesions included bronchopneumonia with trichomonads in the airways. Placentitis was also present (Parsonson et al., 1976; Rhyan et al., 1988). After loss of the fetus, cows may remain infertile for weeks or months, but they usually regain fertility (BonDurant, 1985). Infrequently, very severe uterine inflammation (pyometra) occurs (BonDurant, 1985; Skirrow and BonDurant, 1988). Rarely, cows are infected throughout pregnancy, give birth to a normal calf, and are still infected for several weeks into the postpartum period (Skirrow, 1987). However, the association of bovine trichomoniasis with preterm birth and low-birth-weight calves has not been well studied.

It is likely that immune responses are responsible for clearance of infection, whether the duration of infection is a few weeks or many months. However, protective convalescent-phase immunity appears to be transient, because cows that have cleared the infection are relatively susceptible to reinfection. The resistance to infection associated with convalescent-phase immunity is gradually lost within 2 years (Clark et al., 1983b). Even this short-lived immunity has encouraged studies of host-parasite relationships to determine which specific antigens and immune responses may be protective.

VIRULENCE FACTORS

Several investigators have endeavored to identify virulence factors that may serve as protective immunogens. Since the organism is a flagellated, motile, extracellular pathogen (Fig. 1), motility may be important in penetration of mucus in order to colonize and in movement from the vagina to the uterus. Mucinases (proteinases and glycosidases) are likely to aid in penetration of mucus (Müller, 1973). Our studies with extracellular proteinases of *T. foetus* demonstrated digestion of a number of substrates, such as immunoglobulin G (IgG), that are likely to be important in host defense (Talbot et al., 1991). Sequence comparisons show that the proteinases of *T. foetus* and *T. vaginalis* have very good homology, further supporting the usefulness of *T. foetus* as a model system for human trichomoniasis (Mallinson et al., 1994, 1995; Ikeda and Corbeil, unpublished).

Antigens associated with virulence have been identified in several studies. We used monoclonal antibodies to characterize a highly glycosylated surface "adherence antigen" of *T. foetus* (Hodgson et al., 1990) and later used these antibodies in an immunoaffinity purification of the virulence factor (BonDurant et al., 1993). Other studies showed that the antigen was conserved in 50 strains tested from the United States and other countries (Ikeda et al., 1993). This would be important if the adherence antigen was used for either immunization or immunodiagnosis. Burgess identified another conserved surface antigen (Burgess, 1988). Antibodies to this antigen mediated complement killing and enhanced phagocytosis of trichomonads, suggesting that these antibodies can provide protection (Burgess, 1986).

Trichomonads kill some tissue culture cells. In early studies, Kulda and Honigberg (1969) demonstrated the toxicity of three strains of *T. foetus* for chicken liver cell cultures. Both *T. foetus* cells and culture filtrates were toxic. Although the degree of cell damage differed with each *T. foetus* strain, toxicity did not require adherence of the parasites to the cultured cells, suggesting that soluble secreted toxins are important in bovine trichomoniasis. Later, Burgess and colleagues demonstrated cytotoxic and hemolytic effects of *T. foetus* for mammalian cell lines (Burgess et al., 1990; Burgess and McDonald, 1992). In these studies, monoclonal antibodies were used to identify an adhesion of *T. foetus* of ~190 kDa with ~150- and 65-kDa subunits. This may also be an important protective antigen.

Evasion of the host immune response is another ploy used by many parasites in establishing infection. *T. foetus*, like *T. vaginalis*, apparently has at least two mechanisms for evading host responses. First, the extracellular proteinase, described above, digests bovine IgG1 and IgG2 (Talbot et al., 1991). This should aid in evasion of host defense by IgG1 and IgG2 antibody responses. Second, *T. foetus* binds bovine IgG1, IgG2, and, to a lesser extent, IgM nonspecifically to its surface (Corbeil et al., 1991). This coating with host protein could facilitate evasion by camouflaging surface antigens. Both of these evasion strategies may contribute to the insidious and chronic nature of this infection. However, the host defenses eventually prevail, since infection is ultimately resolved without treatment.

IMMUNIZATION

Studies of the natural history of bovine trichomoniasis suggest that convalescent immunity is partially protective, as indicated above. In addition, a killed *T. foetus* vaccine recently became available commercially and provides some protection (Kvasnicka et al., 1989, 1992).

The concept of systemic immunization to prevent and control a sexually transmitted infection limited to the reproductive tract is supported by several decades of experience with *Campylobacter fetus* subsp. *venerealis* vaccines in cattle. The clinical picture and the pathogenesis of bovine trichomoniasis and campylobacteriosis are very similar in that these two extracellular pathogens (a protozoan and bacterium, respectively) are transmitted exclusively by sexual contact. Both cause insidious chronic infections and are associated with abnormal outcomes of pregnancy. Vaccination of cows against *Campylobacter* infection has virtually controlled this disease. Experimental studies showed that systemic vaccination can also be effective therapeutically in terminating infection in both cows and bulls (Corbeil and Winter, 1978; Schurig et al., 1975, 1978; Winter, 1978). This success with campylobacteriosis encouraged the development of vaccines against trichomoniasis. A recently developed killed-cell vaccine promotes earlier clearance of the infection in immunized cows than in controls (Kvasnicka et al., 1989) and significantly reduces abnormal outcomes of pregnancy (Kvasnicka et al., 1992).

The ability to protect bulls against trichomoniasis has been addressed by other studies. Clark et al. (1983a, 1984) showed that whole-cell or membrane fractions of *T. foetus* in oil adjuvant were effective therapeutically in bulls, as were whole-cell vaccines in oil adjuvant. Vaccination with the whole-cell vaccine also prevented infection in bulls younger than 5 years (Clark et al., 1984).

The mechanisms of protection have also been studied. We have evidence suggesting that vaccination with the purified adherence antigen described above may prevent pregnancy failure (Hodgson et al., 1990). In immunization trials with virgin female cattle (heifers), the antigen-immunized groups (in oil adjuvant with or without dextran sulfate) cleared the infection earlier than did the adjuvant controls (at an average of less than 35 days and greater than 63 days; respectively ($P < 0.005$) (Fig. 2). Most importantly, clearance in most vaccinated animals occurred well before the reported time for initial inflammation and fetal loss (<60 days).

These studies suggest a role for systemic immunization in protection against mucosal infection. Neither *C. fetus* nor *T. foetus* is invasive; they both colonize only the surface of the reproductive mucosa (although *T. foetus*

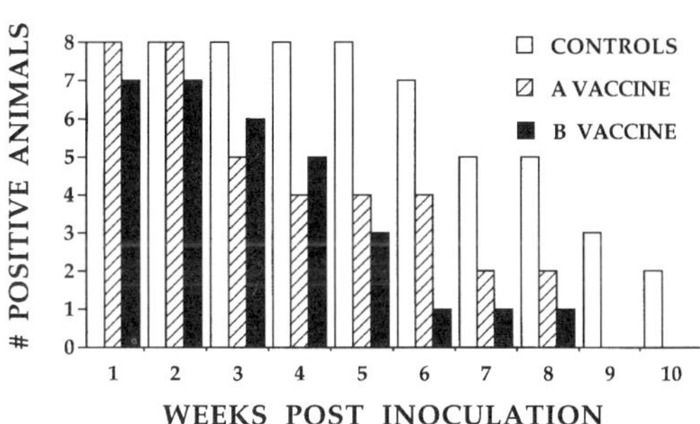

Figure 2 Clearance of *T. foetus* after vaginal inoculation of 10^6 organisms in heifers vaccinated with adherence antigen in Freund's incomplete adjuvant alone (A) or with Freund's incomplete adjuvant and dextran sulfate (B). Controls were vaccinated with adjuvant but no antigen. Positive animals were determined by weekly cultures of vaginal mucus. There were eight animals per group. Modified from BonDurant et al. (1993).

does invade the late-term fetus). Systemic immunization stimulates primarily IgG antibodies in serum (BonDurant et al., 1993; Corbeil et al., 1974a, 1974b). In heifers systemically immunized with purified *T. foetus* adherence antigen, high levels of IgG1 but low levels of IgG2 antibodies were detected in vaginal secretions of only one of two immunized groups, although both groups cleared the infection equally well (Fig. 2) (BonDurant et al., 1993). Clearance occurred as IgA antibody levels increased in the vaginal secretions. Interestingly, IgA antibody levels in vaginal secretions peaked earlier and reached higher levels in systemically immunized animals than in the control group, even though no IgA antibodies were detectable in the serum of immunized animals. These data suggest that systemic immunization primed the host for a memory IgA response at the mucosal surface after challenge with *T. foetus*, suggesting that IgA was important in clearance. Earlier, we had shown that bovine IgG1 antibodies to *T. foetus* inhibited adherence to vaginal epithelial cells (Corbeil et al., 1989). Others have shown that bovine IgG2 is the best opsonin for phagocytes (Desiderio and Campbell, 1980; McGuire et al., 1979; Miller et al., 1988) and that neutrophils kill *T. foetus* (de Azevedo and de Souza, 1993). More recently, Aydintug et al. (1993) showed that bovine neutrophils kill the greatest percentage of a *T. foetus* inoculum in the presence of bovine IgG2 plus complement. Thus, it is likely that both IgA and IgG (including IgG1 and IgG2) play different, isotype-specific roles in protection.

To test the hypothesis that IgG and IgA are both protective but that one class may protect better, we immunized two groups of virgin heifers. An optimal route and dose to produce IgG antibodies and an optimal route and dose to produce IgA antibodies in genital secretions were determined (Corbeil et al., 1998). Both groups were systemically primed twice with the adherence antigen described above; 3 weeks later, one group was given a parenteral booster dose with whole killed cells in Quil A adjuvant while the other group was given an intravaginal booster dose with the same preparation. Both groups cleared the infection earlier than the controls did ($P = 0.02$), but the clearance rates were not significantly different between the two immunized groups (Corbeil et al., 1998). The group that was primed and boosted systemically had higher levels of specific IgG antibodies in vaginal secretions from before challenge until 5 to 7 weeks after challenge than did the group that was boosted intravaginally. After that, the IgG levels in serum and vaginal secretions fell off rather quickly. Vaginally boosted animals, however, had little vaginal IgG antibody and essentially no detectable IgA antibodies to the vaccine antigen at challenge. In these animals, a vaginal anamnestic IgA response was detected by 4 weeks after challenge and remained high until the termination of the experiment at 10 weeks. Controls and parenterally boosted animals had later and much lower vaginal IgA responses. Although both IgG and IgA antibodies to this vaccine antigen appeared to be protective, the greater magnitude and longer duration of the IgA response may be very important in protection in natural cases, when sexual transmission may occur at any time after vaccination.

The detection of high levels of IgA antibodies in vaginal secretions of cattle infected with *C. fetus* or *T. foetus* is noteworthy because vaginal immunization of laboratory animals with other antigens has not usually resulted in much of a local IgA response (McGhee et al., 1992). Perhaps the replicating bacterial or protozoan pathogens induce better IgA responses than soluble antigens do. Others have indicated that the female reproductive tract is not a good inductive site for IgA responses. It has been suggested that oral or nasal immunization may be better than vaginal immunization to induce IgA in the genital tract because of the lack of mucosally associated lymphoid tissue in the female reproductive tract (McGhee et al., 1992). Because high IgA responses occur in the reproductive tracts during trichomoniasis, we examined the vaginal and endometrial mucosa in immunized and control animals for mucosally associated lymphoid tissue, which may have been responsible for induction of local IgA antibodies. Whether heifers mounted an IgA response after immunization and challenge with *T. foetus* or after intravaginal challenge alone, subepithelial mononuclear cell accumulations with underlying lymphoid nodules were seen in the endometrium (Fig. 3) (BonDurant et al., 1993; Anderson et al., 1996; Corbeil et al., 1998). Both immunized and control animals had subepithelial accumulations of mononuclear cells, plasma cells, and eosinophils as well as intraepithelial eosinophils, neutrophils, and mononuclear cells in the vaginal mucosa after challenge. Mucosally associated lymphoid tissue was sometimes detected over mononuclear accumulations (Fig. 4). How-

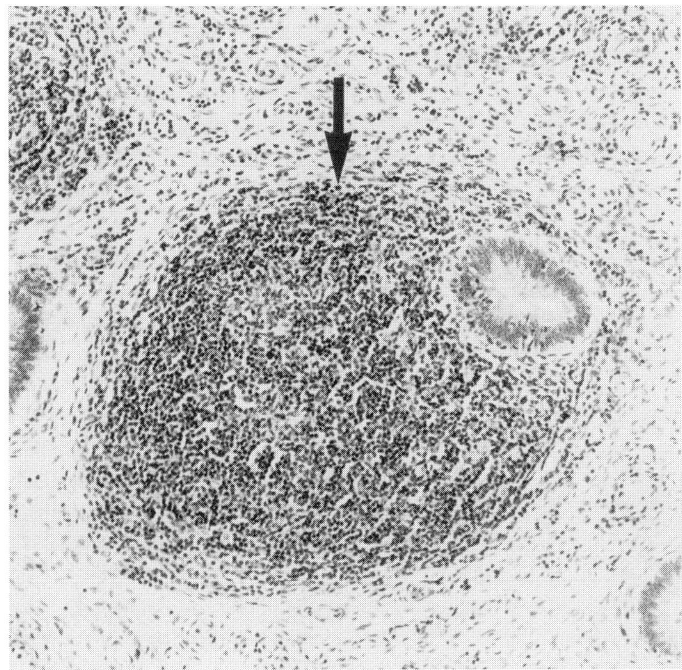

Figure 3 Uterine mucosa of a heifer systemically primed and vaginally boosted with *T. foetus* antigen. Intravaginal challenge with 10^6 *T. foetus* organisms was performed 10 weeks prior to euthanasia. The arrow indicates a lymphoid follicle adjacent to an endometrial gland. *T. foetus*, an anaerobe, is often found in the lumen of such glands, perhaps owing to decreased oxygen tension in this locale. Modified from Corbeil et al. (1998) with the permission of the publisher. Courtesy of M. L. Anderson, University of California, Davis.

ever, vaginal lymphoid aggregates and follicular nodules (Fig. 4) were detected in challenged vaginally boosted and control animals but not in challenged systemically immunized animals (Corbeil et al., 1998), suggesting that systemic immunity (transudated IgG) may prevent the development of local lymphoid nodules. Immunohistochemical studies of infected animals showed that antigen was present in both vaginal and uterine epithelial cells as well as large mononuclear cells below the basement membrane (Rhyan et al., unpublished). These may be antigen-presenting in cells, since Wira and Rossoll (1995a, 1995b) showed that vaginal and uterine epithelial cells can present antigen. Thus, it appears that antigen in epithelial and subepithelial mononuclear cells, the presence of lymphoid nodules or follicles, and diffuse mononuclear infiltrates may form inductive sites that are not present in the naive female reproductive tract. These observa-

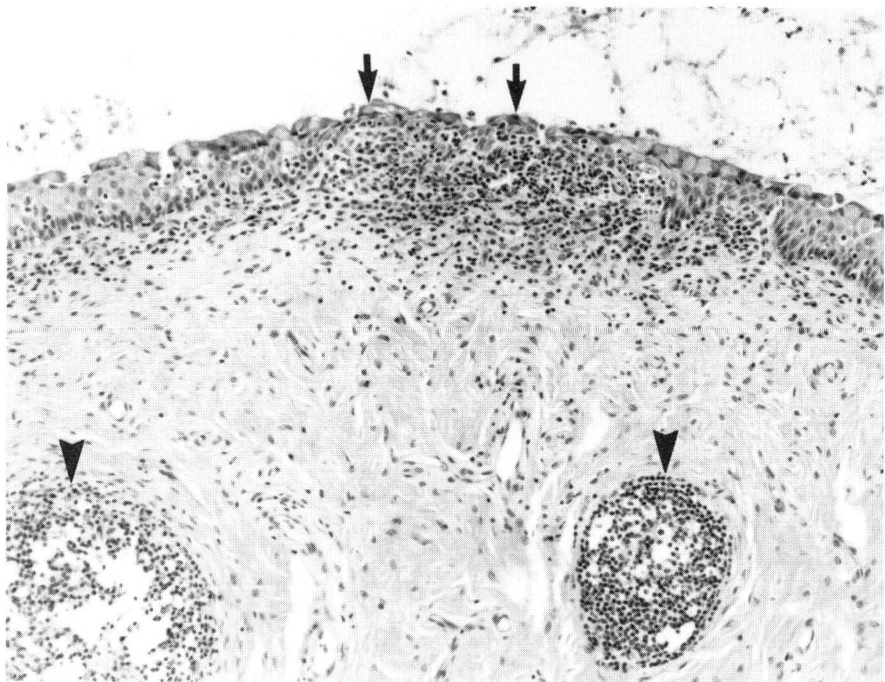

Figure 4 Vaginal mucosa of an animal systemically primed and vaginally boosted with *T. foetus* antigen. Intravaginal challenge with 10^6 *T. foetus* organisms was performed 10 weeks prior to euthanasia and tissue collection. Arrows indicate modified epithelium overlying diffuse infiltration of lymphocytes, as well as plasma cells with fewer neutrophils and eosinophils. Arrowheads show lymphoid follicular nodules in the submucosa. Modified from Corbeil et al. (1998) with permission of the publisher. Courtesy of M. L. Anderson, University of California, Davis.

tions suggest that the infection induced reproductive mucosal lymphoid tissue. In systemically immunized animals, the resolution of infection may have been mediated by vaccine-induced IgG antibodies in secretions before induction of mucosal lymphoid tissue. This hypothesis is supported by the data showing low levels of vaginal IgA in response to systemic immunization with *T. foetus* antigen (Corbeil et al., 1998).

DIAGNOSIS

In the future, control of bovine trichomoniasis may rely on immunoprophylaxis, but currently, accurate diagnosis and management are the basis of prevention and control efforts. Until recently, microscopic examination of wet mounts and culture of reproductive tract secretions have been the only reliable diagnostic methods (Abbitt and Ball, 1978; BonDurant, 1985). However, three negative cultures are necessary to verify that males are not infected, and detectability in females varies with hormonal cycles. Direct microscopic examination is even less sensitive (Skirrow and BonDurant, 1988). Therefore, better diagnostic methods have been a high priority. Early PCR methods were controversial (Appell et al., 1993), but Ho et al. (1994) developed a PCR-based amplification system that could detect as few as 10 organisms in reproductive tract secretions. PCR detected 47 of 52 positive samples (90.4%), whereas culture identified 44 of the 52 positive samples (84.6%). Progress has also been made in the use of antibody-based tests. Conventional serum-based antibody tests have not been useful, since little serum antibody is stimulated by this pathogen (BonDurant et al., 1993; Skirrow and BonDurant, 1990b). We developed an enzyme-linked immunosorbent assay (ELISA) to screen vaginal secretions for IgA antibodies directed against the highly conserved adherence antigen (Corbeil, 1994; Ikeda et al., 1993). Vaginal secretions of experimentally infected heifers were positive by 6 weeks postinfection, and there were no false positives (Ikeda et al., 1995). This test would be useful in individual animals, since fetal loss does not usually occur until after 7 weeks (Parsonson et al., 1976), and also as a herd test. Although conventional serum-based antibody tests have not been useful in the past, a very sensitive hemolytic assay based on *T. foetus* antigen adsorbed to bovine erythrocytes has been described recently (BonDurant et al., 1996). This assay detected antibody in serum by 2 weeks after infection of heifers, and the titers remained high until the termination of the experiment at week 10. The specificity was 95.6%, and sensitivity was 94%. Although culture is still the "gold standard," PCR, vaginal IgA ELISA, and the serum hemolytic assay may also be useful for diagnosis.

CONCLUSIONS

Several observations on bovine trichomoniasis are of interest to researchers investigating the control of human trichomoniasis. First, both diseases are often subclinical. The infections in females continue for weeks or months but are self-limiting. Since the inflammation is not severe, bovine trichomoniasis would not be considered an important problem for the individual infected animal if it were not for abnormal outcomes of pregnancy. However, the embryonic loss usually occurs early (most often toward the end of the first trimester or the beginning of the second trimester) and could go unnoticed if it were not for the return to estrus of individual cows and the decreased pregnancy rate in the herd. Second, the pathogenesis with the two agents may be similar: *T. vaginalis* and *T. foetus* share some virulence factors, including extracellular proteinases, adhesins, and cytotoxins. Nonspecific binding of host Igs and cleavage of IgG probably contribute to temporary evasion of host responses. However, it is possible to overcome this, since convalescent immunity is partially protective and efficacious vaccines have been developed for *T. foetus* infection. The commercially available vaccine for bovine trichomoniasis consists of whole cells. Experimental vaccines containing either membrane proteins or purified surface antigens also stimulate protective immunity. Second-generation subunit vaccines will probably contain antigens and adjuvants that stimulate high levels of protective antibodies; virulence factors that contribute to immune system avoidance will be eliminated.

The relevance of this model for human trichomoniasis is based on both pathogenesis and immunology. The effect of human trichomoniasis infection in first- and second-trimester spontaneous abortion is unstudied. Since *T. foetus* and *T. vaginalis* have such similar virulence factors and metabolisms and such narrow host specificities, it may be that *T. vaginalis* contributes to early abnormal outcomes of pregnancy as well as premature rupture of the membranes and preterm birth/low-birth-weight infants. The role of the male in prevention and control of human trichomoniasis is virtually unstudied because, like bulls, men are usually asymptomatic. Treating infected women without treating their partners is likely to result in reinfection. The success of vaccine-induced immunity in cattle provides hope for the ability of immunoprophylactic or immunotherapeutic approaches to prevent and control human trichomoniasis. These methods might be helpful in preventing reinfection when partners are not treated. Also, if early pregnancy loss is a consequence of human trichomoniasis, primary and secondary prevention strategies are especially important.

Acknowledgments
We thank John Eddow for excellent technical assistance and Sharon McFarlin for preparation of the manuscript. The roles of John Thomford and Mark Anderson in preparation of the material for Figs. 1 and 3, respectively, are also much appreciated. This work is supported in part by USDA grants 9202825 and 8801805 and NIH grants AI32584 and AI33540.

REFERENCES

Abbitt, B., and L. Ball. 1978. Diagnosis of trichomoniasis in pregnant cows by culture of cervico-vaginal mucus. *Theriogenology* **9:**267–270.

Abbitt, B., and G. W. Meyerholz. 1979. *Trichomonas fetus* infection of range bulls in South Florida. *Vet. Med.* **74:**1339–1342.

Akinboade, O. A. 1980. Incidence of bovine trichomoniasis in Nigeria. *Rev. Elev. Med. Vet. Pays Trop.* **33:**381–384.

Anderson, M. L., R. H. BonDurant, R. R. Corbeil, and L. B. Corbeil. 1996. Immune and inflammatory responses to reproductive tract infection with *Tritrichomonas foetus* in immunized and control heifers. *J. Parasitol.* **82:**594–600.

Appell, L. H., W. D. Mickelsen, M. W. Thomas, and W. M. Haromon. 1993. A comparison of techniques used for the diagnosis of *Tritrichomonas foetus* infections in beef bulls. *Agri-Pract.* **14:**30–34.

Aydintug, M. K., P. R. Widders, and R. W. Leid. 1993. Bovine polymorphonuclear leukocyte killing of *Tritrichomonas foetus*. *Infect. Immun.* **61:**2995–3002.
BonDurant, R. H. 1985. Diagnosis, treatment and control of bovine trichomoniasis. *Compend. Contin. Ed. Pract. Vet.* **7:**S179–S188.
BonDurant, R. H., M. L. Anderson, P. Blanchard, D. Hird, C. Danaye-Elmi, C. Palmer, W. M. Sischo, D. Suther, W. Utterback, and B. J. Weigler. 1990. Prevalence of trichomoniasis among California beef herds. *J. Am. Vet. Med. Assoc.* **196:** 1590–1593.
BonDurant, R. H., R. R. Corbeil, and L. B. Corbeil. 1993. Immunization of virgin cows with surface antigen TF1.17 of *Tritrichomonas foetus*. *Infect. Immun.* **61:**1385–1394.
BonDurant, R. H., K. A. Van Hoosear, L. B. Corbeil, and D. Bernoco. 1996. Serological response to in vitro-shed antigen(s) of *Tritrichomonas foetus* in cattle. *Clin. Diagn. Lab. Immunol.* **3:**432–437.
Burgess, D. E. 1986. *Tritrichomonas foetus*: preparation of monoclonal antibodies with effector function. *Exp. Parasitol.* **62:**266–274.
Burgess, D. E. 1988. Clonal and geographic distribution of a surface antigen of *Tritrichomonas foetus*. *J. Protozool.* **35:**119–122.
Burgess, D. E., and C. M. McDonald. 1992. Analysis of adhesion and cytotoxicity of *Tritrichomonas foetus* to mammalian cells by use of monoclonal antibodies. *Infect. Immun.* **60:**4253–4259.
Burgess, D. E., K. F. Knoblock, T. Daughtery, and N. P. Robertson. 1990. Cytotoxic and hemolytic effects of *Tritrichomonas foetus* on mammalian cells. *Infect. Immun.* **58:**3627–3632.
Campero, C. M., N. C. Ballabene, A. C. Cipolla, and A. S. Zamora. 1987. Dual infection of bulls with campylobacteriosis and trichomoniasis: treatment with dimetridazole chlorhydrate. *Aust. Vet. J.* **64:**320–321.
Clark, B. L., I. M. Parsonson, and J. H. Dufty. 1974. Experimental infection of bulls with *Tritrichomonas foetus*. *Aust. Vet. J.* **50:**189–191.
Clark, B. L., J. H. Dufty, and I. M. Parsonson. 1983a. Immunization of bulls against trichomoniasis. *Aust. Vet. J.* **60:**178–179.
Clark, B. L., J. H. Dufty, and I. M. Parsonson. 1983b. The effect of *Tritrichomonas foetus* infection on calving rates in beef cattle. *Aust. Vet. J.* **60:**71–74.
Clark, B. L., D. L. Emery, and J. H. Dufty. 1984. Therapeutic immunization of bulls with the membranes and glycoproteins of *Tritrichomonas foetus* var. *brisbane*. *Aust. Vet. J.* **61:**65–66.
Corbeil, L. B. 1994. Vaccination strategies against *Tritrichomonas foetus*. *Parasitol. Today* **10:**103–106.
Corbeil, L. B. 1995. Use of an animal model of trichomoniasis as a basis for understanding this disease in women. *Clin. Infect. Dis.* **21:**S158–S161.
Corbeil, L. B., and A. J. Winter. 1978. Animal model for the study of genital secretory immune mechanisms: venereal vibriosis in cattle, p. 293–299. *In* G. F. Brooks, E. C. Gotschlich, K. K. Holmes, W. D. Sawyer, and F. E. Young (ed.), *Immunobiology of Neisseria gonorrhoeae.* American Society for Microbiology, Washington, D.C.
Corbeil, L. B., J. R. Duncan, G. G. D. Schurig, C. E. Hall, and A. J. Winter. 1974a. Bovine venereal vibriosis variations in immunoglobulin class of antibodies in genital secretions and serum. *Infect. Immun.* **10:**1084–1090.

Corbeil, L. B., G. D. Schurig, J. R. Duncan, R. R. Corbeil, and A. J. Winter. 1974b. Immunoglobulin classes and biological functions of *Campylobacter (Vibrio) fetus* antibodies in serum and cervicovaginal mucus. *Infect. Immun.* **10:**422–429.

Corbeil, L. B., J. L. Hodgson, D. W. Jones, R. R. Corbeil, P. R. Widders, and L. R. Stephens. 1989. Adherence of *Tritrichomonas foetus* to bovine vaginal epithelial cells. *Infect. Immun.* **57:**2158–2165.

Corbeil, L. B., J. L. Hodgson, and P. R. Widders. 1991. Immunoglobulin binding by *Tritrichomonas foetus. J. Clin. Microbiol.* **29:**2710–2714.

Corbeil, L. B., M. L. Anderson, R. R. Corbeil, J. M. Eddow, and R. H. BonDurant. 1998. Female reproductive tract immunity in bovine trichomoniasis. *Am. J. Reprod. Immunol.* **39:**189–198.

Cotch, M. F., J. G. Pastorek, R. P. Nugent, S. L. Hillier, R. S. Gibbs, D. H. Martin, D. A. Eschenbach, R. E. Delman, J. C. Carey, J. A. Regan, M. A. Krohn, M. A. Klebanoff, A. V. Rao, and G. G. Rhoads. 1997. *Trichomonas vaginalis* associated with low birth weight and preterm delivery. *Sex. Transm. Dis.* **24:**353–360.

de Azevedo, N. L., and W. de Souza. 1993. Fine structure and cytochemistry of *Tritrichomonas foetus* and rat neutrophil interaction. *J. Eukaryot. Microbiol.* **40:**636–642.

Dennett, D. P., R. L. Reece, J. O. Barasa, and R. H. Johnson. 1974. Observations on the incidence and distribution of serotypes of *Tritrichomonas foetus* in beef cattle in North-Eastern Australia. *Aust. Vet. J.* **50:**427–431.

Desiderio, J. V., and S. G. Campbell. 1980. Bovine mammary gland macrophage: isolation, morphologic features, and cytophilic immunoglobulins. *Am. J. Vet. Res.* **41:**1595–1599.

Fleury, F. J., W. S. Van Bergen, R. L. Prentice, J. G. Russell, J. A. Singleton, and J. V. Standard. 1977. Single dose of two grams of metronidazole for *Trichomonas vaginalis* infection. *Am. J. Obstet. Gynecol.* **128:**320–322.

Gibbs, R. S., R. Romero, S. L. Hillier, D. A. Eschenbach, and R. L. Sweet. 1992. A review of premature birth and subclinical infection. *Am. J. Obstet. Gynecol.* **166:** 1515–1528.

Graves, A., and W. A. Gardner, Jr. 1993. Pathogenicity of trichomonas vaginalis. *Clin. Obstet. Gynecol.* **36:**145–152.

Grice, A. C. 1974. Vaginal infection causing spontaneous rupture of the membranes and premature delivery. *Aust. N. Z. J. Obstet. Gynaecol.* **14:**156–158.

Hauth, J. C., R. L. Goldenberg, W. W. Andrews, M. B. DuBard, and R. L. Cooper. 1995. Reduced incidence of preterm delivery with metronidazole and erythromycin in women with bacterial vaginosis. *N. Engl. J. Med.* **333:**1732–1736.

Hillier, S. L., R. P. Nugent, D. A. Eschenbach, M. A. Krohn, R. S. Gibbs, D. H. Martin, M. F. Cotch, R. Edelman, J. G. Pastorek II, A. V. Roa, D. McNellis, J. A. Regan, J. C. Carey, and M. A. Klebanoff, for the Vaginal Infections and Prematurity Study Group. 1995. Association between bacterial vaginosis and preterm delivery of a low-birth-weight infant. *N. Engl. J. Med.* **333:**1737–1742.

Ho, M. S. Y., P. A. Conrad, P. J. Conrad, R. B. LeFebvre, E. Perez, and R. H. BonDurant. 1994. Detection of bovine trichomoniasis with a specific DNA probe and PCR amplification system. *J. Clin. Microbiol.* **32:**98–104.

Hodgson, J. L., D. W. Jones, P. R. Widders, and L. B. Corbeil. 1990. Characterization of *Tritrichomonas foetus* antigens by use of monoclonal antibodies. *Infect. Immun.* **58:**3078–3083.

Hook, R. R., Jr., M. C. St. Claire, L. K. Riley, C. L. Franklin, and C. L. Besch-Williford. 1995. *Tritrichomonas foetus*: comparison of isolate virulence in an estrogenized mouse model. *Exp. Parasitol.* **81:**202–207.

Ikeda, J. S., and L. B. Corbeil. Unpublished data.

Ikeda, J. S., R. H. BonDurant, C. M. Campero, and L. B. Corbeil. 1993. Conservation of a protective surface antigen of *Tritrichomonas foetus*. *J. Clin. Microbiol.* **31:** 3289–3295.

Ikeda, J. S., R. H. BonDurant, and L. B. Corbeil. 1995. Bovine vaginal antibody responses to immunoaffinity-purified surface antigen of *Tritrichomonas foetus*. *J. Clin. Microbiol.* **33:**1158–1163.

Kulda, J., and B. M. Honigberg. 1969. Behavior and pathogenicity of *Tritrichomonas foetus* in chick liver cell cultures. *J. Protozool.* **16:**479–495.

Kvasnicka, W. B., R. E. L. Taylor, J.-C. Huang, D. Hanks, R. J. Tronstad, A. Bosomworth, and M. R. Hall. 1989. Investigations of the incidence of bovine trichomoniasis in Nevada and of the efficacy of immunizing cattle with vaccine containing *Tritrichomonas foetus*. *Theriogenology* **31:**963–971.

Kvasnicka, W. G., D. Hanks, J.-C. Huang, M. R. Hall, D. Sandblom, H.-J. Chu, L. Chavez, and W. M. Acree. 1992. Clinical evaluation of the efficacy of inoculating cattle with a vaccine containing *Tritrichomonas foetus*. *Am. J. Vet. Res.* **53:**2023–2027.

Laga, M., A. Manoka, M. Kivuvu, B. Balele, M. Tuliza, N. Nzila, J. Goeman, F. Behets, V. Batter, M. Alary, W. L. Heyward, R. W. Ryder, and P. Piot. 1993. Nonulcerative sexually transmitted diseases as risk factors for HIV-1 transmission in women: results from a cohort study. *AIDS* **7:**95–102.

Mallinson, D. S., B. C. Lockwood, G. H. Combs, and M. J. North. 1994. Identification and molecular cloning of four cysteine proteinase genes from the pathogenic protozoan *Trichomonas vaginalis*. *Microbiology* **140:**2725–2735.

Mallinson, D. S., J. Livingston, K. M. Appleton, S. J. Lees, G. H. Coombs, and M. J. North. 1995. Multiple cysteine proteinases of the pathogenic protozoan *Tritrichomonas foetus*: identification of seven diverse and differentially expressed genes. *Microbiology* **141:**3077–3085.

McGhee, J. R., J. Mestecky, M. T. Dertzbaugh, and J. H. Eldridge. 1992. The mucosal immune system: from fundamental concepts to vaccine development. *Vaccine* **10:**75–88.

McGroy, T., and G. E. Garber. 1992. Mouse intravaginal infection with *Trichomonas vaginalis* and role of *Lactobacillus acidophilus* in sustaining infection. *Infect. Immun.* **60:**2375–2379.

McGuire, T. C., A. J. Musoke, and T. Kurtti. 1979. Functional properites of bovine IgG1 and IgG2: interaction with complement, macrophages, neutrophils and skin. *Immunology* **38:**249–256.

Miller, R. H., A. J. Guidry, M. J. Paape, A. M. Dulin, and L. A. Fulton. 1988. Relationship between immunoglobulin concentrations in milk and phagocytosis by bovine neutrophils. *Am. J. Vet. Res.* **49:**42–45.

Minkoff, H., A. N. Grunebaum, R. H. Schwarz, J. Feldman, M. Cummings, W. Crombleholme, and W. M. McCormack. 1984. Risk factors for prematurity and premature rupture of membranes: a prospective study of the vaginal flora in pregnancy. *Am. J. Obstet. Gynecol.* **150:**965–972.

Morales, W. J., S. Schorr, and J. Albritton. 1994. Effect of metronidazole in patients with preterm birth in preceding pregnancy and bacterial vaginosis: a placebo-controlled, double-blind study. *Am. J. Obstet. Gynecol.* **171:**345–349.

Müller, M. 1973. Biochemical cytology of trichomonad flagellates. I. Subcellular localization of hydrolases, dehydrogenases, and catalase in *Tritrichomonas foetus*. *J. Cell. Biol.* **57:**453–474.

Parsonson, I. M., B. L. Clark, and J. H. Dufty. 1976. Early pathogenesis and pathobiology of *Tritrichomonas foetus* infection in virgin heifers. *J. Comp. Pathol.* **86:**59–66.

Perez, E., P. A. Conrad, D. Hird, A. Ortuno, J. Chacon, R. BonDurant, and J. Noordhuizen. 1992. Prevalence and risk factors for *Trichomonas foetus* infection in cattle in northeastern Costa Rica. *Prev. Vet. Med.* **14:**155 165.

Read, J. S., and M. A. Klebanoff, for the Vaginal Infections and Prematurity Study Group. 1993. Sexual intercourse during pregnancy and preterm delivery: effects of vaginal microorganisms. *Am. J. Obstet. Gynecol.* **168:**514–519.

Rhyan, J. C., R. H. BonDurant, M. L. Anderson, and L. B. Corbeil. Unpublished data.

Rhyan, J. C., L. L. Stackhouse, and W. J. Quinn. 1988. Fetal and placental lesions in bovine abortion due to *Tritrichomonas foetus*. *Vet. Pathol.* **25:**350–355.

Saurina, G. R., and W. M. McCormack. 1997. Trichomoniasis in pregnancy. *Sex. Transm. Dis.* **24:**361–362.

Schurig, G. D., C. E. Hall, L. B. Corbeil, J. R. Duncan, and A. J. Winter. 1975. Bovine venereal vibriosis: cure of infection in females by systemic immunization. *Infect. Immun.* **11:**245–251.

Schurig, G. G., J. R. Duncan, and A. J. Winter. 1978. Elimination of genital vibriosis in female cattle by systemic immunization with killed cells or cell-free extracts of *Campylobacter fetus*. *J. Infect. Dis.* **138:**463–472.

Skirrow, S. 1987. Identification of trichomonad-carrier cows. *J. Am. Vet. Med. Assoc.* **191:**553–554.

Skirrow, S. Z., and R. H. BonDurant. 1988. Bovine trichomoniasis. *Vet. Bull.* **58:**591–603.

Skirrow, S. Z., and R. H. BonDurant. 1990a. Induced *Tritrichomonas foetus* infection in beef heifers. *J. Am. Vet. Med. Assoc.* **196:**885–889.

Skirrow, S. Z., and R. H. BonDurant. 1990b. Immunoglobulin isotype of specific antibodies in reproductive tract secretions and sera in *Tritrichomonas foetus*-infected heifers. *Am. J. Vet. Res.* **51:**645–653.

Talbot, J. A., K. Neilsen, and L. B. Corbeil. 1991. Cleavage of proteins of reproductive secretions by extracellular proteinases of *Tritrichomonas foetus*. *Can. J. Microbiol.* **37:**384–390.

Wilson, S. K., E. T. Gaudy, and D. Goodwin. 1979. The prevalence of trichomoniasis of Oklahoma beef bulls. *Bovine Pract.* **14:**109–110.

Winter, A. J. 1978. Systemic immunization: efficacy in prevention and termination of venereal vibriosis in cattle, p. 300–302. *In* G. F. Brooks, E. C. Gotschlich, K. K. Holmes, W. D. Sawyer, and F. E. Young (ed.), *Immunobiology of Neisseria gonorrhoeae.* American Society for Microbiology, Washington, D.C.

Wira, C. R., and R. M. Rossoll. 1995a. Antigen-presenting cells in the female reproductive tract: influence of sex hormones on antigen presentation in the vagina. *Immunology* **84:**505–508.

Wira, C. R., and R. M. Rossoll. 1995b. Antigen-presenting cells in the female reproductive tract: influence of the estrous cycle on antigen presentation by uterine epithelial and stromal cells. *Endocrinology* **136:**4526–4534.

Wira, C. R., and C. P. Sandoe. 1987. Specific IgA and IgG antibodies in the secretions of the female reproductive tract: effects of immunization and estradiol on expression of this response *in vivo. J. Immunol.* **138:**4159–4164.

Wira, C. R., and C. P. Sandoe. 1989. Effect of uterine immunization and oestradiol on specific IgA and IgG antibodies in uterine, vaginal and salivary secretions. *Immunology* **68:**24–30.

20
Simian Model for Infection-Associated Preterm Labor

Michael G. Gravett and Miles J. Novy

Preterm labor that results in premature birth is the most common cause of perinatal mortality, accounting for 80% of perinatal deaths which are not attributable to congenital malformations (Rush et al., 1976). A growing body of evidence suggests that maternal genital tract infection, particularly intrauterine and intra-amniotic, may be an important and potentially preventable cause of prematurity. Bacteria indigenous to the lower genital tract have been recovered from the amniotic fluid of 5 to 20% of women in preterm labor with intact fetal membranes (Romero et al., 1991a). Furthermore, a high proportion of women in preterm labor with positive amniotic fluid cultures are refractory to standard tocolytic therapy and experience rapid preterm delivery (62.5%, in contrast to 13% of women with sterile amniotic fluid) (Romero et al., 1991a). This suggests that the pathophysiology of preterm labor associated with intra-amniotic infection is different from that of idiopathic preterm labor.

There is now considerable evidence to suggest that cytokines participate in the pathogenesis of infection-associated preterm labor. These inflammatory mediators include interleukin-1 (IL-1), interleukin-6 (IL-6), interleukin-8 (IL-8), and tumor necrosis factor (TNF) and are produced by macrophages and decidual cells in response to a wide variety of bacteria or bacterial products. A role for selected cytokines in the onset of preterm parturition is based upon the following observations: (i) elevated concen-

Michael G. Gravett, Division of Reproductive Sciences, Oregon Regional Primate Research Center, and Departments of Obstetrics and Gynecology, Legacy Emanuel Hospital and Health Center, and Oregon Health Sciences University, Beaverton and Portland, OR 97227. **Miles J. Novy,** Division of Reproductive Sciences, Oregon Regional Primate Research Center, and Department of Obstetrics and Gynecology, Oregon Health Sciences University, Beaverton and Portland, OR 97227.

Sexually Transmitted Diseases and Adverse Outcomes of Pregnancy
Edited by P. J. Hitchcock, H. T. MacKay, J. N. Wasserheit, and R. Binder
©1999 American Society for Microbiology, Washington, D.C.

trations of IL-1, IL-6, TNF, and prostaglandins are found in the amniotic fluid of patients with intra-amniotic infection and preterm labor (Hillier et al., 1993; Romero et al., 1987, 1989a, 1989b, 1990); (ii) bacterial products stimulate the production of IL-1, IL-6, and TNF by human decidua (Casey et al., 1989; Hillier et al., 1993; Romero et al., 1989c); (iii) these cytokines, in turn, stimulate the production of prostaglandins by in vitro amnion and decidual explants (Mitchell et al., 1991b; Romero et al., 1989b, 1989d); and (iv) systemic administration of recombinant IL-1 to pregnant mice induces preterm labor, which can be prevented by pretreatment with IL-1 receptor antagonist (IL-1ra) protein (Romero et al., 1991b; Romero and Tartakovsky, 1992).

Although the studies cited suggest a connection between intrauterine infection and preterm delivery, no study to date has been sufficiently comprehensive to provide convincing evidence for a causal relationship. The cross-sectional nature of human studies and ethical considerations preclude serial sampling of amniotic fluid in the same patient. This has limited our ability to establish the temporal relationships among bacterial colonization of amniotic fluid, the production of inflammatory mediators, and the evolution of preterm labor in women. As a result, it has been argued by some investigators that accumulation of cytokines and microbial invasion of the amniotic fluid are the consequence of preterm labor rather than its cause (Cox et al., 1993). According to this hypothesis, the accumulation of cytokines and prostaglandins, characteristic of an inflammatory response in amniotic fluid during labor, is the result of exposure of the decidua parietalis and the fetal membranes to bacterial products in the vagina; this occurs after cervical dilatation and not before (MacDonald and Casey, 1993).

Animal models involving pregnant mice (Romero et al., 1991b), rabbits (Dombroski et al., 1990; McDuffie et al., 1992), or sheep (Howie et al., 1989) strengthen the causal link between intrauterine infection and premature birth. However, these studies have largely restricted their design to cross-sectional observations or have relied on pooled amniotic fluid samples obtained from several fetuses. Consequently, they have not clearly defined the sequence of events by which intrauterine infection causes premature contractions, cervical changes, and ultimately preterm delivery. Furthermore, in lower mammalian animal models, both placentation and the hormonal events surrounding parturition differ from humans, thereby limiting generalizations (Challis and Olson, 1988).

PRIMATE MODEL IN INTRA-AMNIOTIC INFECTION

Nonhuman primates have been used to study a wide range of lower (Moller and Freundt, 1983; Street et al., 1983) and upper (Patton et al., 1987) genital tract infections in the nonpregnant state. During pregnancy, both the rhesus macaque, *Macaca mulatta* (Larson et al., 1981), and the pigtail macaque, *Ma-*

caca nemestrina (Rubens et al., 1991), have been used to study intra-amniotic infection and resultant neonatal sepsis. To examine the temporal and quantitative relationships between intra-amniotic infection and preterm labor, we have developed a simian model involving chronically catheterized rhesus monkeys (*M. mulatta*) with timed gestations. The model provides a useful means of studying the in vivo immune, endocrine, and even paracrine interactions in the intrauterine space. It offers several advantages over experimental models in lower mammalian species (Table 1). Rhesus placentation is hemochorial, and the endocrine events surrounding parturition are qualitatively similar to those in human pregnancy (Challis et al., 1988; Novy and Haluska, 1988). Samples of maternal and fetal blood and amniotic fluid can readily be obtained in a serial fashion from individual animals. Uterine activity can be continuously monitored and correlated with indices of infection and inflammatory mediators. Finally, the cervical-vaginal microbial flora of rhesus monkeys is remarkably similar to that of women.

In collaboration with Sharon Hillier, we have performed preliminary studies of the cervical-vaginal flora of 31 pregnant rhesus monkeys at the Oregon Regional Primate Research Center (Gravett, unpublished). A mean of 8 (range, 3 to 14) bacterial species were recovered from each animal. Facultative microorganisms were recovered from 29 (94%) of the 31 animals, and anaerobes were also recovered from 29 (94%). The species of bacteria recovered, and their isolation rates, were similar to the human cervical-

Table 1 Advantages and disadvantages of a nonhuman primate model for preterm delivery and intrauterine infection[a]

- Advantages
  - Similarities to human pregnancy
    - Adequate amniotic fluid volume
    - Singleton gestation
    - Long gestational period (167 days)
    - Hemochorial placentation
    - Similar endocrinology of parturition
    - Circadian uterine activity rhythm
  - Experimental
    - Longitudinal sampling of individuals
    - Simultaneous sampling of maternal, fetal, and amniotic compartments
    - Continuous quantitative assessment of uterine activity
- Disadvantages
  - Expensive
  - Limited availability

[a] Reproduced from Gravett et al. (1994b) with permission of the publisher.

vaginal flora (Table 2). Interestingly, potentially pathogenic bacteria implicated in human intra-amniotic infection (including streptococci, *Escherichia coli*, and anaerobes) were recovered from the monkeys with similar isolation rates to those in humans. Bacterial vaginosis, previously associated with preterm labor (Gravett et al., 1986; Hillier et al., 1995) and intra-amniotic infection (Silver et al., 1989) in women, was identified by Gram stain criteria (Nugent et al., 1991) in 8 of 31 monkeys (26%), a prevalence similar to that reported in women, and was likewise associated with increased intravaginal concentrations of *Gardnerella vaginalis*, *Mobiluncus* spp., and anaerobes.

Table 2 Cervicovaginal microbial flora among 31 pregnant rhesus macaques at the Oregon Regional Primate Research Center

Microorganism	No. with isolate	% of total no. (n = 31)
Facultative bacteria		
Diphtheroids	28	90
Lactobacillus sp.	10	32
Streptococcus, viridans group	26	84
Streptococcus, beta-hemolytic	2	6
Enterococcus sp.	6	19
Staphylococcus, coagulase negative	14	45
Staphylococcus aureus	4	13
Gardnerella vaginalis	9	29
Escherichia coli	1	3
Haemophilus sp.	1	3
Other gram-negative rods	2	6
Anaerobic bacteria		
Bacteroides sp.	20	65
Bacteroides, black pigmented	12	39
Bacteroides ureolyticus	11	35
Prevotella bivia	4	13
Bacteroides fragilis group	4	13
Prevotella disiens	3	10
Clostridium sp.	4	13
Eubacterium sp.	4	13
Fusobacterium nucleatum	1	3
Mobiluncus curtisii sp.	6	19
Peptostreptococcus prevotii	10	32
Peptostreptococcus asaccharolyticus	6	19
Peptostreptococcus anaerobius	11	35
Peptococcus niger	5	16
Propionibacterium sp.	4	13

In our model, on approximately day 110 of gestation (with term being 167 days), pregnant animals are conditioned to a jacket-and-tether system (Ducsay et al., 1988). After conditioning, intrauterine surgery is performed at or near 120 days gestation under halothane anesthesia (Haluska et al., 1987). Maternal femoral arterial and venous catheters, fetal arterial and venous catheters, two open-ended intra-amniotic pressure catheters, myometrial electromyographic electrodes, and fetal electrocardiographic electrodes are surgically implanted (Fig. 1). All animals receive terbutaline sulfate (1 mg intravenously over 3 to 5 h, twice daily) for 1 to 5 days after surgery to control postoperative uterine irritability. The animals also receive cefazolin (250 mg intravenously, every 12 h), which is discontinued at least 72 h prior to infection or other experimentation.

Intra-Amniotic Inoculation of Bacteria

After postoperative stabilization for 10 days (approximately day 135 of gestation), we have reproducibly established intra-amniotic infection by inoculation, through one of the intra-amniotic pressure catheters, of 10^6 CFU of group B streptococci, type III (Gravett et al., 1994a). Both before and after inoculation, amniotic fluid samples are collected serially from all animals for quantitative bacterial cultures, Gram stain of uncentrifuged fluid, leukocyte analysis by hemocytometer, cytokine (IL-1β, IL-6, and TNF) (by enzyme-linked immunoassay or bioassay) and prostaglandin (by enzyme-linked immunoassay) concentrations, and sex steroid hormone concentrations by radioimmunoassay. Fetal and maternal blood are also serially sampled for a complete blood cell analysis and for sex steroid hormone concentrations. The fetal electrocardiogram and uterine activity (electromyelographic and intra-amniotic pressure) are continuously recorded from the time of surgery until delivery. The uterine contractility is recorded as the area under the contraction curve per hour and is expressed as the hourly contraction area (HCA) in mmHg · seconds per hour. Consistency, effacement, and dilatation of the maternal cervix and maternal rectal temperature are also determined.

We used group B streptococci in our initial experiments because they are indigenous to both humans and rhesus monkeys and are important contributors to both human intra-amniotic infection and neonatal infectious morbidity.

Uterine Activity during Intra-Amniotic Infection

Following intra-amniotic inoculation with 10^6 group B streptococci, there is rapid exponential growth within the amniotic fluid. Associated with this infection, there are sequential increases in the levels of cytokines and prostaglandins in amniotic fluid and uterine activity. Increases in uterine contractility from preinoculation HCA levels of 0 to 100 mmHg · s/h rise to

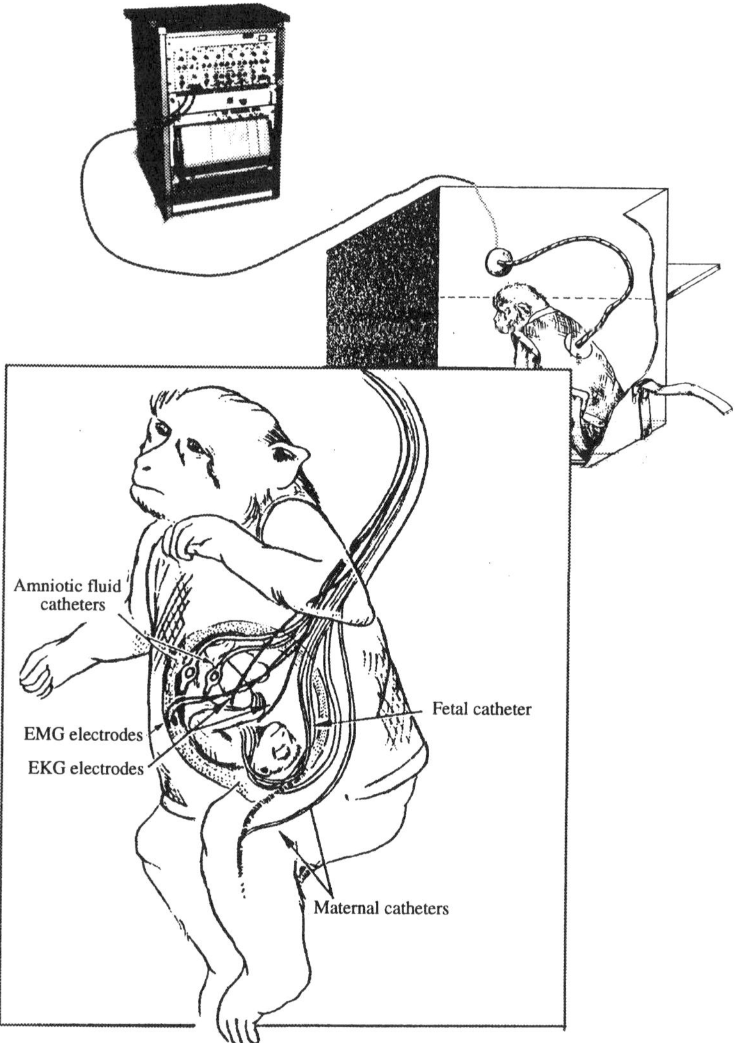

Figure 1 Diagrammatic representation of the chronic jacket-and-tether system utilized to study intrauterine infection in the rhesus macaque.

peak levels of 10,000 to 20,000 mmHg · s/h at a mean of 28 h (range, 14 to 40 h) after inoculation (Table 3). The marked increase in uterine contractility led to progressive cervical effacement and dilatation in infected animals. To illustrate these temporal relationships, data from a single representative monkey with intra-amniotic infection are depicted in Fig. 2. In contrast, inoculation with 10^6 CFU of heat-inactivated group B streptococci does not

Table 3 Summary of bacterial counts and cytokine and prostaglandin concentrations in amniotic fluid and uterine activity in experimental intra-amniotic infection

Parameter	Value at:			
	Preinoculation	Inoculation	Onset of contractions	Delivery
GBS (CFU/ml)[a]	n.g.	5×10^6	8×10^9	1×10^{10}
HCA (mmHg · s/h)[b]	100	150	4,600	12,500
TNF (pg/ml)[b]	52	29	>20,000	>20,000
IL-1β (pg/ml)[b]	<20	<20	1,504	2,467
IL-1ra (ng/ml)[b]	14.8	13	66.4	102.4
IL-6 (ng/ml)[b]	12.9	9.9	49.6	46
PGE_2 (pg/ml)[b]	494	510	16,046	15,274
$PGF_{2\alpha}$ (pg/ml)[b]	215	280	5,547	5,490

[a] Geometric mean titer of group B streptococci (GBS).
[b] Expressed as median values.

result in an increase in uterine activity, suggesting that an active infection which elicits a progressive inflammatory response is necessary to induce preterm labor.

Clinical Correlation and Histopathologic Findings

We have also evaluated the relationships of common clinical parameters of intra-amniotic infection and the onset of uterine contractions and delivery in four animals (Gravett et al., 1994a). None of four mothers with intra-amniotic infection were febrile ($T > 102°F$) or had leukocytosis (defined as a peripheral leukocyte count of >15,000 or the presence of greater than 1% immature neutrophils) at the onset of contractions. At the time of delivery, only one of four mothers had become febrile, but all had developed leukocytosis. No fetus developed tachycardia, periodic heart rate decelerations, or leukocytosis by the onset of labor, but two fetuses did develop leukocytosis near the time of delivery. Despite the absence of clinical indicators of infection, necropsy revealed bacteremia and pneumonitis in all four fetuses and meningitis in three of the four. Group B streptococci were cultured from fetal lungs and blood in four fetuses and from the meninges in three of the four fetuses.

These data closely parallel earlier work by Larson et al. (1981), in which none of 19 rhesus monkeys given experimental intra-amniotic infection by intra-amniotic inoculation of group B streptococci became "clinically ill." These data also parallel the experience in humans, in which nearly half of otherwise asymptomatic women with intact fetal membranes in preterm

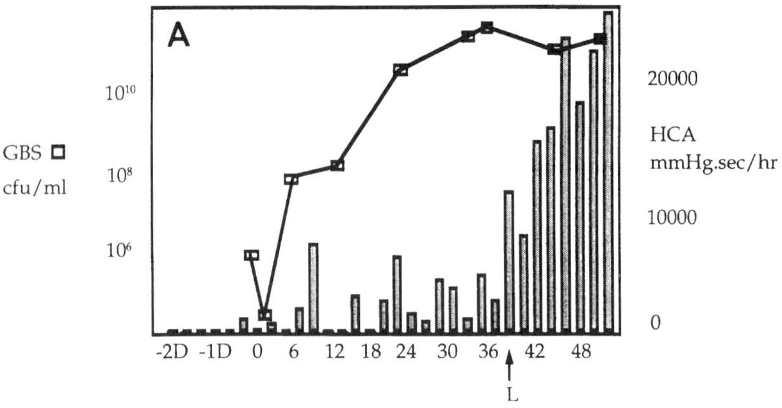
A
GBS
cfu/ml
10¹⁰
10⁸
10⁶
20000
HCA
mmHg.sec/hr
10000
0
-2D -1D 0 6 12 18 24 30 36 42 48
L
Hours After Inoculation (hrs)

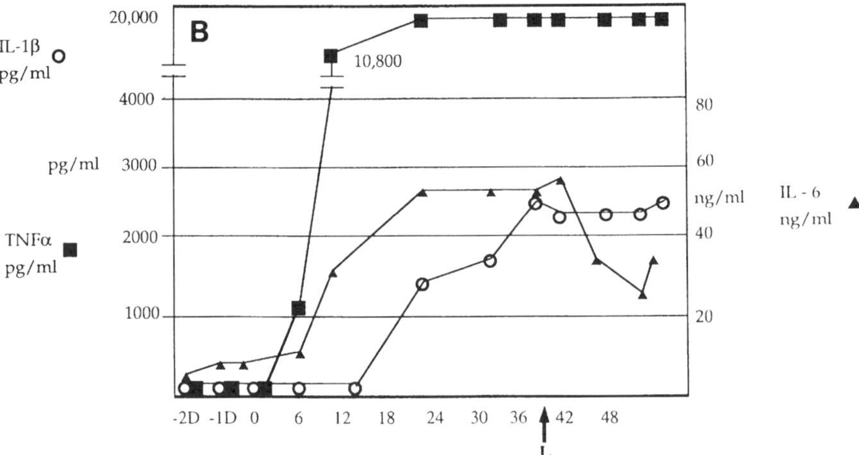
B
IL-1β
pg/ml
20,000
10,800
4000
pg/ml
3000
2000
1000
TNFα
pg/ml
80
60
ng/ml
40
20
IL - 6
ng/ml
-2D -1D 0 6 12 18 24 30 36 42 48
L
Hours After Inoculation (hrs)

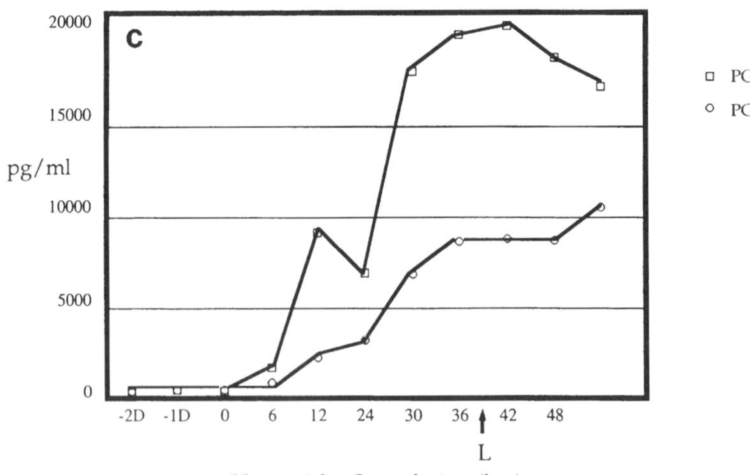
C
20000
15000
pg/ml
10000
5000
0
PGE₂
PGF₂α
-2D -1D 0 6 12 24 30 36 42 48
L
Hours After Inoculation (hrs)

labor with positive amniotic fluid cultures develop clinical chorioamnionitis by the time of delivery (Romero et al., 1991a). Together, these data point to the need to develop more sensitive and specific noninvasive tests for intra-amniotic infection.

Cytokines in Intra-Amniotic Infection

The concentrations of TNF, IL-1β, and IL-6 in amniotic fluid all rise dramatically following experimental intra-amniotic infection and prior to increases in uterine contractility, as we have reported (Gravett et al., 1994a). These temporal relationships are illustrated for a single animal in Fig. 2B. TNF concentrations in amniotic fluid rose from 52 pg/ml (range, 0 to 81 pg/ml) prior to inoculation to greater than 20,000 pg/ml at an average of 9 h (range, 6 to 14 h) after inoculation and 20 h (range, 8 to 34 h) before increases in uterine contractility (Table 3). Increases in TNF concentrations in amniotic fluid preceded increases in IL-1β or IL-6 concentrations in amniotic fluid by 4 to 8 h in all infected animals and represented the earliest marker of infection in our study.

After the rise in TNF concentrations in amniotic fluid, there were increases in both IL-1β and IL-6 concentrations in amniotic fluid. An initial rise in IL-6 concentrations occurred an average of 15 h (range, 12 to 22 h) after inoculation and 13 h (range, 2 to 28 h) prior to increases in uterine contractions. Similar elevations in the IL-1β concentration occurred 18 h (range, 12 to 24 h) after inoculation and preceded increases in uterine contractility by an average of 10 h (range, 2 to 18 h). Further increases in IL-1β concentrations to 2,467 pg/ml (range, 1,417 to 2,708 pg/ml) occurred at delivery. These data are summarized in Table 3. The elevations in cytokine levels in amniotic fluid observed after experimental infection are consistent with those reported in pregnant women with infection-associated labor (Hillier et al., 1993; Romero et al., 1989a, 1989b, 1990).

In contrast to preterm labor induced by intra-amniotic infection in our model, spontaneous parturition near term in control animals was not as-

Figure 2 Temporal relationship between intra-amniotic infection, cytokine and prostaglandin concentrations in amniotic fluid, and uterine activity for a single representative monkey. The clinical onset of labor is denoted by an arrow and L. Reproduced from Gravett et al. (1994a) with permission of the publisher. (A) Quantitative relationship between group B streptococcus (GBS) concentrations in amniotic fluid and uterine contractility, expressed as the HCA under the amniotic fluid-pressure curve. (B) Concentrations of IL-1β, TNF, and IL-6 in amniotic fluid before and after infection. (C) Concentrations of PGE_2 and $PGF_{2\alpha}$ in amniotic fluid before and after infection.

sociated with increases in concentrations of either interleukin-1β or TNF in amniotic fluid above low basal levels, and only modest increases in IL-6 were observed (Gravett et al., 1994a).

Prostaglandins and Their Regulation by Cytokines

Following intra-amniotic infection, increases in prostaglandin E_2 (PGE_2) and $PGF_{2\alpha}$ concentrations in amniotic fluid occur in parallel with increases in cytokine concentrations in amniotic fluid and precede increases in uterine contractility (Fig. 2C). The most striking increase is in the PGE_2 concentration, which rises >15,000 pg/ml at delivery (Table 3). Similar but smaller increases in the $PGF_{2\alpha}$ concentration also occur. These prostaglandin concentrations are severalfold higher than the prostaglandin concentrations seen among comparison animals in spontaneous parturition near term (Fig. 3). These results are consistent with human in vitro studies that have demonstrated that levels of PGE_2 and $PGF_{2\alpha}$ are higher in the fetal membrane, decidua, and placenta during chorioamnionitis (Bernal et al., 1989; van der Elst et al., 1991). The more striking increase in the PGE_2 concentration dur-

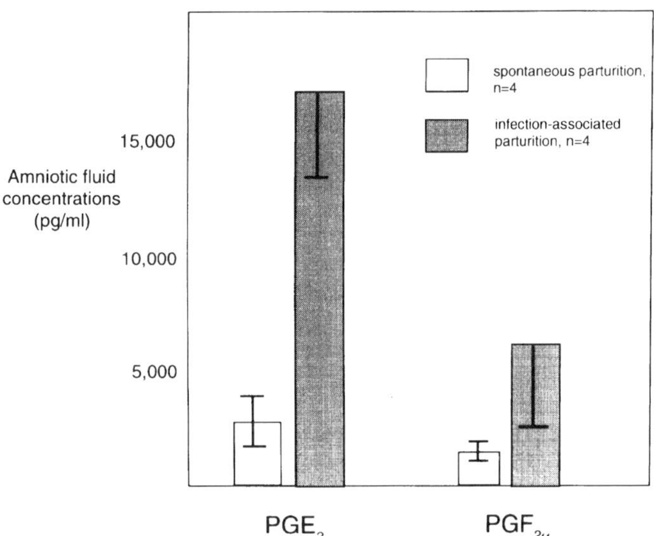

Figure 3 Prostaglandin concentrations in amniotic fluid for spontaneous ($n = 4$) and infection-induced parturition ($n = 4$). Data are expressed as mean and standard deviation. Concentrations observed among animals with infection-induced labor were greater than those with spontaneous labor for both PGE_2 (17,851 ± 4,548 and 2,765 + 782 pg/ml, respectively; $P < 0.05$) and for $PGF_{2\alpha}$ (6,431 ± 4,026 and 708 ± 89 pg/ml, respectively; $P < 0.05$). Comparisons were made by the Mann-Whitney U test. Reproduced from Gravett et al. (1994b) with permission of the publisher.

ing chorioamnionitis may reflect the preferential production of PGE_2 by the infected amnion and accumulation within amniotic fluid (Novy and Liggins, 1980). In contrast, $PGF_{2\alpha}$ is preferentially synthesized by the decidua.

The mechanisms responsible for the increased prostaglandin concentrations in amniotic fluid observed during intrauterine infection have been the subject of investigations (Mitchell et al., 1991a). The clinical and experimental elevation of prostaglandin and cytokine levels supports the theory that infection induces preterm labor by mechanisms that involve the synthesis and release of prostaglandins or leukotrienes. Direct stimulation of prostaglandin synthesis in the amnion, chorion, and decidua by proinflammatory cytokines (e.g., IL-1β and TNF), as has been demonstrated in vitro (Mitchell et al., 1991a, 1991b; Romero et al., 1989b, 1989d), is probably responsible for the increased prostaglandin concentrations in amniotic fluid. The enhanced expression of IL-1 receptors may also be an important step in regulating the effects of cytokines on amnion PGE_2 production (Bry et al., 1993).

Although relatively high concentrations of cytokines are required to stimulate amnion or decidual prostaglandin release, these concentrations can be found in the amniotic fluid of infected patients and in our experimental intra-amniotic infection model in rhesus monkeys. Since there is little or no evidence that cytokines directly stimulate myometrial contractions (Oshiro et al., 1993), it follows that IL-1, IL-6, and TNF contribute to the generation of uterine contractions by stimulating the production of prostaglandins or lipoxygenase products by intrauterine tissues.

INTERLEUKIN-1β INTRA-AMNIOTIC INFUSION

To clarify the temporal sequence of events and the quantitative relationships among IL-1β, TNF, prostaglandins, and uterine contractility in the absence of infection, we have used chronically instrumented rhesus monkeys in which myometrial contractility was induced by the intra-amniotic infusion of graded doses of human recombinant IL-1β (Baggia et al., 1996). On days 128 to 138 of gestation, four monkeys underwent serial intra-amniotic infusions of 2, 5, and 10 to 20 μg of recombinant human IL-1β. Each infusion was continued for 2 h, and subsequent infusions were at least 48 h later. Amniotic fluid was serially sampled, both before and after infusion, for IL-1β, TNF, and PGE_2 and $PGF_{2\alpha}$ by specific assays, and uterine activity was continuously recorded.

Intra-amniotic concentrations of IL-1β rose dramatically following infusion (Fig. 4). This was rapidly followed by the appearance of TNF in the amniotic fluid, with maximal levels reached 5 h after initiation of the infusion. Both IL-1β and TNF were rapidly cleared from the amniotic fluid and returned to baseline concentrations by 24 to 48 h. Increases in the PGE_2 and $PGE_{2\alpha}$ concentrations paralleled those of the two cytokines. Stimulation

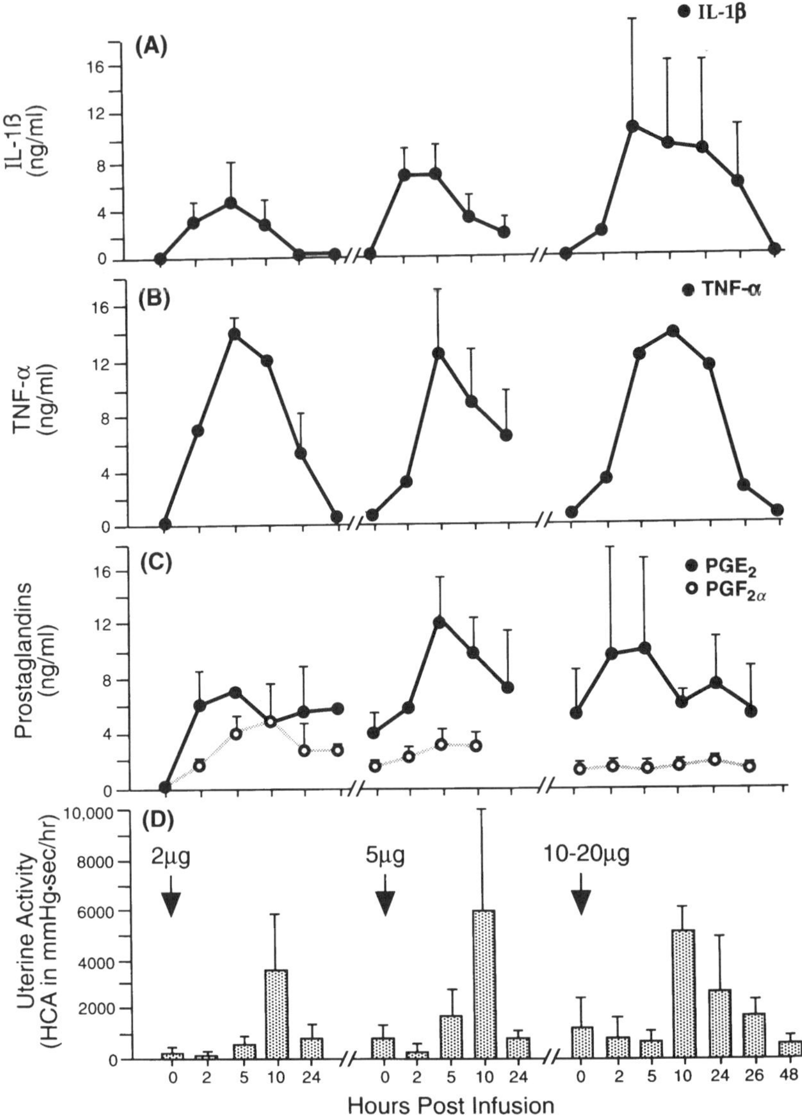

Figure 4 Concentrations of IL-1β (A), TNF (B), and PGE_2 and $PGF_{2\alpha}$ (C) in amniotic fluid and uterine activity (D) after serial intra-amniotic infusions of 2, 5, 10, or 20 μg of recombinant human IL-1α in four catheterized uninfected animals. Uterine activity is expressed as the HCA under the amniotic fluid-pressure curve. Reproduced from Baggia et al. (1996) with permission of the publisher.

of uterine contractility from preinfusion levels of 200 HCA to peak levels of 7,000 HCA occurred an average of 6 to 10 h after IL-1β infusion, usually abated by 22 h after infusion, and did not result in frank labor. These data provide direct in vivo evidence that IL-1β (and/or TNF) is a prime agonist in inducing prostaglandin production within the amniotic cavity.

To further clarify the role of prostaglandins and cytokines in uterine activity, we have recently repeated these studies in three monkeys with indomethacin pretreatment to inhibit prostaglandin synthesis (Sadowsky et al., 1996). IL-1β was infused into each animal twice: (i) with indomethacin pretreatment (50 mg orally twice daily for 5 days) and (ii) without indomethacin pretreatment. Following IL-1β infusion, the concentrations of IL-1β in amniotic fluid increased similarly in the animals with and without indomethacin treatment (Table 4). However, increases in prostaglandin concentrations in amniotic fluid did not occur, nor were there increases in uterine activity with indomethacin treatment. These data further support the hypothesis that increases in uterine activity with IL-1β infusion (and presumably intra-amniotic infection) are mediated through prostaglandins or other cyclooxygenase derivatives and suggest that indomethacin or other cyclooxygenase inhibitors may be useful in inhibiting cytokine-induced uterine activity in the setting of infection.

Interleukin-1 Receptor Antagonist

Because infection-associated preterm birth appears to be initiated by cytokine activation, the presence within the amniotic sac of modulators capable of down-regulating cytokine production may be an essential component of immunoregulatory mechanisms operational during pregnancy. Several such naturally occurring down-regulating modulators have been described (Di-

Table 4 Mean IL-1β and prostaglandin concentrations in amniotic fluid and uterine activity following intra-amniotic IL-1β infusion with and without indomethacin pretreatment[a]

Parameter	Value with:	
	Indomethacin pretreatment	No indomethacin pretreatment
IL-1β (pg/ml)	15,187 ± 3,602	12,112 ± 3,354
PGE_2 (pg/ml)	569 ± 410	7,591 ± 4,109[b]
$PGF_{2\alpha}$ (pg/ml)	237 ± 125	1,480 ± 659[b]
Uterine activity (HCA, mmHg · s/h)	285 ± 50	5,135 ± 989[b]

[a] Adapted from Sadowsky et al. (1996).
[b] $P < 0.05$ (ANOVA).

narello et al., 1993). These include soluble receptors to IL-1 and to TNF, transforming growth factor β (TGF-β), and IL-1ra. IL-1ra is a naturally occurring inhibitor of both IL-1α and IL-1β. IL-1ra competes with IL-1α and IL-1β for binding to IL-1 receptors and can inhibit IL-1-induced responses such as IL-G, collagenase, and PGE_2 production and T-lymphocyte proliferation (McIntyre et al., 1991). However, since only a small percentage of occupied IL-1 receptors are needed to elicit a biological response, a 100- to 1,000-fold molar excess of IL-1ra is necessary to inhibit IL-1 bioactivity.

We have been able to detect IL-1ra by enzyme-linked immunoassay in the amniotic fluids of all monkeys tested (Witkin et al., 1994). The median concentration was 15 ng/ml (range, 7.5 to 28 ng/ml). Human amniotic fluid also contains IL-1ra at a similar concentration (Romero et al., 1992). In the monkey model, intra-amniotic IL-1ra production was readily inducible by intra-amniotic IL-1β infusion or by intra-amniotic infection with 10^6 CFU of group B streptococci (for infection, refer to Table 3). In both cases, the IL-1ra/IL-1 ratio in amniotic fluid decreased from >6,000:1 prior to treatment to <40:1 after treatment. This change was accompanied by the initiation of myometrial contractions (Table 5). A recent study has documented an increase in IL-1ra concentrations in human fetal and amniotic fluid compartments with microbial invasion, thus confirming our results obtained with rhesus monkeys (Greig et al., 1995).

To assess the maternal and fetal contributions to IL-1ra concentrations in amniotic fluid, the levels of this compound in maternal and fetal plasma were also determined. Il-1ra was not detected in maternal plasma at any time before or after IL-1β infusion or streptococcal infection. In marked contrast, both treatments resulted in the rapid appearance of IL-1ra, but not IL-1β, in the fetal plasma. The subsequent drop in IL-1ra levels in the fetal circulation was followed by a rise in the IL-1ra concentration in amniotic fluid.

Table 5 Median concentrations of IL-1β and IL-1ra in amniotic fluid and uterine activity following experimental intra-amniotic infection[a]

Stage	IL-1β concn (ng/ml)	IL-1ra concn (ng/ml)	IL-1ra/IL-1β ratio[b]	HCA (mmHg · s/h)
Preinoculation	0.002	13.4	>6,000:1	100
Onset of contractions	1.5	45.3	30:1	6,150
Delivery	2.5	83.9	34:1	12,260

[a]Reprinted from Gravett et al. (1994b) with permission of the publisher.
[b]1,000:1 ratio necessary to inhibit IL-1β.

Thus, two opposing mechanisms appear to be in place during pregnancy. During an uneventful pregnancy, the large excess of IL-1ra in amniotic fluid inhibits induction of the cytokine cascade and PGE_2 production and thereby prevents premature expulsion of the fetus. Small perturbations in the intra-amniotic cytokine response, due to a low-level infection or to an immune response between the semi-allogeneic fetus and its mother, are prevented from inducing premature contractions by the presence of high levels of IL-1ra. The ability of the fetus to produce additional IL-1ra in response to IL-1β or a bacterial infection further suggests that the fetus plays an active role in down-regulating immune system activation within the amniotic cavity. In contrast, in the face of an overwhelming intra-amniotic infection or high levels of IL-1, the inhibitory capacity of IL-1ra is exceeded and labor is rapidly initiated to remove the fetus from a hostile environment. The threshold for the triggering of these two opposing events undoubtedly varies among individuals and would be expected to be influenced by differences in the immune system capacity for IL-1ra production relative to IL-1 production. Whether pregnant women who are low producers of IL-1ra and/or high producers of IL-1 would benefit from administration of exogenous IL-1ra remains to be determined. In mice, injection of a large excess of IL-1ra prior to injection of IL-1 inhibits cytokine-induced preterm labor (Romero and Tartakovsky, 1992).

FETOPLACENTAL STEROIDOGENESIS

The rhesus macaque placenta, like the human placenta, contains steroid aromatase but not 17α-hydroxylase activity. Thus, estrogen production during pregnancy is dependent upon an intact fetoplacental unit, with fetal adrenal androgens as precursors of placentally derived estrogens. Unlike in sheep or other animals, parturition in rhesus monkeys and in humans is not signaled by declining peripheral progesterone levels. Spontaneous parturition is preceded by increased fetal adrenal synthesis of C_{19} androgens and rising concentrations of dehydroepiandrosterone sulfate and androstenedione in the fetal blood. In turn, these are converted by the placenta into estrogens, so that increasing concentrations of estradiol appear in maternal blood and rising estrone levels appear in maternal blood, fetal blood, and amniotic fluid. The rise in estrone concentrations precedes or coincides with the rise in prostaglandin concentrations in amniotic fluid, which also begin to increase several days prior to parturition (Walsh et al., 1984). The peripheral cortisol and progesterone concentrations remain relatively unchanged.

As discussed above, preterm labor induced by infection, in contrast to spontaneous parturition, is associated with rapid and large elevations of cytokine and prostaglandin concentrations in amniotic fluid. A complex interplay of both positive and negative feedback effects exists among the various cytokines, prostaglandins, and steroid hormones. There is increasing evidence for important interactions between the immune system and the endocrine system, at the hypothalamic and pituitary levels as well as locally (Aoki et al., 1990; Besedovsky and Del Rey, 1996; Reichlin, 1993). From a teleological standpoint, such interactions are relevant, considering the important functions of the adrenocortical system and the immune system in responding to stress. It is noteworthy that IL-1, IL-2, IL-6, and presumably TNF can stimulate the release of adrenocorticotropin (Reichlin, 1993) and that IL-1 directly stimulates adrenocortical cells to release cortisol (Aoki et al., 1990). Glucocorticoids are well-established immunosuppressants (in part by inhibiting the release of these cytokines), but other steroid hormones elaborated within the fetoplacental unit may also modulate cytokine function. High concentrations of estrogens or progesterone have been reported to inhibit spontaneous IL-1 production in monocytes (Polan et al., 1988). Dehydroepiandrosterone has also been demonstrated to reduce TNF production and to protect mice from endotoxin toxicity (Danenberg et al., 1992).

We hypothesized, therefore, that normal steroid biosynthesis by the fetoplacental unit may be altered or impaired in the presence of intrauterine infection. To investigate this, we have measured, by specific radioimmunoassay, the concentrations of adrenal androgens (androstenedione, dehydroepiandrosterone, and dehydroepiandrosterone sulfate), estrogens (estrone and estradiol), progesterone, and cortisol in rhesus monkeys with experimental intra-amniotic ($n = 4$) or choriodecidual ($n = 2$) infection and in four monkeys with spontaneous parturition near term (Gravett et al., 1996). Spontaneous parturition was characterized by initial increases in fetal adrenal biosynthesis of progesterone and the androgens androstenedione, dehydroepiandrosterone, and dehydroepiandrosterone sulfate which occurred 8 to 10 days prior to the onset of labor. These changes are summarized in Table 6. Increases in placental estrogen biosynthesis, beginning 6 to 8 days before spontaneous parturition, followed the increases in fetal adrenal androgen biosynthesis. There were no significant changes in the concentrations of the glucocorticoid cortisol in the fetus, mother, or amniotic fluid.

In contrast to spontaneous parturition, infection-induced preterm parturition was characterized by abrupt increases in fetal adrenal steroid biosynthesis but no corresponding increases in placental estrogen biosynthesis, as summarized in Table 7. In all instances, these increases in fetal steroid biosynthesis occurred concurrently with or following increases in uterine contractility. Progesterone concentrations increased significantly in the fetal artery, maternal artery, and amniotic fluid (Table 7). Significant increases in the concentration of the androgen androstenedione were also observed in all three compartments. Significant increases in dehydroepiandrosterone

Table 6 Median steroid hormone concentrations in rhesus monkeys (n = 4) undergoing spontaneous parturition near term[a]

Hormone	Concn[b] in:					
	Fetal artery		Maternal artery		Amniotic fluid	
	Basal	Delivery	Basal	Delivery	Basal	Delivery
Estrogens						
Estrone (pg/ml)	223	805[c]	314	520[c]	115	706[c]
Estradiol (pg/ml)	33	120[c]	378	579[c]	8	63[c]
Androgens						
Androstenedione (ng/ml)	0.98	4.39[c]	0.71	1.18	0.63	0.73
Dehydroepiandrosterone (ng/ml)	11.42	17.77[c]	22.9	28.8	3.22	11.0[c]
Dehydroepiandrosterone sulfate (ng/ml)	338	2,083[c]	357	367	51	159
Glucocorticoids						
Cortisol (ng/ml)	89	138	204	237	107	150
Progesterone (ng/ml)	2.8	15.6[c]	3.2	5.4[c]	0.10	0.21[c]

[a] Adapted from Gravett et al. (1996).

[b] Basal concentrations were determined from samples obtained 14 to 24 days prior to parturition. Delivery concentrations were identified as those in the last sample (no more than 1 day prior to delivery).

[c] $P < 0.05$ with respect to basal concentration by the Mann-Whitney U test. Data are medians.

Table 7 Median steroid hormone concentrations in rhesus monkeys ($n = 4$) undergoing infection-induced preterm parturition near term[a]

Hormone	Concn[b] in:					
	Fetal artery		Maternal artery		Amniotic fluid	
	Basal	Delivery	Basal	Delivery	Basal	Delivery
Estrogens						
Estrone (pg/ml)	156	170	147	172	34	114[c]
Estradiol (pg/ml)	26	39	277	279	7.75	24.5
Androgens						
Androstenedione (ng/ml)	0.96	2.44[c]	0.64	1.00[c]	0.08	0.29[c]
Dehydroepiandrosterone (ng/ml)	8.81	20.24[c]	23.02	39.48	2.35	5.61[c]
Dehydroepiandrosterone sulfate (ng/ml)	284	850[c]	188	189	18.5	22.9
Glucocorticoids						
Cortisol (ng/ml)	91	221[c]	257	349	112	162
Progesterone (ng/ml)	2.58	8.75[c]	2.56	5.53[c]	0.04	0.20[c]

[a] Adapted from Gravett et al. (1996).

[b] Basal concentrations were determined from samples obtained for several days prior to infection. Delivery concentrations were identified as those in the last sample obtained prior to delivery.

[c] $P < 0.05$ with respect to basal concentration by the Mann-Whitney U test. Data are medians.

concentrations were observed in the fetal artery and in amniotic fluid, and increases in dehydroepiandrosterone sulfate concentrations were observed only in the fetal artery. Despite these increases in the concentrations of C19 androgens, increases in estrogen concentrations were observed only for amniotic fluid estrone, which increased modestly from 34 pg/ml (range, 10 to 63 pg/ml) prior to infection to 114 pg/ml (range, 42 to 426 pg/ml) at delivery ($P < 0.05$). No changes in the concentration of estradiol were observed in any compartment.

In contrast to spontaneous parturition, increases in cortisol concentrations occurred in the fetal artery in infection-induced parturition (Table 7). Fetal concentrations of cortisol increased significantly from 91 ng/ml (range, 74 to 148 ng/ml) to 221 ng/ml (range, 103 to 268 ng/ml) following infection ($P < 0.05$). Similar but smaller increases in cortisol concentrations in amniotic fluid were also noted. Concentrations of cortisol in the maternal artery did not change significantly following infection.

Since the endocrine changes observed during infection-induced parturition occur at the same time as or soon after the onset of contractions, it is unlikely that they play a major role in the initiation of preterm labor in the setting of infection. Nevertheless, selected steroid hormones may modulate immune system function in the amniotic cavity and in fetal membranes, as mentioned above. The endocrine profiles which we have observed during intra-amniotic infection are consistent with acute fetal stress and resultant activation of the fetal pituitary-adrenal axis and placental dysfunction in estrogen biosynthesis. At present, it is not clear to what extent stimulation of the fetal adrenal gland is due to adrenocorticotropin secretion secondary to fetal hypoxemia or directly to cytokine-mediated effects. However, activation of the fetal hypothalamic-pituitary-adrenal axis by stress or directly by proinflammatory cytokines may play a role in fetal immunomodulation and down-regulation of the cytokine prostaglandin cascade initiated by infection.

FUTURE PERSPECTIVES

We have established a nonhuman primate experimental model which involves the use of chronically catheterized rhesus monkeys to study the pathophysiology of intra-amniotic infection. The presence of a single fetus, the hormonal control of parturition, and hemochorial placentation with an abundant amniotic fluid cavity all approximate the human situation. Our chronic preparation has the advantage of allowing frequent serial sampling of maternal blood, fetal blood, and amniotic fluid on individual animals. Thus, it allows for a more precise and complete description of the temporal relationships among indices of intra-amniotic infection and mediators of preterm labor that are necessary to establish causal relationships and to develop rational treatment strategies.

Our experimental results indicate that increases in bacterial counts and in cytokine and prostaglandin levels in amniotic fluid precede the clinical recognition of infection and the onset of labor by many hours. We suggest that interventions to prevent infection-associated preterm delivery should take into account these well-defined pathophysiologic mechanisms and that aggressive treatment should be initiated early.

Ideally, prevention of prematurity should be directed toward identification and eradication of the offending microorganism while it is still confined to the lower genital tract, as has been demonstrated for certain lower genital tract infections. Nevertheless, most human clinical trials of empirical antibiotic therapy during pregnancy have not reduced the incidence of premature labor. The next logical step for intervention would be the treatment and eradication of choriodecidual infection before there is intra-amniotic infection. However, more sensitive and specific diagnostic tests for bacterial infection will have to be developed before this approach will become a reality. New immunologic or biochemical assays or molecular probes for bacterial and leukocyte products, as well as for cytokines and eicosanoids, show promise as markers for infection. Finally, once intra-amniotic infection exists, it is important to recognize that preterm labor results from a complex interplay among microbial products, cytokines, prostaglandins, steroid hormones, and immunomodulators. A multifactorial approach directed toward each component of this cascade is desirable in our view. It is well known that single-agent tocolysis (as with β-agonists) for preterm labor is largely ineffective in the setting of infection and has done little to reduce the rate of preterm births (Romero et al., 1991a).

It is possible that in the near future, effective comprehensive therapy will include administration of a general tocolytic agent (e.g., β-agonists) together with cyclooxygenase and lipoxygenase inhibitors to reduce eicosanoid effects, immunomodulators (such as IL-1ra, TGF-β, soluble receptors to IL-1 and TNF, anti-inflammatory cytokines such as IL-10, and glucocorticoids) to counteract cytokine-induced prostaglandin production, and broad-spectrum antibiotics to eradicate specific microorganisms.

In the meantime, there are still many basic questions to be answered. What are the effects of different microorganisms and specific sites of inoculation? By what mechanisms do sexually transmitted microorganisms generally confined to the lower genital tract cause or contribute to preterm birth? What are the sites of synthesis of IL-1ra, and how is it regulated? How do steroid hormones influence the function of cytokines? How does the fetus respond to infection and participate in the immune response? It is certain that many more immune, endocrine, and paracrine interactive functions will be discovered.

Acknowledgments
This study was supported by NIH grants AI42490, RR00163, RR05412, HD-06159, and HD-18185.

REFERENCES

Aoki, N., Y. Ohno, and M. Imamura. 1990. Physiological interactions between the immune and endocrine systems: are cytokines hormones? *Med. Sci. Res.* **18:**195–201.

Baggia, S., M. G. Gravett, S. S. Witkin, G. J. Haluska, and M. J. Novy. 1996. Interleukin-1β intraamniotic infusion induces tumor necrosis factor-α, prostaglandin production, and preterm contractions in pregnant rhesus monkeys. *J. Soc. Gynecol. Invest.* **3:**121–126.

Bernal, A. L., D. J. Hansell, T. Y. Khong, and J. W. Keeling. 1989. Prostaglandin E production by the fetal membranes in unexplained preterm labor and preterm labor associated with chorioamnionitis. *Br. J. Obstet. Gynecol.* **96:**1133–1139.

Besedovsky, H. O., and A. Del Rey. 1996. Immune-neuro-endocrine interactions: facts and hypothesis. *Endocr. Rev.* **17:**64–102.

Bry, K., V. Lappalainen, and M. Hallman. 1993. Interleukin-1 binding and prostaglandin E2 synthesis by amnion cells in culture: regulation by tumor necrosis factor-α, TFG-β, and interleukin-1 receptor antagonist. *Biochim. Biophys. Acta* **1181:** 31–36.

Casey, M. L., S. M. Cox, B. Beutler, L. Milewich, and P. C. MacDonald. 1989. Cachectin/tumor necrosis factor-alpha formation in human decidua. Potential role for cytokines in infection-induced preterm labor. *J. Clin. Invest.* **83:**430–436.

Challis, J. R. G., and D. M. Olson. 1988. Parturition, p. 2177–2216. *In* E. Knobil, J. Neill, L. Ewing, G. Greenwald, C. Market, and D. Pfaff (ed.), *The Physiology of Reproduction.* Raven Press, New York, N.Y.

Cox, S. M., M. R. King, M. L. Casey, and P. C. MacDonald. 1993. Interleukin-1β, and -6, and prostaglandins in vaginal/cervical fluids of pregnant women before and during labor. *J. Clin. Endocrinol. Metab.* **77:**805–815.

Danenberg, H. D., G. Alpert, S. Lustig, and D. Ben-Nathan. 1992. Dehydroepiandrosterone protects mice from endotoxin toxicity and reduces tumor necrosis factor production. *Antimicrob. Agents Chemother.* **36:**2275–2279.

Dinarello, C. A., J. A. Gelfand, and S. M. Wolff. 1993. Anticytokine strategies in the treatment of the systemic inflammatory response syndrome. *JAMA* **269:**1829–1835.

Dombroski, R. A., D. S. Woodard, M. J. K. Harper, and R. S. Gibbs. 1990. A rabbit model for bacterial-induced preterm pregnancy loss. *Am. J. Obstet. Gynecol.* **163:** 1938–1943.

Ducsay, C. A., M. J. Cook, and M. J. Novy. 1988. Simplified vest and tether system for maintenance of chronically catheterized rhesus monkeys. *Lab. Anim. Sci.* **38:** 343–344.

Gravett, M. G. Unpublished data.

Gravett, M. G., H. P. Nelson, T. DeRouen, C. Critchlow, D. A. Eschenbach, and K. K. Holmes. 1986. Independent associations of bacterial vaginosis and *Chlamydia trachomatis* infection with adverse pregnancy outcome. *JAMA* **256:**1899–1903.

Gravett, M. G., S. S. Witkin, G. J. Haluska, J. L. Edwards, M. J. Cook, and M. J. Novy. 1994a. An experimental model for intraamniotic infection and preterm labor in rhesus monkeys. *Am. J. Obstet. Gynecol.* **171:**1660–1667.

Gravett, M. G., S. S. Witkin, and M. J. Novy. 1994b. A nonhuman primate model for chorioamnionitis and preterm labor. *Semin. Reprod. Endocrinol.* **12:**246–262.

Gravett, M. G., G. J. Haluska, M. J. Cook, and M. J. Novy. 1996. Fetal and maternal endocrine responses to experimental intrauterine infection in rhesus monkeys. *Am. J. Obstet. Gynecol.* **174:**1725–1733.

Greig, P. C., W. N. P. Herbert, B. L. Robinette, and L. A. Teot. 1995. Amniotic fluid interleukin-10 concentrations increase through pregnancy and are elevated in patients with preterm labor associated with intrauterine infection. *Am. J. Obstet. Gynecol.* **173:**1223–1227.

Haluska, G. J., F. Z. Stanczyk, M. J. Cook, and M. J. Novy. 1987. Temporal changes in uterine activity and prostaglandin response to RU486 in rhesus macaques in late gestation. *Am. J. Obstet. Gynecol.* **157:**1487–1495.

Hillier, S. L., S. S. Witkin, M. A. Krohn, D. H. Watts, N. B. Kiviat, and D. A. Eschenbach. 1993. The relationship of amniotic fluid cytokines and preterm delivery, amniotic fluid infection, histologic chorioamnionitis, and chorioamnion infection. *Obstet. Gynecol.* **81:**941–948.

Hillier, S. L., R. P. Nugent, D. A. Eschenbach, M. A. Krohn, R. S. Gibbs, D. H. Martin, M. F. Cotch, R. Edelman, J. G. Pastorek II, V. Rao, D. McNellis, J. A. Regan, J. C. Carey, and M. A. Klebanoff. 1995. Association between bacterial vaginosis and preterm delivery of a low-birth-weight infant. *N. Engl. J. Med.* **333:** 1737–1742.

Howie, A., H. A. Leaver, I. D. Aitken, L. A. Hay, I. E. Anderson, G. E. Williams, and G. Jones. 1989. The effect of chlamydial infection on the initiation of premature labor: serial measurements of intrauterine prostaglandin E_2 in amniotic fluid, allantoic fluid and utero-ovarian vein, using catheterized sheep experimentally infected with an ovine abortion strain of *Chlamydia psittaci. Prostaglandins Leukotrienes Essent. Fatty Acids* **37:**203–211.

Larson, J. W., Jr., W. T. London, C. J. Baker, B. L. Curfman, and J. L. Sever. 1981. Intraamniotic infection due to group B *Streptococcus*: treatment and antibody response. *Obstet. Gynecol.* **58:**222–226.

MacDonald, P. C., and M. L. Casey. 1993. The accumulation of prostaglandins (PG) in amniotic fluid is an aftereffect of labor and not indicative of a role for PGE2 or PGF2a in the initiation of human parturition. *J. Clin. Endocrinol. Metab.* **76:**1332–1339.

McDuffie, R. S., Jr., M. P. Sherman, and R. S. Gibbs. 1992. Amniotic fluid tumor necrosis factor-α and interleukin-1 in a rabbit model of bacterially induced preterm pregnancy loss. *Am. J. Obstet Gynecol.* **167:**1583–1588.

McIntyre, K. W., G. J. Stepan, K. D. Kolinsky, W. R. Benjamin, J. M. Plocinski, K. L. Kaffa, C. A. Campen, R. A. Chizzonite, and P. L. Kilan. 1991. Inhibition of interleukin (IL-1) binding and bioactivity *in-vitro* and modulation of acute inflammation *in-vivo* by IL-1 receptor antagonist and anti-IL-1 receptor antibody. *J. Exp. Med.* **173:**931–939.

Mitchell, M. D., D. W. Branch, S. Lundin-Schiller, R. J. Romero, R. A. Daynes, and D. J. Dudley. 1991a. Immunologic aspects of preterm labor. *Semin. Perinatol.* **15:**210–224.

Mitchell, M. D., D. J. Dudley, S. S. Edwin, and S. L. Schiller. 1991b. Interleukin-6 stimulates prostaglandin production by human amnion and decidual cells. *Eur. J. Pharmacol.* **192:**189–191.

Moller, B. R., and E. A. Freundt. 1983. Monkey animal model for study of mycoplasmal infections of the urogenital tract. *Sex. Transm. Dis.* **11**(Suppl.):359–362.

Novy, M. J., and G. J. Haluska. 1988. Endocrine and paracrine control of parturition in rhesus monkeys, p. 321–334. *In* D. McNellis, J. R. G. Challis, P. C. Macdonald, P. W. Nathanielsz, and J. M. Roberts (ed.), *The Onset of Labor: Cellular and Integrative Mechanisms.* Perinatology Press, New York, N.Y.

Novy, M. J., and G. C. Liggins. 1980. Role of prostaglandins, prostacyclin, and thromboxanes in the physiologic control of the uterus and in parturition. *Semin. Perinatol.* **4**:45–66.

Nugent, R. P., M. A. Krohn, and S. L. Hillier. 1991. Reliability of diagnosing bacterial vaginosis is improved by a standardized method of Gram stain interpretation. *J. Clin. Microbiol.* **29**:297–301.

Oshiro, B. T., M. Monga, N. L. Eriksen, J. M. Graham, N. W. Weisbrodt, and J. D. Blanco. 1993. Endotoxin, interleukin-1β, interleukin-6, or tumor necrosis factor-α do not acutely stimulate isolated murine myometrial contractile activity. *Am. J. Obstet. Gynecol.* **169**:1424–1427.

Patton, D. L., C. C. Kuo, S. P. Wang, and S. A. Halbert. 1987. Distal tubal obstruction induced by repeated *Chlamydia trachomatis* salpingeal infection in pig-tail macaques. *J. Infect. Dis.* **155**:1292–1299.

Polan, M. L., A. Damele, and A. Kuo. 1988. Gonadal steroids modulate human monocyte interleukin-1 (IL-1) activity. *Fertil. Steril.* **49**:964–968.

Reichlin, S. 1993. Neuroendocrine-immune interactions. *N. Engl. J. Med.* **329**:1246–1253.

Romero, R., and B. Tartakovsky. 1992. The natural interleukin-1 receptor antagonist prevents interleukin-1 induced preterm delivery in mice. *Am. J. Obstet. Gynecol.* **167**:1041–1045.

Romero, R., M. Wan, M. Emamian, R. Quintero, J. C. Hobbins, and M. D. Mitchell. 1987. Prostaglandin concentrations in amniotic fluid of women with intra-amniotic infection and preterm labor. *Am. J. Obstet. Gynecol.* **157**:1461–1467.

Romero, R., D. T. Brody, E. Oyarzun, M. Mazur, Y. K. Wu, J. C. Hobbins, and S. K. Durum. 1989a. Infection and labor. III. Interleukin-1: a signal for the onset of parturition. *Am. J. Obstet. Gynecol.* **160**:1117–1123.

Romero, R., K. R. Manogue, M. D. Mitchell, Y. K. Wu, E. Oyarzun, J. C. Hobbins, and A. Cerami. 1989b. Infection and labor. IV. Cachetin-tumor necrosis factor in the amniotic fluid of women with intraamniotic infection and preterm labor. *Am. J. Obstet. Gynecol.* **161**:336–341.

Romero, R., Y. K. Wu, D. T. Brody, E. Oyarzun, G. W. Duff, and S. K. Durum. 1989c. Human decidua: a source of interleukin-1. *Obstet. Gynecol.* **73**:31–34.

Romero, R., S. Durum, C. A. Dinarello, E. Oyarzun, J. C. Hobbins, and M. D. Mitchell. 1989d. Interleukin-1 stimulated prostaglandin biosynthesis by human amnion. *Prostaglandins* **37**:13–22.

Romero, R., C. Avila, U. Santhanam, and P. G. Sehgal. 1990. Amniotic fluid interleukin-6 in preterm labor: association with labor. *J. Clin. Invest.* **85**:1392–1400.

Romero, R., C. Avila, C. A. Brekus, and R. Morotti. 1991a. The role of systemic and intrauterine infection in preterm parturition. *Ann. N. Y. Acad. Sci.* **85**:355–375.

Romero, R., M. Mazur, and B. Tartakovsky. 1991b. Systemic administration of interleukin-1 induces preterm parturition in mice. *Am. J. Obstet. Gynecol.* **165**:969–971.

Romero, R., W. Sepulveda, M. Mazor, F. Brandt, D. B. Cotton, C. Dinarello, and M. Mitchell. 1992. The natural interleukin-1 receptor antagonist in term and preterm parturition. *Am. J. Obstet. Gynecol.* **167:**863–872.

Rubens, C. E., H. V. Raff, C. Jackson, E. Y. Chi, J. T. Bielitzki, and S. L. Hillier. 1991. Pathophysiology and histology of Group B streptococcal sepsis in *Macaca nemestrina* primates induced after intraamniotic inoculation: evidence for bacterial cellular invasion. *J. Infect. Dis.* **164:**320–330.

Rush, R. W., M. G. Keirse, P. Howat, J. D. Baum, A. B. M. Anderson, and A. C. Trunbull. 1976. Contribution of preterm delivery to perinatal mortality. *Br. J. Med.* **2:**965–968.

Sadowsky, D. W., G. J. Haluska, M. J. Cook, and M. J. Novy. 1996. Indomethacin (INDO) blocks interleukin-1α (IL-1α) induced myometrial contractions in pregnant rhesus monkeys. *J. Soc. Gynecol. Invest.* **3**(Suppl. 2)**:**321A (abstr. 528).

Silver, H. M., R. S. Sperling, P. J. St. Clair, and R. S. Gibbs. 1989. Evidence relating bacterial vaginosis to intra-amniotic infection. *Am. J. Obstet. Gynecol.* **161:**808–812.

Street, D. A., D. Taylor-Robinson, and C. M. Hetherington. 1983. Infection of female squirrel monkeys (*Saimiri sciureus*) with *Trichomonas vaginalis* as a model of trichomoniasis in women. *Br. J. Vener. Dis.* **59:**249–254.

van der Elst, C. W., A. L. Bernal, and C. C. Sinclair-Smith. 1991. The role of chorioamnionitis and prostaglandins in preterm labor. *Obstet. Gynecol.* **77:**672–676.

Walsh, S. W., F. Z. Stanczyk, and M. J. Novy. 1984. Daily hormonal changes in the maternal, fetal, and amniotic fluid compartments before parturition in a primate species. *J. Clin. Endocrinol. Metab.* **58:**629–639.

Witkin, S. S., M. G. Gravett, G. J. Haluska, and M. J. Novy. 1994. Induction of interleukin 1 receptor antagonist in rhesus monkeys following intraamniotic infection with group B streptococci or interleukin 1 infusion. *Am. J. Obstet. Gynecol.* **171:**1668–1672.

INDEX

R

COLLEGE